# Workbook to Accompany
# Medical Assisting:
## Administrative and Clinical Competencies

## Fifth Edition

*Angela Kave*

Lucille Keir, CMA-A
Barbara A. Wise, BSN, RN, MA(Ed)
Connie Krebs, CMA-C, BGS

D1403766

**THOMSON**

**DELMAR LEARNING**    Australia    Canada    Mexico    Singapore    Spain    United Kingdom    United States

## THOMSON

### DELMAR LEARNING

**Workbook to Accompany**

**Medical Assisting: Administrative and Clinical Competencies, Fifth Edition**

by Lucille Keir, Barbara A. Wise, and Connie Krebs

**Executive Director:**
William Brottmiller

**Executive Editor:**
Cathy L. Esperti

**Acquisitions Editor:**
Rhonda Dearborn

**Developmental Editor:**
Deb Flis

**Executive Marketing Manager:**
Dawn F. Gerrain

**Channel Manager:**
Jennifer McAvey

**Editorial Assistant:**
Jill O'Brien

**Executive Production Manager:**
Karen Leet

**Art and Design Coordinator:**
Robert Plante

**Project Editor:**
Sherry McGaughan

**Production Coordinator:**
Nina Lontrato

ISBN 0-7668-4150-2
Library of Congress Catalog Number 2002025907

### NOTICE TO THE READER

# CONTENTS

# TO THE LEARNER

This Workbook has been written to help you review the concepts and information presented in the textbook and provide a means for you to achieve competency in performance of various procedures. Each unit in the text is correlated to a unit in this Workbook. The material in the Workbook contains many different types of exercises.

Assignment sheets have been developed to help you review the theory and skill contents, general technical content, and basic anatomy content. These sheets ask you to answer various types of questions (brief answer, multiple choice, true/false, and critical thinking scenarios), identify correctly spelled words, fill in blanks, match answers, label figures, and word puzzles (unscrambles, word puzzles, word searches, and crossword puzzles). When you have completed the sheets for each chapter, remove them and give them to your teacher for evaluation. Always be sure to fill in your name and the date. (The answers to the questions have been included in your teacher's Instructor's Manual.)

Another feature of your Workbook is Performance Evaluation Checklists. You will find one in the back of this Workbook for each procedure in your textbook. These sheets provide a means for you to achieve a measurement of your ability to perform the procedures. You should practice the procedures following the steps identified in your text, keeping the performance objectives in mind. You will notice procedure competency involves using the correct equipment and materials, accurately performing the procedure steps, and completing the procedure within an acceptable period of time. In procedures where a period of time for completion has not been identified in the objective, it is because of the great amount of variability involved in the task or availabilitiy of equipment and materials. Spaces have been provided on the Performance Evaluation Checklists to document the time required to complete the procedure, as well as the time the procedure began and ended. In procedures where no standards for time and accuracy are provided, your instructor will inform you of the required standards based on the actual classroom situation.

When you feel you have mastered a given skill, ask one of your classmates (if you are in a school situation) to observe your technique following the procedure evaluation requirements. When you are confident of your ability, sign the evaluation form and give it to your teacher. This will inform the teacher that you are ready for evaluation. The teacher will then observe your performance of the procedure (or may delegate the responsibility to another person).

In many units, you will find "situations" to which you are asked to respond. There are no specific right or wrong answers. Think about the things you have read in your text in order to arrive at your answer. You will encounter many similar actual situations both in and out of the office. When family members, friends, and neighbors know you are a medical assistant, they will come to you for information and advice. These simulated situations will be very helpful, but remember, you are not qualified to diagnose an illness or prescribe treatment. Your role is to recognize potential problems, advise, facilitate care and treatment, and provide information within the limits of your knowledge and experience.

It is suggested that you obtain a large three-ring notebook in which to keep your completed assignment and evaluation sheets. Insert the sheets into their original position and maintain your complete Workbook for reference and review.

The authors hope you will find the Workbook to be both challenging and interesting. It is our desire that you master the content of the text to the best of your ability, and we believe this Workbook will assist you in that process. We wish you success as you complete your assignments and prepare to be a medical assistant.

## ASSIGNMENT SHEET

### Section 1:  MEDICAL HEALTH CARE ROLES AND RESPONSIBILITIES

### Chapter 1:  HEALTH CARE PROVIDERS

Review the objectives and text for each unit before completing the assignment sheet for that unit. When you have completed all sheets for the chapter, remove them from this Workbook and give them to the instructor for evaluation.

### Unit 1:  A BRIEF HISTORY OF MEDICINE

**A.  Spelling:  Each line contains three different spellings of a word. Underline the correctly spelled word.**

1. anesthesha     anesthesia     anethesha
2. aprenticeship     apprentiship     apprenticeship
3. aceptic     aseptic     aseptec
4. caughtery     cauterey     cautery
5. disease     desease     deseace
6. epedemic     epidemic     epidemik
7. ethere     ether     ethir
8. gilds     guelds     guilds
9. infectious     infectuous     enfectuous
10. physican     psychian     physician
11. plaque     plage     plague
12. practitioners     practioners     practitoners
13. scintific     scientific     sientific
14. surgeon     sirgin     sergeon
15. vakcination     vaccination     vacsination

**B.  Matching:  Match the pre-19th-century medical pioneer in column II with his or her correct description in column I.**

COLUMN I

_____  1. Father of modern medicine
_____  2. A physician in Rome who wrote over 500 books
_____  3. First reported studies of circulation of blood by heart
_____  4. Built over 200 microscopes and first to see RBCs
_____  5. Founder of scientific surgery
_____  6. Developed the smallpox vaccine
_____  7. Early female physician; author of *Diseases of Women*
_____  8. Greatest French surgeon, who served four kings
_____  9. Developed first mercury thermometer

COLUMN II

a. Anton van Leeuwenhoek
b. William Harvey
c. Edward Jenner
d. Galen
e. Pare
f. Hippocrates
g. John Hunter
h. Gabriel Fahrenheit
i. Trotula Platearius

**C. Matching:** Match the 19th- or 20th-century medical pioneer in column II with his or her correct description in colunm I.

COLUMN I

     1. Invented the stethoscope
     2. First successful heart transplant
     3. Discovered a red dye that resulted in sulfa drugs
     4. Determined cause of yellow fever
     5. Developed oral polio vaccine
     6. Developed the pap test
     7. Introduced the use of ether as an anesthesia
     8. Discovered the process of pasteurization
     9. Developed the foundation for aseptic technique
     10. Discovered X-rays
     11. Nobel Prize in 1912 for joining blood vessels
     12. Nurse who founded the American Red Cross
     13. First woman to qualify as Physician in the US
     14. Founder of modern nursing
     15. Discovered polio and developed a vaccine
     16. Woman scientist whose work led to radium treatments for cancer
     17. Instituted first nutrition program for medical students in the world.
     18. Discovered a mold that later led to penicillin
     19. Used tubing to replace arteries

COLUMN II

a. George Papaniolaou
b. Wilhelm Roentgen
c. W.T.G. Morton
d. Alexis Carrel
e. Louis Pasteur
f. Sir Alexander Fleming
g. Elizabeth Blackwell
h. A.B. Sabin
i. Christian Bernard
j. Jonas Salk
k. Rene Laennec
l. Marie Curie
m. Gerhard Domagk
n. Walter Reed
o. Clara Barton
p. Michael DeBakey

q. Joseph Lister

r. Grace Goldsmith
s. Florence Nightengale

**D. Brief Answer**

During the ancient medical history period, several things were believed responsible for illness and some unusual treatments were used.

1. What was credited as the cause of disease? _____

2. How were migraines, epilepsy, insanity, and head injuries treated? _____

3. How did the Egyptians solve "clogged" body canals? _____

4. The Greeks believed in a god of healing. What did they use for treatments? _____

_____

In medieval history, other beliefs and methods of treatment were prevalent.

5. What did Anglo-Saxons in Britain believe caused illness? _____

_____

6. How did the priests cure the sick in about 400 AD? _____

_____

7. In 1277 AD, how was tuberculosis treated? _____

8. In 1352, what different things were believed to be the cause of the plagues? _____

_____

9. The practice of medicine at the beginning of the 17th century was divided among three guilds. Name and briefly describe their education and area of practice.

a. _____

b. _____

_____

c. _____

10. As late as the 1600s, what were some of the old practices still being used in the colonies and what was the unusual prescription ordered for Queen Anne? _____

_____

11. What sciences aided medical science in making rapid advances in the 18th century? _____

_____

12. Name the two people who developed polio vaccine and identify the type they developed. What are three reasons the second type was more desirable? _____

_____

_____

13. During the 1950s, what changed the way human bodies could be seen inside? _____

14. Name eight types of "artificial" body parts that have been developed.

a. _____  b. _____  c. _____  d. _____

e. _____  f. _____  g. _____  h. _____

15. Congress has enacted several laws concerning health care. What did the following laws provide?

a. Hill–Burton Act: _____

b. What did the combined Public Health Services and the Food and Drug Administration originally and then later become? _____

_____

c. What did the National Cancer Institute and the Public Health Services Hygienic Lab become? _____

_____

d. What two health programs were enacted in 1965? _____

16. Women had a difficult time being accepted as physicians. Briefly identify the major contribution of the following female physicians.

a. Trotula Platearius _____

b. Elizabeth Garrett Anderson _____

c. Elizabeth Blackwell _____

_____

d. Aletta Jacobs _____

e. Elsie Strang L'Esperance _____

f. Dorothy Hansine Anderson _____

g. Grace Arabell Goldsmith _____

h. Dorothy Hodgkins _____

17. What did *Ebony* Magazine report in 1993 regarding the accomplishments of Drs. Alexa Canady and M. Deborah Hyde-Rowan? _____

18. Refer to the Role Delineation Chart in Appendix A of the textbook. Within the area of *Instruction,* which role relates to the content of this unit? _____

After your instructor has returned your work to you, make all necessary corrections and place in a three-ring notebook for future reference.

**ASSIGNMENT SHEET**

**Chapter 1: HEALTH CARE PROVIDERS**

**Unit 2: THE HEALTH CARE TEAM**

**A. Multiple Choice: Place the correct letter on the blank line for each question.**

_____ 1. One whose primary duty is obtaining a medical history and other important information from patients in the hospital is termed a(n)

    a. registered nurse               c. dietitian

    b. admissions clerk            d. office manager

_____ 2. A _____ performs specialized chemical, microscopic, and bacteriological tests of blood, tissue, and other body fluids.

    a. nurse practitioner           c. laboratory technician

    b. physician assistant          d. accessioning technician

_____ 3. One who practices skills most often in the hospital setting to assist patients in many ways through purposeful activity is called a(n)

    a. physician assistant          c. physical therapist

    b. pharmacist                  d. occupational therapist

_____ 4. A member of the health care team who helps patients with their diets, usually in a hospital or clinic, is called a

    a. nurse practitioner           c. dietitian

    b. pharmacist                  d. nutritionist

_____ 5. One who is trained by physicians, instructed in certain aspects of medicine, and practices under their direct supervision is called a

    a. registered nurse              c. physician assistant

    b. licensed practical nurse      d. paramedic

_____ 6. The _____ is trained in the art of drawing blood for diagnostic purposes.

    a. paramedic                   c. physician assistant

    b. physical therapist           d. phlebotomist

_____ 7. A qualified person who has been trained in assisting patients in rehabilitation programs following accident or injury is called a(n)

    a. occupational therapist        c. registered nurse

    b. physical therapist           d. podiatrist

_____ 8. One who is a licensed specialist in formulating and dispensing medications is a

    a. pharmacist                 c. registered nurse

    b. paramedic                 d. physician

_____ 9. A professional who is highly trained and skilled in mechanical manipulation of the spinal column is a(n)

    a. occupational therapist        c. licensed practical nurse

    b. chiropractor                d. physical therapist

_____ 10. A member of the health care team who performs procedures to improve the ventilatory functions of a patient is a(n)

    a. phlebotomist              c. radiology technician

    b. electrocardiogram technician   d. respiratory therapist

_____ 11. A _____ provides testing and counseling services to patients in private or group practice.

        a. podiatrist                       c. paramedic

        b. dietitian                        d. psychologist

**B. Spelling: Each line contains four different spellings of a word. Underline the correctly spelled word.**

| | | | |
|---|---|---|---|
| 1. dietitian | dietician | deititian | dietision |
| 2. phlebatomist | plebotamist | phlebotomist | pflebotomist |
| 3. therapast | theirapist | therapist | tharapist |
| 4. technicien | technician | technision | tecnician |
| 5. chiropractor | chiropracter | chyroprakder | chirupractor |
| 6. nutricionist | nutrionist | nutritionist | newtritionist |
| 7. ocupational | occupattional | occupational | occupationale |
| 8. licensed | licenced | licensced | licensead |
| 9. professional | preffessional | profesional | professionel |
| 10. physiciaan | physichian | pysican | physician |

**C. Matching: Match the subspecialty in column I with the correct description in column II.**

COLUMN I

_____ 1. Immunology

_____ 2. Preventive medicine

_____ 3. Acupuncture

_____ 4. Hypnosis

_____ 5. Rheumatology

_____ 6. Nutrition

_____ 7. Surgery

_____ 8. Cardiovascular disease

_____ 9. Hypertension

_____ 10. Aerospace medicine

COLUMN II

a. Mainly used in psychotherapy

b. Treats high blood pressure

c. How the body utilizes nutrients

d. Deals with allergies

e. Originated in the Far East

f. Stresses keeping healthy

g. Research effects of space environment

h. Treats inflammatory disorders

i. Many specialized areas

j. Heart and circulatory problems

**D. Fill in the Blank**

1. The podiatrist or _____ deals with diseases and disorders of the _____

2. The business office manager should have good _____ skills.

3. The licensed practical nurse may perform basic nursing skills under the direct supervision of a physician or _____

4. The _____ is one who specializes in the microscopic identification of cells and tissues.

5. Emergency Medical Technicians must _____ every two years.

6. An R.N. is defined as a _____ nurse who has completed a school of nursing and passed the NCLEX-RN.

7. A _____ is sometimes called an administrative specialist or a ward secretary.

8. A registered nurse who has acquired expert knowledge in a special branch of practice is called a nurse _____

9. The _____ acts as an assistant to, or in place of, the physician, especially in the military and in emergency services.

10. The _____ of the X-ray technician must be proved by the American Registry of Radiologic Technologists.

11. A _____ has graduated from a school with CAAHEP approval and has successfully passed the certification exam of the AAMA.

12. The _____ assists women throughout pregnancy, childbirth, and the postpartum period.

13. The _____ must have met pre-med requirements and successfully completed a two-year program, and works under the direct supervision of the physician.

14. A degree in business administration is desirable to be a _____

After your instructor has returned your work to you, make all necessary corrections and place in a three-ring notebook for future reference.

**ASSIGNMENT SHEET**

**Chapter 1: HEALTH CARE PROVIDERS**

**Unit 3: MEDICAL PRACTICE SPECIALTIES**

**A. Fill in the Blank**

1. _____ dedicate their lives to the practice of medicine or to acquiring skills in the art and science of treating disease and maintaining health.

2. A physician may have an area of special interest that may be referred to as a _____

3. The term _____ is derived from the Latin word meaning "to teach."

4. Persons who hold _____ or _____ are entitled to be addressed as "doctor."

5. A _____ contributes specific expert skills and knowledge in serving patients.

6. The type of practice that covers the broadest spectrum is called _____

7. Three types of medical specialties that are hospital based are _____ _____ and emergency or traumatic medicine.

8. In the practice of _____ manipulation therapy may be used to alleviate illness.

9. Refer to the Role Delineation Chart in Appendix A of the textbook. Within the area of *Allied Health* Professions and Credentialing, which two roles relate to the content of this unit? _____

_____

**B. Matching: Match the specialty in Column II with the correct abbreviation in column I.**

COLUMN I               COLUMN II
_____   1. OD        a. Doctor of Osteopathy
_____   2. PhD       b. Doctor of Dental Surgery
_____   3. DPM       c. Doctor of Medicine
_____   4. DC        d. Doctor of Divinity
_____   5. DO        e. Doctor of Optometry
_____   6. DDS       f. Doctor of Veterinary Medicine
_____   7. MD        g. Doctor of Philosophy
                       h. Doctor of Chiropractic
                       i. Doctor of Podiatric Medicine

**C. Multiple Choice: Place the correct letter on the blank line for each question.**

_____ 1. One who specializes in the treatment of diseases and disorders of the stomach and intestines is a(an)
    a. gerontologist                 c. gastroenterologist
    b. endocrinologist             d. allergist

_____ 2. The field of medicine that deals with diagnosing and treating diseases and disorders of the female reproductive tract is
    a. gerontology                 c. nephrology
    b. gynecology                 d. obstetrics

_____ 3. Measuring the accuracy of vision to determine if corrective lenses (eyeglasses) are needed describes the field of
    a. orthopedics                 c. optometry
    b. oncology                  d. obstetrics

_____ 4. A specialty that deals with the diagnosis and treatment of diseases and disorders of the CNS (central nervous system) is
    a. psychology                 c. nuclear medicine
    b. neurology                  d. nephrology

_____ 5. Treatment and diagnosis of acute illnesses or injuries is a specialty called
    a. surgery                     c. pathology
    b. physical medicine          d. traumatic medicine

_____ 6. One who specializes in the treatment and diagnosis of pronounced manifestation of emotional problems or mental illnesses that may have an organic causative factor is called a
    a. psychiatrist                c. neurologist
    b. psychologist              d. podiatrist

_____ 7. Analysis of tissue samples to confirm diagnosis is performed by a
    a. urologist                  c. pathologist
    b. hematologist             d. nephrologist

_____ 8. One who specializes in the diagnosis and treatment of the foot is called a
    a. surgeon                   c. pathologist
    b. podiatrist                d. chiropractor

_____ 9. Sports medicine is a medical specialty that deals with diagnosing and treating
    a. emotional problems        c. disorders and diseases of the urinary system
    b. injuries sustained in athletic events      d. conditions of altered immunological reactivity

_____ 10. A radiologist specializes in diagnosing and treating diseases and disorders
    a. by manual or operative methods      c. with roentgen rays and other forms of radiant energy
    b. with the use of radionuclides         d. with manipulative treatment

_____ 11. Dermatology is the specialty of medicine that deals with diagnosis and treatment of diseases and disorders of the
   a. glands of internal secretion
   b. skin
   c. teeth and gums
   d. kidneys

_____ 12. Nephrology is the medical specialty that deals with the diagnosis and treatment of
   a. blood and blood-forming tissue
   b. the internal organs
   c. stomach and intestines
   d. the kidneys

_____ 13. One who is a specialist in the diagnosis and treatment of problems in conceiving and maintaining pregnancy is a(n)
   a. pediatrician
   b. family practitioner
   c. endocrinologist
   d. infertility specialist

_____ 14. A hematologist specializes in the diagnosis and treatment of disorders and diseases of
   a. the internal organs
   b. bones
   c. blood and blood-forming tissue
   d. the central nervous system

_____ 15. The field of medicine that provides direct care to pregnant females during pregnancy, childbirth, and immediately thereafter is called
   a. obstetrics
   b. infertility
   c. pediatrics
   d. gynecology

_____ 16. Anesthesiology is the medical specialty that deals with
   a. manual or operative methods
   b. the use of radionuclides
   c. administering anesthetic agents prior to and during surgery
   d. altered immunological reactivity

_____ 17. A cardiologist specializes in the diagnosis and treatment of abnormalities, diseases, and disorders of the
   a. glands
   b. aging
   c. heart
   d. central nervous system

_____ 18. One who specializes in diagnosing and treating diseases and malfunctions of the glands of internal secretion is called a(an)
   a. cardiologist
   b. chiropractor
   c. endocrinologist
   d. otorhinolaryngologist

Name _____

## D. Crossword Puzzle

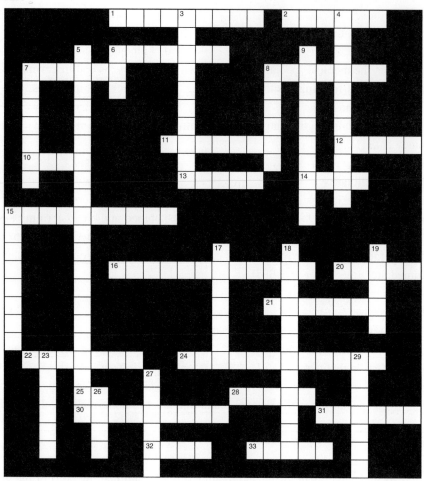

ACROSS

1. Urgency
2. Responsibilities
6. Altered immune reaction
7. Common name for physician
8. Branch of medicine that uses radionuclides
10. A dermatologist treats problems of the _____
11. Renewed periodically
12. Pulmonary specialists treat diseases and disorders of the _____
13. Expertise in a certain area
14. A surgeon cuts _____ skin
15. Field of medicine dealing with small children
16. Deals with pregnancy/childbirth
20. Anesthetics make you _____
21. Pathology is the study of _____
22. Operation
24. Commonly known as a counselor
25. Abbreviation for symptoms
28. Opposite of chronic
30. _____ medicine is practiced in the emergency room
31. Prefix that refers to the heart
32. The health care _____ works together
33. Orthopedics

DOWN

3. Field of medicine that deals with senior citizens
4. Specialist who helps childless couples
5. ENT specialist
6. Practicing medicine is an _____ and science
7. Deals with problems of the teeth and gums
8. A neurologist is expert in this specific anatomical area
9. Career/work
15. Branch of medicine that treats problems of the feet
17. Field of medicine that treats genitourinary problems
18. Chiropractic
19. From general practice to a specialist
23. Emergency
26. Radiologists use these in diagnosing
27. Prefix that refers to blood
29. Endocrinologists study about what glands _____

10

**E. Spelling: Each line contains four different spellings of a word. Underline the correctly spelled word.**

| | | | |
|---|---|---|---|
| 1. allargist | allergest | allergist | alergist |
| 2. anesthesiology | annesthesiology | anesthisology | anasthesiology |
| 3. gastrointerologist | gastroenterologist | gastronterologist | gastranologist |
| 4. geriatricks | gariacktrics | giractrics | geriatrics |
| 5. ophthalmology | opthalmology | optamology | ophthalamalagy |
| 6. obstitrician | obstetrician | obstatrician | obstetrecian |
| 7. psychiatrist | psychiotrist | psyciatrist | psychatrist |
| 8. pediatrist | padiatrist | podiatrist | podatrist |
| 9. pediatician | pediatrician | peditrician | pedeatrician |
| 10. urologist | uriologist | urologest | urolgist |

**CRITICAL THINKING SCENARIOS: What would your response be in the following situations?**

1. Your neighbor asks you the difference between an internal medicine specialist and an endocrinologist.

   _____

   _____

2. You are attending a family reunion and overhear a discussion where there is an obvious uncertainty about the use of the title "Doctor" _____

   _____

3. A female patient, whom the physician has never seen before, phones to ask about the possibility of having a food allergy. This patient tells you that she has a fine red rash all over her body. _____

   _____

   _____

   After your instructor has returned your work to you, make all necessary corrections and place in a three-ring notebook for future reference.

**ASSIGNMENT SHEET**

**Chapter 2:  THE MEDICAL ASSISTANT**

Review the objectives and text for each unit before completing the assignment sheet for that unit. When you have completed all sheets for the chapter, remove them from this Workbook and give them to the instructor for evaluation.

**Unit 1:  TRAINING, JOB RESPONSIBILITIES, AND EMPLOYMENT OPPORTUNITIES**

**A.  Brief Answer**

1.  Why did health care occupations develop? _____

2.  Name the fourteen fastest-growing occupations in the health service industry. _____

3.  Why have health occupations grown? _____

4.  Looking at Table 2-2 on page 31 in the textbook, identify the following:
    a.  Which occupation showed a surplus in 1998 and is projected in 2008? _____
    b.  Which occupation shows the greatest number of job openings? _____
    c.  How many projected new medical assistants will be needed by 2008? (Remember, the listings are in thousands.) _____
    d.  How many medical secretaries were employed in 1998 and how many more will be needed by 2008? _____
    e.  What is the most significant source of training for medical records technicians? _____
5.  Where can training for medical assisting be obtained? _____

6.  In the discussion of jobs under *Career Laddering* in the textbook, determine the amount of training and licensure (if needed) required to obtain the following jobs:
    a.  Licensed practical nurse _____
    b.  Emergency medical technician _____
    c.  Recreational therapist _____
    d.  Respiratory therapist _____
    e.  Dental hygienist _____
    f.  Nuclear medicine technologist _____
    g.  Physician assistant _____
    h.  Pharmacy technician _____
    i.  Occupational therapy assistant _____
7.  Refer to the CAAHEP Standards in Appendix B of the textbook. Within the area of *Professional Components*, which curriculum standards are discussed in this unit _____

**B. Fill in the Blank:** For each task below, identify if it is considered administrative or clinical by placing an "A" or "C" in the space provided.

_____ 1. Complete insurance forms

_____ 2. Maintain medical records

_____ 3. Take vital signs

_____ 4. Schedule appointments

_____ 5. Take medical histories

_____ 6. Prepare and give injections

_____ 7. Assist with medical procedures

_____ 8. Prepare medications

_____ 9. Handle mail

_____ 10. Prepare correspondence

_____ 11. Perform ECGs

_____ 12. Handle telephone calls

**C. Matching:** Match the definition in column II with the correct term in column I.

| COLUMN I | COLUMN II |
|---|---|
| _____ 1. Administrative | a. Conformity to formal or official requirements |
| _____ 2. Analysis | b. Following a plan or method |
| _____ 3. Clinical | c. One trained and skilled in the methods of a profession |
| _____ 4. Competency | d. A person trained in the technical aspect of an area of study |
| _____ 5. Compliance | e. Business and management tasks of a practice |
| _____ 6. Confidential | f. Non-public educational institutions |
| _____ 7. Methodical | g. An examination to determine something's content |
| _____ 8. Professional | h. Tasks dealing with patient examination and treatment |
| _____ 9. Proprietary | i. Having medicinal or healing properties |
| _____ 10. Technologist | j. A person who provides restorative treatments |
| _____ 11. Therapist | k. Being capable, able to perform at an acceptable level |
| _____ 12. Therapeutic | l. Held in strict confidence, secretive |

**D.  Word Puzzle:  Use the clues below to spell out these health occupations.**

1.                    _ _ O _ _ _ _ _ _ _
2.          _ _ _ _ _ C _ _ _
3.              _ _ C _ _ _ _
4.            _ _ _ U _
5.          _ _ _ _ P _ _ _ _ _ _
6.              _ _ A _ _ _
7.          _ _ _ _ _ T _ _ _
8.  _ _ _ _ _ _ I _ _
9.          _ _ _ _ _ O _ _ _ _ _ _
10.                  N _ _ _ _
11.  _ _ _ _ _ _ S _ _ _ _ _

1. Individual responsible for maintaining financial records
2. A doctor
3. Legal permit to engage in a certain activity
4. AAMA occupational analysis
5. A person who greets or welcomes
6. A state of freedom from disease
7. Individual responsible for office correspondence
8. An individual who provides a remedy
9. A person who applies scientific or mechanical methods
10. A person who provides care for the sick or injured
11. A person trained and skilled in a profession

After your instructor has returned your work to you, make all necessary corrections and place in a three-ring notebook for future reference.

**ASSIGNMENT SHEET**

**Chapter 2: THE MEDICAL ASSISTANT**

**Unit 2: PERSONAL CHARACTERISTICS**

**A. Matching: Match the definition in column II with the correct term in column I.**

COLUMN I

_____ 1. Accuracy
_____ 2. Adaptable
_____ 3. Conservative
_____ 4. Courteous
_____ 5. Dependable
_____ 6. Discreet
_____ 7. Empathy
_____ 8. Enthusiasm
_____ 9. Honesty
_____ 10. Initiative
_____ 11. Patience
_____ 12. Perseverance
_____ 13. Punctual
_____ 14. Reliable
_____ 15. Respectful
_____ 16. Self-control
_____ 17. Tact

COLUMN II

a. Can be relied upon, responsible
b. Ambition, hustle; set something in motion
c. Detailed correctness, exactness
d. Trustworthy, the quality of being truthful
e. Show restraint
f. Calmness in waiting; tolerant
g. Delicate skill in saying or doing the right thing
h. In exact agreement with appointed time
i. Zeal, intense interest
j. The ability to adjust
k. Showing regard for, considerate
l. Trying to identify one's feelings with those of another
m. To be cautious, handle with care, not wasteful
n. Prudent, cautious, especially in speech
o. To be polite, well-mannered
p. Trustworthy, dependable, responsible
q. Persistent effort, prolong

**B. Brief Answer**

1. Five personality qualities were identified in the text. List each one and give a brief definition.

   a. _____
   b. _____
   c. _____
   d. _____
   e. _____

2. Refer to the Role Delineation Chart in Appendix A of the textbook. Within the area of *Professionalism,* which role relates to your appearance? _____

**C. True or False:** Place a "T" for true or "F" for false in the space provided. For false statements, explain why they are false.

To be perceived as a professional, you must look like a professional. The following statements apply to your image. Indicate if they are true or false.

_____ 1. A skin rash on your body should not cause concern to a patient.

_____ 2. Being grossly overweight is beneficial when dealing with dieting patients who need to identify with a role model.

_____ 3. Personal illness requires prompt attention.

_____ 4. Deodorant will cover the odor from old perspiration.

_____ 5. Refrain from using hand cream because it attracts organisms.

_____ 6. Care should be taken to keep your hands out of your hair.

_____ 7. Chewing gum while working is unprofessional.

_____ 8. It is best to wear white underwear under a white uniform.

_____ 9. Your posture affects your energy level.

_____ 10. Chapped, cracked hands may allow organisms to enter the body.

_____ 11. Wearing a fragrance with a strong aroma helps soften the medicinal environment in the physician's office.

_____ 12. For women, vivid cosmetics and nailpolish are nice accents to a white uniform.

**D. Word Puzzle:** Use the clues below to spell out these terms.

```
 1.            _ _ C _ _ _ _ _
 2.        _ _ _ _ _ H _
 3.    _ _ _ _ _ _ A _ _ _
              _ _ R _ _ _ _ _
 4.        _ _ _ _ A _ _ _
 5.          _ _ _ C _ _ _ _ _
 6.          _ _ T _ _ _ _ _
 7.      _ _ _ _ _ E _ _ _
 8.      _ _ _ _ _ R _ _ _
 9.        _ _ _ _ I _ _ _ _ _
10.    _ _ _ _ _ S _ _ _ _
11.        _ _ T _ _ _ _ _ _
12.      _ _ _ _ I _ _ _
13.    _ _ _ _ _ C _ _ _ _
14.      _ _ _ _ S _ _
```

1. Correct
2. Identify with the feelings of another
3. Visible presence
4. Dependable
5. Prudent, cautious
6. Show tolerance
7. Polite

8. Act together
9. Set in motion
10. Intense interest
11. Feelings toward
12. Willing to adjust
13. Show regard for
14. Trustworthy

After your instructor has returned your work to you, make all necessary corrections and place in a three-ring notebook for future reference.

**ASSIGNMENT SHEET**

**Chapter 2: THE MEDICAL ASSISTANT**

**Unit 3: PROFESSIONALISM**

**A. Fill in the Blank**

1. The pioneers in medicine often were paid with a family's goods or valuables, which is called _____

2. _____ of every transaction between physician and patient is a must.

3. In _____ medical assistants from _____ states met in Kansas City, and adopted the name _____

4. The primary purpose of the AAMA was to raise the standards of the medical assistant to a _____

    _____

5. The Maxine Williams Scholarship fund was established to assist those interested in pursuing a career in medical assisting; scholarships are based on _____

6. The American Registry of Medical Assistants (ARMA) was established in _____ and operates with continual support and guidance from the _____

7. The purpose of the ARMA is to advance the standards and profession of medical assisting and to

    _____

8. A _____ year revalidation process has been developed through the American Medical Technologists Institute for Education (AMTIE) for ARMA members.

9. One who interprets and transcribes patient information from oral to printed form by typing or with the use of a word processor is known as a _____

10. In _____ the American Association for Medical Transcription (AAMT) was incorporated in _____ for the advancement of medical transcription.

11. _____ is the registered service mark for the rating that has become the recognized standard of measurement of secretarial proficiency.

12. The American Medical Technologists outline the requirements of professionalism in their

    _____

13. Both the AAMA national certification exam and the ARMA registry exam are designed to evaluate _____ competency in medical assisting.

14. Continuing education is available through professional medical assistant organizations that offer _____ to those who successfully complete seminars, workshops, publications, and home-study programs.

**B. Matching: Match the definition in column II with the correct term in column I.**

COLUMN I

_____ 1. Evaluation
_____ 2. Competent
_____ 3. Professionalism
_____ 4. Accreditation
_____ 5. Registry

_____ 6. Revalidation
_____ 7. Certification
_____ 8. Reputation
_____ 9. Initiative

COLUMN II

a. Process of evaluating competency in a specific area of expertise
b. Reconfirmation of one's competency in a specific area of expertise
c. To start on one's own; to begin
d. Assessment; judgment concerning worth of a person
e. The assignment of credentials; approval given for meeting established standards
f. What is generally believed about one's character
g. One who is trained and skilled in the methods of the profession
h. Place where the listing of competent individuals is kept
i. Fit, able, capable in a specific area

**C. Brief Answser**

1. When, where, and why did the medical assistant profession begin? _____

_____

2. a. Write the AAMA-approved definition of medical assisting: _____

_____

_____

   b. Write the ARMA approved definition of medical assisting: _____

_____

3. State the purpose of the AMT Standards of Practice and what members must recognize in themselves. _____

_____

_____

_____

4. List the nine competencies outlined in the AAMA Role Delineation Chart that demonstrate professionalism.

_____

_____

5. Explain why it is important for professionals to certify or recertify according to the guidelines set by the professional medical assistant organizations. _____

_____

_____

6. List the professional organizations that would be beneficial to the medical assistant.

   a. _____

   b. _____

   c. _____

   d. _____

**D. True or False: Place a "T" for true or "F" for false in the space provided. For false statements, explain why they are false.**

_____ 1. The AAPC *Coding Edge* is the professional magazine of the AAMA.

_____ 2. Many employers require current certification or registration for medical assistants to be considered for employment.

_____ 3. To stay current with the field of medicine, medical assistants should participate in continuing education programs to earn CEUs toward recertification.

_____ 4. Medical assistants as well as physicians have a code of ethics to follow in their professions.

_____ 5. The competency of medical assistant programs is determined by the accrediting board of the American Medical Association.

After your instructor has returned your work to you, make all necessary corrections and place in a three-ring notebook for future reference.

**ASSIGNMENT SHEET**

## Chapter 3: MEDICAL ETHICS AND LIABILITY

Review the objectives and text for each unit before completing the assignment sheet for that unit. When you have completed all sheets for the chapter, remove them from this Workbook and give them to the instructor for evaluation.

## Unit 1: ETHICAL AND LEGAL RESPONSIBILITIES

**A. Multiple Choice: Place the correct letter or letters on the blank line for each question.**

_____ 1. Which item is *not* a requirement for a physician to be licensed?

 a. be of good moral character     c. be of legal age

 b. completed approved residency program     d. has no allergies

_____ 2. The exceptions to the need for a license to practice medicine are

 a. an emergency situation     c. treating family members

 b. physician in military     d. school physician

_____ 3. The two basic elements that constitute the practice of medicine are

 a. diagnosis     c. prescribing

 b. scheduling     d. accounting

_____ 4. Areas of medical ethics that are of concern to the medical assistant are

 a. honesty     c. competency

 b. confidentiality     d. all of these

_____ 5. When the medical assistant improves skills and acquires additional knowledge in the field of medicine, who benefits?

 a. the medical assistant     c. the patient

 b. colleagues     d. all of these

## B. Brief Answer

1. How can DRGs cause ethical issues for physicians? _____

_____

2. What is the most common transplant? _____

3. Explain what the term emancipated minor means. _____

_____

4. What is the recommended statement that should be made to the patient by the medical assistant responsible for obtaining a signature on the consent form for invasive, experimental, and high-risk medical services?

_____

5. What does *privileged communication* mean? _____

_____

6. Describe the conditions for revocation or suspension of a medical license. _____

_____

7. Describe unprofessional conduct. _____

_____

_____

**B. Matching:** Match the definition in column II with the correct term in column I.

COLUMN I

_____ 1. Offer
_____ 2. Contract law
_____ 3. Reciprocity
_____ 4. Ethics
_____ 5. Tort
_____ 6. Implied consent
_____ 7. Civil laws
_____ 8. Endorsement
_____ 9. Acceptance
_____ 10. Consideration

COLUMN II

a. Deals with what is morally right and wrong
b. Deals with findings of negligence; most common basis for lawsuits against physicians
c. Takes place when appointment is given and the doctor examines the patient
d. Written consent for medical services
e. Pass exam administered by the National Board of Medical Examiners
f. Takes place when a competent individual indicates desire to be a patient
g. Payment given in exchange for services
h. License granted in new state because of equal requirements of original license
i. Patient enters into agreement by coming to see physician
j. Patient-physician relationship considered contract
k. Defines powers of government and its citizens
l. Deals with laws governing property ownership, corporation, and inheritance

**D. Fill in the Blank**

1. A medical license may be revoked for _____

2. A license may be revoked because of proven _____ in the application for the license.

3. Physicians who are found to be incompetent to practice because of _____ may have their license revoked.

4. The ethical standards established by a profession are administered by _____

5. The physician must release patient information when the patient authorizes the release or if the release of information is _____

6. With proper documentation, any person of sound mind and legal age may give any part of the body after death for _____

7. Human organs should never be _____

8. Copies of the living will document should be filed with the _____
_____

9. Every member of the medical care team should be currently certified in _____

10. Under the _____ patients must receive written information explaining their right-to-die options according to their state laws.

11. A _____ is defined as any number of actions done by one person or group of persons that causes injury to another or others.

12. The negligent causing of an injury, when committed by a physician in the course of professional duties, is commonly referred to as _____

13. Libel and slander are two forms of _____

14. A deliberate attempt or threat to touch without consent is called _____

15. _____ is the unauthorized touching of another person.

**E. Word Puzzle:** Use the clues below to spell out these terms.

```
 1.              __ __ P __ __ __ __ __
 2.                 __ R __ __ __ __
 3.  __ __ __ __ __ __ __ O __
 4.              __ __ C __ __ __ __ __
 5.     __ __ __ __ __ R __ __ __
 6.           __ __ __ A __ __ __ __ __
 7  __ __ __ __ __ __ __ S __
 8.    __ __ __ __ __ __ T __
 9.        __ __ __ I __ __ __ __
10.                 N __ __ __ __ __ __ __ __ __
11.           __ __ A __ __ __ __ __ __ __
12.           __ __ __ T
13.           __ I __ __ __ __ __ __
14.        __ __ __ O __ __ __ __ __
15.     __ __ __ __ N __ __ __ __
```

1. Definite, specific
2. Violation of a law, contract, or other agreement
3. A standard of criticism or judgment
4. The principles of any branch of knowledge
5. To count separately; name one by one
6. Injury done to a person's reputation by or through slanderous statements
7. To surround, enclose
8. To bind legally or morally
9. Feebleness of body or mind caused by old age
10. Malpractice
11. Characterized by cheating and deceit; obtaining by dishonest means
12. An injurious, harmful action, not involving a breach of contract, for which a civil action can be brought
13. Anything to which a person is liable, responsible, legally bound
14. To cancel; withdraw; take back
15. A legal permit to engage in an activity

After your instructor has returned your work to you, make all necessary corrections and place in a three-ring notebook for future reference.

**ASSIGNMENT SHEET**

**Chapter 3: MEDICAL ETHICS AND LIABILITY**

**Unit 2: PROFESSIONAL LIABILITY**

**SUGGESTED RESPONSES TO CRITICAL THINKING CHALLENGE IN TEXTBOOK**

1. What should Lisa have done? _____

_____

2. Who is responsible for the patient's record? _____

_____

_____

3. What would you have done? _____

4. Should the supervisor, physician, or office manager be called about this? If so, why? _____

_____

_____

**A. Brief Answer**

1. Describe the correct procedure for terminating the physician-patient contract.

_____

_____

_____

_____

_____

2. Explain the term *abandonment,* and give an example.

_____

_____

_____

3. What is professional negligence? Give an example.

_____

_____

4. In what situations could a medical assistant be charged with malpractice?

_____

5. What is the purpose of the Good Samaritan Act?

_____

6. List the reasons for keeping medical records.

_____

7. Who owns medical office records?

_____

8. Do patients have the right to the information in their medical records?

_____

_____

9. What special precautions should be taken when giving written instructions to a patient?

_____

_____

10. What kinds of notes are inappropriate in a patient's chart? Why?

_____

_____

_____

11. Describe the acceptable method for making changes in medical records.

_____

_____

12. List and discuss the guidelines for reducing the number of forged prescription orders.

_____

_____

13. Discuss with other class members the issue of manipulated stem cell and cultivated donor tissue
    experimentation and research. Then write your concerns and your opinion about this controversial topic.

_____

_____

_____

**B. True or False:** **Place a "T" for true or "F" for false in the space provided. For false statements, explain
why they are false.**

_____ 1. Physicians have no right to determine whom they will see as patients.

_____ 2. Patients have the right to receive care equal to the standards of care in the community as a
whole.

_____ 3. A physician may choose to withdraw from the care of a patient who does not follow
instructions for treatment or follow-up appointments or who leaves a hospital against advice
to stay.

_____ 4. The medical assistant has the right to be free from sexual discrimination.

_____ 5. The victim of sexual harassment must be of the opposite sex.

_____ 6. The testimony of a physician as an expert medical witness is never necessary in a case of
negligence.

_____ 7. The doctrine, *res ipsa loquitur,* means the thing speaks for itself.

_____ 8. The physician's liability is expressed in the doctrine of *respondeat superior.*

_____ 9. The medical assistant is considered an agent for the physician under the law of agency.

_____ 10. The Good Samaritan law covers physicians even if they receive compensation for the
emergency care given.

_____ 11. An implied agreement is considered to be a legal contract in a medical office.

_____ 12. The medical assistant should never attempt to perform a procedure without having been
properly trained.

## C. Fill in the Blank

1. Derogatory statements regarding patients may be considered _____ of character and a breach of confidentiality.

2. An attorney may agree to take the testimony of the physician by _____

3. A medical assistant may receive a _____ to appear in court with patient records.

4. A _____ is a law that designates a specific time limit during which a claim may be filed in malpractice suits or in the collection of bills.

5. _____ cannot be tolerated in handling medical records.

6. Each office should have a _____ regarding the release of information from a medical record.

7. The requirement of confidentiality regarding the medical record is no longer recognized when the patient _____ against the physician.

8. When in doubt about disclosing patient information, _____ by not disclosing rather than by disclosing.

9. The _____ to disclose information should be placed in the patient's chart with a copy of the information released.

10. Corrections in the medical record should appear in _____

After your instructor has returned your work to you, make all necessary corrections and place in a three-ring notebook for future reference.

**ASSIGNMENT SHEET**

**Chapter 4: INTERPERSONAL COMMUNICATIONS**

Review the objectives and text for each unit before completing the assignment sheet for that unit. When you have completed all sheets for the chapter, remove them from this Workbook and give them to the instructor for evaluation.

**Unit 1: VERBAL AND NONVERBAL MESSAGES**

**SUGGESTED RESPONSES TO CRITICAL THINKING CHALLENGE IN TEXTBOOK**

1. What is going on here? _____

2. Does Jackie have a reason to be upset? _____

_____

_____

3. What should Kelly and Sabrina have done to alleviate the brewing situation? _____

_____

**A. Unscramble**

1. _ _ _ _ _ _ _ _ _ _ _ _     RTMINTRSIEPE
2. _ _ _ _ _ _ _ _ _ _     TIAGBELNN
3. _ _ _ _ _ _ _     SDRTOIT
4. _ _ _ _ _ _ _ _ _     IUINONITT
5. _ _ _ _ _ _ _ _ _ _     OIPPETNREC
6. _ _ _ _ _ _ _ _ _ _ _     ICOGOUNNRSU
7. _ _ _ _ _ _ _ _ _ _ _ _     UOUSSRUCLLYP
8. _ _ _ _ _ _ _ _ _ _     NDTICARTCO
9. _ _ _ _ _ _ _ _ _ _ _     PIEMRIYLALC
10. _ _ _ _ _ _ _ _ _ _     CUETLTIARA
11. _ _ _ _ _ _ _ _ _ _ _ _ _     ENZCEOPCUTALI

**B. Labeling:** Add labels to each boxed section of this communication process model. Refer to Figure 4-1 in the textbook.

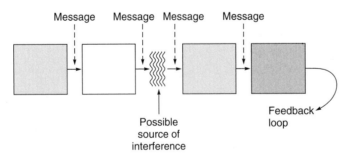

**C. Brief Answer**

1. Describe the basic pattern of communication. _____

_____

_____

2. Give examples of nonverbal communication. _____
_____
_____

3. Explain how verbal and nonverbal communication can sometimes be misinterpreted. _____
_____
_____

4. How can tone and speed of speech affect a message? _____
_____
_____

5. Why is it important to wear appropriateattire when working with patients? _____
_____
_____
_____

6. Explain what perception is. _____
_____

7. Why is it important to develop the skill of perception? _____
_____
_____

8. Why is silence such a powerful nonverbal message (communication)? _____
_____
_____

9. What benefit does the communication of touch provide to patients? _____
_____
_____

**D. True or False: Place a "T" for true or "F" for false in the space provided. For false statements, explain why they are false.**

_____ 1. The medical assistant can be instrumental in providing comfort and compassion to patients in need.

_____ 2. A harmonious team effort makes for an efficient and pleasant work environment.

_____ 3. Becoming perceptive can only be attained by reading.

_____ 4. Your overall appearance sends out messages to anyone who looks at you.

_____ 5. Setting a good example is not part of your responsibility in the care of others.

_____ 6. Your attitude has nothing to do with your overall appearance.

_____ 7. Gestures are body movements that can help the receiver understand the message being communicated.

_____ 8. Studies show that a caring touch can elicit better response in treatment of patients.

_____ 9. It is possible to contradict a verbal message by an inappropriate facial expression.

_____ 10. Your attitude shows in your facial expression.

_____ 11. Active listening during triage involves repeating back to the patient what was said to you to verify the problem.

_____ 12. There are some expressions, remarks, and hand gestures that may be offensive to those who are from different cultures, backgrounds, or countries.

_____ 13. The proper distance between people who are having a personal conversation is from 10 to 18 feet.

_____ 14. It is very important to be courteous with patients when communicating information to them.

**E. Crossword Puzzle**

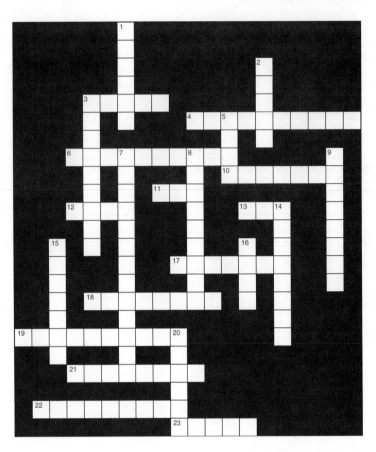

ACROSS

3. How you project this is of utmost importance
4. You must speak this way if you are to be understood
6. Being aware of your own and others' feelings
10. You should set a good _____
11. Effective communication is an _____
12. _____ work
13. Conveys feelings of affection
17. To twist or mess up
18. Efficient use of time comes from _____
19. Good rapport
21. To send a message
22. Unspoken
23. Conveys a positive message

DOWN

1. Spoken
2. Gives patients a sense of security and caring
3. To come between
5. You should speak in a pleasant _____
7. Exchange of information
8. Perception
9. Everyone has them
14. Body movements that send messages
15. What a team gives each other
16. A strong communication (language)
20. You must continually strive to master _____

**CRITICAL THINKING SCENARIOS: What would your response be in the following situations?**

1. A 25-year-old female patient arrives a half hour early for her appointment. You notice that she is sitting off by herself and is sobbing. _____
_____

2. A middle-aged male patient has just finished a consultation with the doctor. The patient tells you that it is getting harder all the time taking care of his invalid father. _____
_____

3. You notice that a co-worker has made several charting errors in the past few days. It bothers you, for you are worried about quality patient care and the legal ramifications. _____
_____

4. Your physician-employer asks you to help an elderly patient overcome procrastination about taking his medication and eating regularly. _____
_____

5. A young mother of four (ranging in age from 6 months to 5 years) complains to you that she has no time for herself, is always exhausted, and is a nervous wreck. _____
_____

After your instructor has returned your work to you, make all necessary corrections and place in a three-ring notebook for future reference.

**ASSIGNMENT SHEET**

**Chapter 4: INTERPERSONAL COMMUNICATIONS**

**Unit 2: BEHAVIORAL ADJUSTMENTS**

**A. Matching: Match the definition in column II with the correct term in column I.**

COLUMN I

_____ 1. Adjustment
_____ 2. Analytical
_____ 3. Ardently
_____ 4. Displacement
_____ 5. Intellectualization
_____ 6. Malinger
_____ 7. Projection
_____ 8. Rationalization
_____ 9. Repression
_____ 10. Stratagem
_____ 11. Sublimation
_____ 12. Unobtrusive
_____ 13. Procrastination

COLUMN II

a. To keep down or hold back
b. Devotedly
c. To pretend to be ill
d. To settle or bring into accord
e. Below the threshold of consciousness
f. Rationalism; reasoning without regard to feelings
g. A plan to deceive
h. Question/examine
i. Unconsciously blaming another for one's own inadequacies
j. putting things off
k. Modest; unpretending
l. Transfer of feelings about another to an innocent person
m. Devising a socially acceptable explanation for inadequate behavior
n. Discord; confusion

**B. Brief Answer**

1. List the commonly used defense mechanisms and give an example of each. _____

_____

_____

_____

_____

_____

_____

_____

_____

_____

_____

_____

_____

2. What could happen to a person who habitually uses one or more of the commonly used defense mechanisms?

_____

_____

_____

_____

3. Why is it necessary to know oneself before one can relate effectively with others? _____

_____

_____

_____

_____

4. What are the problem-solving steps outined in this unit?

   a. _____

   _____

   b. _____

   c. _____

   d. _____

   _____

5. Apply the problem-solving steps to a particular problem you may have. _____

_____

_____

_____

6. Explain the importance of one's mental and emotional status to overall health. _____

_____

_____

_____

## C. Fill in the Blank

1. Problem-solving skills can help one eliminate _____

2. How we view ourselves is our _____

3. Our response to others is dealt with by our _____

4. Unfortunately, many of us never come close to reaching our true _____

5. Making a list of our strengths and weaknesses is a good way to begin a _____ of ourselves.

6. Two good times to take a look at ourselves for evaluation and renew our goals and aspirations are _____ and _____

7. _____ is a complex process in which one has to be aware of all facets for complete information exchanges to occur.

8. The perceptive medical assistant should be able to decide what _____ to ask a patient to determine whether the look on that patient's face matches the patient's demeanor.

9. The medical assistant must impart a genuine _____ for the patient's well-being.

10. Patients may open up about their problems or preoccupations if the medical assistant shows an _____ and takes the _____ with them that they need.

11. _____ take the blame away from the person you are speaking to and places it on the thing being discussed.

**D. Word Search:** **(1) Find the following words hidden in the puzzle. (2) Use each even-numbered word in a sentence.**

1. ACTS
2. AVOID
3. DEFENSE MECHANISMS
4. SELF
5. REGRESSION
6. ACCEPT
7. MALINGER
8. BLAME
9. KIND
10. INFLUENCE

11. ANXIETY
12. RATIONALIZATION
13. CONCERN
14. BEHAVIOR
15. PROBLEM
16. DENIAL
17. PATIENTS
18. EMOTIONS
19. CARE
20. EXPRESS

```
A N L V A Z E S P T V O F T K Q P R O E N
O B S O A C T S A C P S R T L Z M Y M R Y
D R W Z V T A L T S G W L P T O A A B A L
P Z E A O P N S E Q R O A E E S L Z Q C G
A Q R N I N T L Q S R Z P C L B I L R A B
N O V E D E F E N S E M E C H A N I S M S
T D D I O E P G T P G S M A D N G O T Z X
I N F L U E N C E D R A O D L M E B N W O
N I V A L B F I Y Z E D B H M E R L E B T
D K N X C W L T A A S L E F E L A A I L S
I S W A F B E O J L S M H T J B O M T F V
S Z R A T I O N A L I Z A T I O N Z A K A
O P R O X G Z C Q A O T V K B R P F P I L
P C O N C E R N L Z N H I A H P O E R N R
D A A X O W B J E K S N O S S E R P X E Q
Z M B E M O T I O N S A R S S R D M S C B
```

1. _____
2. _____
3. _____
4. _____
5. _____
6. _____
7. _____
8. _____
9. _____
10. _____

After your instructor has returned your work to you, make all necessary corrections and place in a three-ring notebook for future reference.

## ASSIGNMENT SHEET

**Chapter 4: INTERPERSONAL COMMUNICATIONS**

**Unit 3: PATIENTS AND THEIR FAMILIES**

**A. Matching: Match the definition in column II with the correct term in column I.**

COLUMN I

_____ 1. Marginal
_____ 2. Holistic
_____ 3. Terminal
_____ 4. Absurd
_____ 5. Incomprehensible
_____ 6. Nonchalant
_____ 7. Hostility
_____ 8. Inevitable
_____ 9. Devastate
_____ 10. Plight

COLUMN II

a. Cannot be understood
b. Showing no interest
c. A sad situation
d. Certain to happen
e. Overwhelm
f. Close to a limit
g. Pertaining to whole
h. Apprehension
i. Ridiculous
j. Antagonistic
k. Final

**B. Brief Answser**

1. Why is it important to develop good rapport with patients?_____
_____
_____

2. How can the medical assistant safeguard the patient's right to confidentiality?_____
_____
_____
_____

3. What are the patient's options in relation to the physician's treatment plan?_____
_____
_____

4. Describe the stages that patients experience following the diagnosis of terminal illness. _____
_____
_____
_____

5. What is the medical assistant's role in dealing with terminally ill patients? _____
_____
_____

6. What is the purpose of the living will (also referred to as advance directives)? _____
_____
_____

7. What is the purpose of the hospice movement? _____

_____

_____

8. List the services the hospice movement provides. _____

_____

_____

_____

_____

## C. Fill in the Blank

1. The first responsibility for the medical professional is to the _____

2. Facing unfamiliar surroundings and unfamiliar medical language adds to the patient's _____

3. Tact and good communication skills help promote _____ with patients.

4. The patient's _____ must be obtained to release information about him or her to unauthorized persons.

5. The physician must be informed of a patient's _____ for it may have some bearing on the condition of the patient.

6. The medical assistant plays an integral part in _____ the physician's orders.

7. _____ is the key in helping patients accept and comply with treatment.

8. By being a good _____ the medical assistant reinforces the physician's advice.

9. A copy of the living will is filed with the physician, the _____ and the family of a terminally ill patient.

10. Terminally ill patients and their families may need _____ guidance more at this time than ever before in their lives.

11. When communicating with patients who speak a different language than you do, an _____ should be scheduled for the time of the patient's appointment.

12. A defense mechanism that protects one from reaching a set goal because it seems too difficult to complete is called _____ behavior.

13. Patients who have documentation stating they do not wish for extreme life-saving efforts should have _____ or _____ written in their chart.

After your instructor has returned your work to you, make all necessary corrections and place in a three-ring notebook for future reference.

**ASSIGNMENT SHEET**

## Chapter 4:  INTERPERSONAL COMMUNICATIONS

## Unit 4:  OFFICE INTERPERSONAL RELATIONSHIPS

### SUGGESTED RESPONSES TO CRITICAL THINKING CHALLENGE IN TEXTBOOK

1. What should Marcia do about this situation? _____

_____

2. Should Marcia tell the doctor about Julie's behavior? _____

_____

3. Is there any way that Marcia can suggest that Julie needs a refresher course on professionalism? _____

_____

4. What would you do in this situation? _____

_____

### A.  Unscramble

1. _ _ _ _ _          YETPT
2. _ _ _ _ _ _ _ _ _ _ _          LATNEAOIVU
3. _ _ _ _ _ _ _ _ _ _          RLXGNIPEPE
4. _ _ _ _ _          IRMTE
5. _ _ _ _ _ _ _ _ _ _ _          PDSECITRINO
6. _ _ _ _ _ _ _          ULISERE
7. _ _ _ _ _ _ _ _ _ _          VRJETENAUE

### B.  Brief Answer

1. What are the most important factors in the relationships among medical assistant, employers, and co-workers? _____

_____

_____

2. List positive factors of externship. _____

_____

3. What are the reasons for staff meetings? _____

_____

4. List some methods of intraoffice communication. _____

_____

5. What is the purpose of the employee evaluation? _____

_____

_____

_____

**C. Matching:  MATCH the definition in column II with the correct term in column I.**

COLUMN I

_____ 1. Annual evaluations
_____ 2. Positive attitude
_____ 3. Self-discipline
_____ 4. Medical assistant
_____ 5. Break-time
_____ 6. Cooperation
_____ 7. Intraoffice memo
_____ 8. Teamwork
_____ 9. Job descriptions
_____ 10. Good rapport
_____ 11. AAMA and ARMA

COLUMN II

a.  Means of communicating important information to staff
b.  Continuing education
c.  Results in quality patient care
d.  Promote efficiency
e.  Necessary to accomplish objectives of physician and patient
f.  Regular exercise
g.  Creates pleasant work environment
h.  Necessary in a professional setting
i.  Essential in smooth office operation
j.  Motivate employees and keep communication lines open
k.  Must relate well to others
l.  Essential to well-being

After your instructor has returned your work to you, make all necessary corrections and place in a three-ring notebook for future reference.

**ASSIGNMENT SHEET**

**Chapter 5:  THE OFFICE ENVIRONMENT**

   Review the objectives and text for each unit before completing the assignment sheet for that unit. When you have completed all sheets for the chapter, remove them from this Workbook and give them to the instructor for evaluation.

**Unit 1:  SAFETY, SECURITY, AND EMERGENCY PROVISIONS IN THE MEDICAL OFFICE**

**A.  Brief Answer**

1. List four things to check every morning to assure a safe environment in the medical office.

   a. _____     c. _____

   b. _____     d. _____

2. Identify four hazards to which you should be alert in the business area of an office.

   a. _____     c. _____

   b. _____     d. _____

3. Name five things in an examination room that might cause an unsafe situation.

   a. _____     d. _____

   b. _____     e. _____

   c. _____

4. What does the term *fire triangle* mean? _____

   _____

   _____

5. Name seven things that might start a fire in an office.

   a. _____     e. _____

   b. _____     f. _____

   c. _____     g. _____

   d. _____

6. What types of natural disasters require an established office policy regarding appropriate action to take?

   _____

   _____

7. Why are severe weather drills necessary? _____

8. How does knowing what to do or how to act affect a person's response to a crisis? _____

   _____

   _____

   _____

9. How would you clean up the following?

   a. Body fluids _____

   b. Glass fragments _____

10. Name the eight telephone numbers that should be posted near each office telephone.

   a. _____     e. _____

   b. _____     f. _____

   c. _____     g. _____

   d. _____     h. _____

11. Using your local phone directory, complete the "card" below listing the service and its appropriate number.

```
┌─────────────────────────────────────────────────────────────────────┐
│                        EMERGENCY NUMBERS                            │
│                                                                     │
│   SERVICE        NUMBER           SERVICE        NUMBER             │
│                                                                     │
│   _____      _____       _____      _____          │
│                                                                     │
│   _____      _____       _____      _____          │
│                                                                     │
│   _____      _____       _____      _____          │
│                                                                     │
│   _____      _____       _____      _____          │
│                                                                     │
└─────────────────────────────────────────────────────────────────────┘
```

12. What can you do to protect yourself from skin and mucous membrane exposure to harmful organisms? List six examples of protective items. _____

_____

13. Refer to the Role Delineation Chart in Appendix A of the textbook. Within the area of *Legal Concepts,* which three roles relate to the content of this unit? _____

_____

_____

## B. Crossword Puzzle

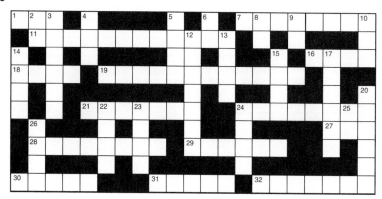

**ACROSS**

1. A pair
7. To leave
11. Device to put out fire
16. Entranceway
18. Floor coverings
19. Contaminated material
21. Obstruction, a guard
24. Potentially dangerous
28. Holder for soap
29. Reducing danger
30. Remains, left over
31. Covering for hand
32. A disease prevention substance

**DOWN**

2. Us
3. An essential element for life and combustion
4. The virus associated with AIDS
5. A federal agency
6. Myself
8. Virginia (abbreviation)
9. California (abbreviation)
10. Assists with hearing
12. Dangers
13. Unusual, not common
14. A section, place
15. Combustible material
17. Place of employment
20. Safe, protected from dange
22. The eventual result of HIV
23. Dangerous chance
24. Able to see
25. Learning disabled (abbreviation)
26. A federal agency

After your instructor has returned your work to you, make all necessary corrections and place in a three-ring notebook for future reference.

**ASSIGNMENT SHEET**

**Chapter 5:  THE OFFICE ENVIRONMENT**

**Unit 2:  EFFICIENT OFFICE DESIGN**

**A.  Word Puzzle:  Use the clues below to spell out these terms.**

1.         _ _ _ I _ _
2.         _ _ _ _ _ M _ _ _
3.   _ _ _ _ _ _ P _ _ _ _ _
4.   _ _ _ _ _ _ L _ _ _
5.         _ _ _ E _ _ _ _ _ _ _
6.        _ _ _ _ M _ _ _ _ _ _
7         _ E _ _ _ _ _ _
8.   _ _ _ _ _ N _ _ _ _ _
9.         _ _ _ T _ _ _ _
10.       _ _ _ _ A _ _
11.       _ _ _ T _ _ _ _ _ _ _ _ _
12.       _ _ _ I _ _ _
13.       _ _ _ O _ _ _ _
14.       _ _ _ N _ _

1. Layout, arrangement
2. To act out
3. Foresight
4. Limitation, physical handicap
5. Translator
6. To serve
7. Practicable/workable
8. Infectious
9. Nurture
10. Order by law
11. To infect
12. Printing/writing system for the blind
13. Sleeplessness
14. Actions/gestures used to convey information

**B. Brief Answer**

1. Explain the ADA and state when it became effective.

   _____
   _____
   _____
   _____

2. What specifically is mandated by the ADA?

   _____
   _____
   _____

3. Where in a medical facility should provisions be made for persons with disabilities?

   _____

4. Explain in your own words what is meant by "efficient office design."

   _____
   _____

5. Discuss what can make patients feel comfortable and satisfied when visiting a medical facility.

   _____

6. Discuss the reasons for separating well-visit and sick patients in the reception area.

   _____

7. Where shouldrest rooms, public phones, and water fountains be located for patient use in the medical facility?

   _____

8. Explain the proper way to speak to a hearing-impaired (deaf) person.

   _____
   _____

9. What may happen if the daily schedule is more often than not backed up? Why?

   _____

10. Describe how one should speak to a person in a wheelchair.

    _____

11. Where can information be obtained regarding regulations concerning persons with disabilities?

    _____
    _____

**C. True or False:** **Place a "T" for true or "F" for false in the space provided. For false statements, explain why they are false.**

_____ 1. Patients who are hearing-impaired or deaf should have a signer available to communicate their needs

_____ 2. You should talk directly to the interpreter to communicate information for the patient with disabilities.

_____ 3. Proper ventilation and moderate temperature are necessary for comfort in a public facility.

_____ 4. All patients waiting for appointments are placed at-risk for possible exposure to communicable diseases.

_____ 5. The management of the schedule is not a vital part of the medical practice.

_____ 6. All office furniture should be arranged to accommodate wheelchairs.

_____ 7. Educational programs on television for patients to view in the reception room should be very loud so that the hearing-impaired can also benefit from them.

_____ 8. It is a sensible practice when walking in hallways to keep to the right to create and maintain an orderly traffic pattern.

After your instructor has returned your work to you, make all necessary corrections and place in a three-ring notebook for future reference.

**ASSIGNMENT SHEET**

**Chapter 5: THE OFFICE ENVIRONMENT**

**Unit 3: ERGONOMICS IN THE MEDICAL OFFICE**

**A. Multiple Choice: Place the correct letter or letters on the blank line for each question.**

_____ 1. The science that applies to the physician and staff in the workplace is
    a. physics                 c. ecology
    b. psychiatry           d. ergonomics

_____ 2. Considerations that should be taken when planning a medical office layout are
    a. floor plan/blueprints     c. room space
    b. environmental factors    d. all of these

_____ 3. The way to keep the medical facility free of foul odors is to
    a. remove trash as needed    c. use an air freshener
    b. clean routinely         d. all of these

_____ 4. Items that can absorb sound to keep noise at a moderate level are
    a. furniture              c. carpet
    b. reading materials      d. silk flower arrangements

_____ 5. Ergonomists recommend that computer operators
    a. wear wrist supports     c. use special keyboard
    b. vary their duties       d. all of these

**B. Brief Answer**

1. Why is ergonomics important?

_____

_____

2. What are the two most important points to consider in a medical office layout design?

_____

_____

3. Comment on room size in an office plan.

_____

_____

4. Discuss lighting and how it relates to safety.

_____

_____

5. What is ocular accommodation, and what can be done to prevent it?

_____

_____

6. How is a TV best used in a medical office reception room (if at all)?

_____

_____

7. Refer to Figure 5-13. Why is the work station in this picture ergonomically correct?

_____

_____

_____

**C. True or False:  Place a "T" for true or "F" for false in the space provided. For false statements, explain why they are false.**

_____    1. A medical office with problems in patient flow and scheduling can be helped by an ergonomist.

_____    2. Room temperature can affect work performance.

_____    3. Soft instrumental music can be comforting and relaxing to both staff and patients.

_____    4. A pleasant decor in the latest color and style in the medical office is meant to impress patients with the physician's success.

_____    5. The goal of ergonomics is to make jobs as easy and efficient as possible for optimum use of time and space.

**D. Unscramble**

1. _ _ _ _ _          KOVEE

2. _ _ _ _ _ _ _ _     RMETLANI

3. _ _ _ _ _          REGLA

4. _ _ _ _ _ _        MARUAT

5. _ _ _ _ _ _ _ _ _ _  SDIICEILNP

6. _ _ _ _ _ _        NUTLEN

7. _ _ _ _ _ _ _      YLASPDI

8. _ _ _ _ _ _ _ _    VANOREET

**E. Fill in the Blank**

1. A varied schedule of duties can help you stay _____

2. The avoidance of _____ is advised with all lighting, as it can impair vision and is uncomfortable as well.

3. _____ may signal problems such as overheating of equipment, chemical leaks, or other serious potential health hazards.

4. The proper _____ of the computer monitor will prevent glare from incoming light from windows and artificial lights in the room.

5. For those who work with computers routinely, a _____ should be used.

6. People feel more _____ in bright and colorful rooms.

7. For those who sit most of the day at work, _____ is necessary to prevent back and other work-related conditions.

8. An adjustable chair is desirable for comfort and _____ of the back.

9. Using a _____ may help in avoiding posture problems.

10. The _____ is the most critical for an ergonomically sound workplace.

After your instructor has returned your work to you, make all necessary corrections and place in a three-ring notebook for future reference.

**ASSIGNMENT SHEET**

**Chapter 5: THE OFFICE ENVIRONMENT**

**Unit 4: PREPARING FOR THE DAY**

**SUGGESTED RESPONSES TO CRITICAL THINKING CHALLENGE IN TEXTBOOK**

1. Can you put yourself in Mrs. Diaz's place? _____

   _____

2. How would you feel? _____

   _____

   _____

   _____

   _____

3. Does a person's nationality or skin color affect how he or she are perceived? _____

   _____

   _____

   _____

4. Do you think the office manager should mention this situation to the physician so that other people are not treated the same? _____

   _____

   _____

   _____

   _____

5. What could be done in the office to assure that this type of situation does not occur again? _____

   _____

**Brief Answer**

1. Prepare a checklist for opening the office. (Refer to Procedure 5-1.) _____

   _____

   _____

2. What is the role of the receptionist? _____

3. Why is the reception room atmosphere important? _____

   _____

4. Name six things to check in the reception room. _____

   _____

5. List information that might be included in a practice information brochure. _____

   _____

6. Complete the new patient information form on the following page as if you are the patient. Then role-play being a receptionist and interview another student.

7. Why should social climate be monitored? _____

   _____

## PATIENT INFORMATION                                        DATE:

| PATIENT'S NAME | MARITAL STATUS | DATE OF BIRTH | SOCIAL SECURITY NO. |
|---|---|---|---|
| | S \| M \| W \| DIV \| SEP | | |

| STREET ADDRESS ☐ PERMANENT ☐ TEMPORARY | CITY AND STATE | | ZIP CODE | HOME PHONE NO. |
|---|---|---|---|---|

| PATIENT'S EMPLOYER | OCCUPATION (INDICATE IF STUDENT) | HOW LONG EMPLOYED? | BUSINESS PHONE NO. |
|---|---|---|---|

| EMPLOYER'S STREET ADDRESS | CITY AND STATE | ZIP CODE |
|---|---|---|

| IN CASE OF EMERGENCY CONTACT: | | DRIVERS LIC. NO. |
|---|---|---|

| SPOUSE'S NAME |
|---|

| SPOUSE'S EMPLOYER | OCCUPATION (INDICATE IF STUDENT) | HOW LONG EMPLOYED? | BUSINESS PHONE NO. |
|---|---|---|---|

| EMPLOYER'S STREET ADDRESS | CITY AND STATE | ZIP CODE |
|---|---|---|

| WHO REFERRED YOU TO THIS PRACTICE? |
|---|

## IF THE PATIENT IS A MINOR OR STUDENT

| MOTHER'S NAME | STREET ADDRESS, CITY, STATE AND ZIP CODE | HOME PHONE NO. |
|---|---|---|

| MOTHER'S EMPLOYER | OCCUPATION | HOW LONG EMPLOYED? | BUSINESS PHONE NO. |
|---|---|---|---|

| EMPLOYER'S STREET ADDRESS | CITY AND STATE | ZIP CODE |
|---|---|---|

| FATHER'S NAME | STREET ADDRESS, CITY, STATE AND ZIP CODE | HOME PHONE NO. |
|---|---|---|

| FATHER'S EMPLOYER | OCCUPATION | HOW LONG EMPLOYED? | BUSINESS PHONE NO. |
|---|---|---|---|

| EMPLOYER'S STREET ADDRESS | CITY AND STATE | ZIP CODE |
|---|---|---|

## INSURANCE INFORMATION

| PERSON RESPONSIBLE FOR PAYMENT, IF NOT ABOVE | STREET ADDRESS, CITY, STATE AND ZIP CODE | HOME PHONE NO. |
|---|---|---|

| ☐ COMPANY   NAME & ADDRESS | NAME OF POLICYHOLDER | CERTIFICATE NO. | GROUP NO. |
|---|---|---|---|
| ☐ COMPANY   NAME & ADDRESS | NAME OF POLICYHOLDER | POLICY NO. | |
| ☐ COMPANY   NAME & ADDRESS | NAME OF POLICYHOLDER | POLICY NO. | |

| ☐ MEDICARE | MEDICARE NO. | ☐ MEDICAID | PROGRAM NO. | COUNTY NO. | ACCOUNT NO. |
|---|---|---|---|---|---|

In order to control our cost of billing, we request that office visits be paid at the time service is rendered. We would rather control our billing costs than be forced to raise our fees.

**AUTHORIZATION:** I hereby authorize the physician indicated above to furnish information to insurance carriers concerning this illness/accident, and I hereby irrevocably assign to the doctor all payments for medical services rendered. I understand that I am financially responsible for all charges whether or not covered by insurance.

_____
Responsible Party Signature

New patient information form

8. List desirable characteristics for a receptionist. _____
_____
_____

9. Complete the charge form on page 48 to reflect the following situation. Use yourself as the patient.
   Insurance company—Health Care One
   Insurance ID—123-45-6789-A  Coverage Code S—Group-II
   You have been ill for the past week: fever, chills, coughing, pain over LL chest area, expectorating, blood-tinged mucus
   Description Section: new patient, high complexity ($110), culture for strep ($35), therapeutic injection ($25), ECG ($50), respiratory function ($70), misc. drugs ($20)
   Diagnosis: acute bronchitis; pneumonia (viral), otitis media
   Doctor: use your physician's name—office visit accept assignment

10. Complete the charge form on page 49 to reflect the following situation. Use yourself as the patient, today's date, and the same insurance information as in question 9.
    For interview—about one week ago, you began having abdominal discomfort and occasional diarrhea. The pain and frequency of diarrhea have intensified.
    Diagnosis: abdominal pain; diarrhea; diverticulitis
    Description: extended exam—established patient ($85), antibiotic injection ($25)
    Procedure: high sigmoidoscopy ($90)
    Misc.: Review X-ray report ($15)
    Next appt.: one month
    Doctor: use your personal physician

11. What tasks should you do when closing the office for the day? _____
_____
_____
_____

**ACHIEVING SKILL COMPETENCY**

Reread the performance objective for each procedure and then practice the skills listed below, following the procedure in your textbook.
Procedure 5-1:  Open the Office
Procedure 5-2:  Obtain New Patient Information
Procedure 5-3:  Close the Office

After your instructor has returned your work to you, make all necessary corrections and place in a three-ring notebook for future reference.

Name _____

| Patient First Name | | Patient Last Name | | DATE OF ONSET FOR ILLNESS OR ACCIDENT |
|---|---|---|---|---|
| Responsible Party Last Name | | Patient Last Name (If Different) | Date / / | |

**CHANGE OF:** ☐ NAME ☐ ADDRESS ☐ PHONE ☐ INSURANCE ☐ EMPLOYER

| DIAGNOSIS: | CODE | DIAGNOSIS: | CODE | DIAGNOSIS: | CODE | DIAGNOSIS: | CODE | DIAGNOSIS: | CODE |
|---|---|---|---|---|---|---|---|---|---|
| __ Abdominal Pain | 789.0 | __ Chest Pain | 786.50 | __ Enteritis | 008.0 | __ Impetigo | 684 | __ Pneumonia | 486 |
| __ Abrasion | 959.9 | __ CHF | 428.0 | __ Esophagitis | 530.1 | __ Insomnia | 780.51 | __ Post Menopaus. Atr. Vag. | 627.3 |
| __ Abscess | 682.9 | __ Cholecystitis | 575.1 | __ Fatigue | 780.7 | __ Irritable Bowel Synd. | 564.1 | __ Pregnancy | V22 |
| __ Acne | 706.1 | __ Cirrhosis | 571.5 | __ Flu Syndrome | 487.1 | __ Keratosis | 701.1 | __ Prostatis Hypertrophy | 600 |
| __ Alcoholism | 303.9 | __ Colitis | 558.9 | __ FUO | 780.6 | __ Labyrinthitis | 386.3 | __ Prostatitis | 601.9 |
| __ Allergic Reaction | 995.3 | __ Concussion | 850.9 | __ Furuncle | 680.9 | __ Laceration | 882.0 | __ Pyelonphritis | 590.10 |
| __ Allergic Rhinitis | 477.9 | __ Conjunctivitis | 372.3 | __ Gastritis | 535.5 | __ Laryngitis | 464.0 | __ Radiculitis | 729.2 |
| __ Amenorrhea | 626.0 | __ Constipation | 564.9 | __ Gastroenteritis | 558.9 | __ Low Back Pain | 847.9 | __ Renal Failure | 586 |
| __ Anemia | 281.9 | __ Costochondritis | 733.6 | __ GI Bleeding | 578.9 | __ Lumbar Disc Dis. | 847.2 | __ Rheum. Arthritis | 714.0 |
| __ Angina Pectoris | 413.9 | __ Contusion | 924.9 | __ Gingivitis | 523.1 | __ Lumbar Strain | 846.7 | __ Sebaceous Cyst | 706.2 |
| __ Anxiety State | 300.00 | __ COPD | 496 | __ Gout Unspecified | 274.9 | __ Menopausal Syndr. | 672.2 | __ Seborrhea | 690 |
| __ Appendicitis | 541. | __ Corneal Abrasion | 918.1 | __ Headache, Migraine | 346.9 | __ Menorrhagia | 626.2 | __ Seizure Disorder | 345.1 |
| __ Arrhythmia | 427.9 | __ Cough | 786.2 | __ Headache, Tension | 307.81 | __ Mult. Contusions | 924.0 | __ Sinusitis | 473.9 |
| __ ASHD | 414.0 | __ CVA | 431 | __ Hematuria | 599.7 | __ Myocard. Inf | 429.1 | __ Sprain | 848.9 |
| __ Asthma | 493.9 | __ Cystitis | 595.9 | __ Hemorrhoids | 455.6 | __ Myositis | 729.1 | __ Suture Removal | V58.3 |
| __ Atrial Fibrillation | 427.31 | __ Dementia | 331.0 | __ Hernia Hiatal | 553.3 | __ Nephrosclerosis | 403.9 | __ Tendonitis | 726.90 |
| __ Back Pain | 724.2 | __ Depression | 296.2 | __ Hernia Ventral | 553.20 | __ Nose Bleed | 784.7 | __ Thrombophleb | 451.9 |
| __ Breast Fibrocystic Dis. | 610.1 | __ Derangement Knee | 717.9 | __ Hernia, Inguinal | 550.9 | __ Obesity | 278 | __ Tonsillitis | 463 |
| __ Breast Tumor | 239.3 | __ Dermatitis | 692.5 | __ Herpes Simplex | 054.9 | __ Osteoarthritis | 715.9 | __ Urethritis | 597.80 |
| __ Bronchitis Nos. | 493.9 | __ Diabetes Mellitus | 250.00 | __ Herpes Zoster | 053.9 | __ Otitis Externa | 380.12 | __ URI | 460 |
| __ Bursitis | 727.3 | __ Diarrhea | 558.9 | __ Hypercholesteremia | 272.0 | __ Otitis Media | 382.9 | __ Vaginitis No. 5 | 616.1 |
| __ CAD | 746.85 | __ Diverticulitis | 562.11 | __ Hyperlipidemia | 272.4 | __ Ovarian Cyst | 620.2 | __ Vaginitis Trich | 131.01 |
| __ Cellulitis | | __ Duodenal Ulcer | 532.1 | __ Hypertension | 401.9 | __ Pancreatitis | 577 | __ Vaginitis Candida | 112.1 |
| __ Cerv. Disc. Disease | 722.9 | __ Dysfunct. Uterus Bid. | 626.8 | __ Hyperventilation | 786.01 | __ Paronychia, Finger | 681.02 | __ Vertigo | 780.4 |
| __ Cervical Strain Syndr. | 723.8 | __ Dysmenorrhes | 625.3 | __ Hypoestrogenism | 256.3 | __ Paronychia, Toe | 681.11 | __ Warts, Viral | 078.1 |
| __ Cervicitis Chronic | 616.0 | __ Electrolyte Imb. | 276.9 | __ Hypothyroidism | 244.9 | __ Pharyngitis | 462 | | |
| __ CHD | 414.9 | __ Endometriosis | 617.9 | __ Impacted Cerumen | 380.4 | __ PID | 614.9 | | |

DIAGNOSIS: (IF NOT CHECKED ABOVE)

| ✓ | DESCRIPTION | CODE/MD | DX | FEE | ✓ | DESCRIPTION | CODE/MD | DX | FEE | ✓ | DESCRIPTION | CODE/MD | DX | FEE |
|---|---|---|---|---|---|---|---|---|---|---|---|---|---|---|
| | **OFFICE VISIT - ESTABLISHED PATIENT** | | | | | **LABORATORY** | | | | | **DIAGNOSTIC PROCEDURES (Cont'd)** | | | |
| | Minimal Exam | 99211 | | | | Venipuncture-DR. | 36410 | | | | Spirometry | 94010YB | | |
| | Limited Exam | 99212 | | | | Venipuncture | 36415 | | | | Holter Recording | 93224YB | | |
| | Intermediate Exam | 99213 | | | | Handling | 99000 | | | | Sigmoidoscopy | 45330 | | |
| | Extended Exam | 99214 | | | | Throat Culture | 87060 | | | | High Sigmoidoscopy | 45360 | | |
| | Comprehensive Exam | 99215 | | | | Monilia Culture | 87086 | | | | Sigmoidoscopy w/ Biopsy | 45331 | | |
| | | | | | | Urinalysis | 81000 | | | | | | | |
| | **OFFICE VISIT - NEW PATIENT** | | | | | Urine Culture | 87086 | | | | **PHYSICAL THERAPY** | | | |
| | Limited Exam | 99202 | | | | | | | | | Hydrocollator | 97010 | | |
| | Intermediate Exam | 99203 | | | | **PROCEDURES** | | | | | Ultrasound | 97128 | | |
| | Extended Exam | 99204 | | | | Arthrocentesis Small Joint | 20600 | | | | PT Unlisted | 97039 | | |
| | Comprehensive Exam | 99205 | | | | Arthrocentesis Interm. Joint | 20605 | | | | | | | |
| | Accident Work-up | 90020 | | | | Arthrocentesis Major Joint | 20610 | | | | **SUPPLIES** | | | |
| | | | | | | Trigger Point Injection | 20550 | | | | Surgical Tray A4550 | 99070 | | |
| | **INJECTIONS** | | | | | Cryosurgery Cervix | 57511 | | | | Sterile Kit | 84550 | | |
| | B12 J3420 | 90782 | | | | Face Cryosurgery | 17000 | | | | | | | |
| | Cortisone J0810 | 90782 | | | | Not Face, 1st | 17100 | | | | **MISCELLANEOUS** | | | |
| | Flu | 90724 | | | | Not Face, 2nd | 17101 | | | | Special Reports | 99080 | | |
| | Pneumovax | 90732 | | | | Not Face 3 or More, Each | 17102 | | | | Emergency O.V. | 99058 | | |
| | Tetanus Toxoid | 90703 | | | | Ear Lavage | 69210 | | | | Review X-Ray Report | 76140-26 | | |
| | DPT | 90701 | | | | | | | | | | | | |
| | Polio | 90712 | | | | | | | | | | | | |
| | MMR | 90707 | | | | | | | | | | | | |
| | HIB | 90729 | | | | | | | | | | | | |
| | Estrogen J0970 | 90782 | | | | **DIAGNOSTIC PROCEDURES** | | | | | | | | |
| | Lidocaine J2000 | 90782 | | | | Audiometry | 92552 | | | | | | | |
| | Skin Test (TB, Cocci, Histo) | 86585 | | | | ECG | 93000YB | | | | | | | |
| | Therapeutic Inj. | 90782 | | | | ECG (Medicare) | 93005 | | | | | | | |
| | Drug: Dose: | | | | | | | | | | | | | |
| | Antibiotic Inj. | 90788 | | | | | | | | | | | | |
| | Drug: Dose: | | | | | | | | | | | | | |

| REC'D BY: | | |
|---|---|---|
| ☐ CASH | **TOTAL FEE** | |
| ☐ CK. #_____ | | |
| ☐ CO-PAY | **AMT. REC'D** | |
| ☐ MC/VISA | | |

**Authorization/Responsibility Agreement**

I hereby authorize any insurance company to pay the proceeds of any benefits due me directly to: JAY RICHARD HODES, M.D. A copy of this can be considered as an original for insurance purposes.

Signed: _____ Date: _____

I hereby agree to pay my account as services are provided. If for any reason there is a balance owing on my account, I agree to pay promptly upon receipt of the monthly statement.

Signed: _____ Date: _____

I acknowledge and understand that I am responsible for all of the charges for all of the services rendered to me or any member of my family.
Although I have requested the doctor to bill my insurance company on my behalf, I clearly understand that it is still my responsibility to make sure the bill is paid in a reasonable time. If for any reason any portion of my bill is not paid by my insurance, I further agree to make arrangements for prompt payment of the bill.

Signed: _____ Date: _____

**NEXT APPOINTMENT**

| MON | TUES | WED | THUR | FRI | SAT |
|---|---|---|---|---|---|
| 2 WKS | | 1 M | | 2 M | |
| 3 M | | 6 M | | 12 M | |

**DOCTOR'S SIGNATURE & DATE**

Charge form for question 9.

**PATIENT INFORMATION**

| PATIENT'S LAST NAME | FIRST | INITIAL | BIRTHDATE | | SEX □ MALE □ FEMALE | TODAY'S DATE |
|---|---|---|---|---|---|---|

| ADDRESS | CITY | STATE | ZIP | RELATIONSHIP TO SUBSCRIBER | INJURY DATE |
|---|---|---|---|---|---|

| SUBSCRIBER OR POLICYHOLDER | | INSURANCE CARRIER |
|---|---|---|

| ADDRESS | CITY | STATE | ZIP | INS. I.D. | COVERAGE CODE | GROUP |
|---|---|---|---|---|---|---|

**ASSIGNMENT AND RELEASE**: I HEREBY AUTHORIZE MY INSURANCE BENEFITS TO BE PAID DIRECTLY TO THE UNDERSIGNED PHYSICIAN. I AM FINANCIALLY RESPONSIBLE FOR NON-COVERED SERVICES. I ALSO AUTHORIZE THE PHYSICIAN TO RELEASE ANY INFORMATION REQUIRED.

OTHER HEALTH COVERAGE □ YES □ NO          IDENTIFY

DISABILITY RELATED TO:
□ ACCIDENT   □ INDUSTRIAL   □ ILLNESS   □ OTHER

SIGNED _____ Date _____
(PATIENT, OR PARENT, IF MINOR)

DATE SYMPTOMS APPEARED, INCEPTION OF PREGNANCY, OR ACCIDENT OCCURRED:

| ✓ | DESCRIPTION | CPT/MD | FEE | ✓ | DESCRIPTION | CPT/MD | FEE | ✓ | DESCRIPTION | CPT/MD | FEE |
|---|---|---|---|---|---|---|---|---|---|---|---|
| | OFFICE VISITS | NEW PT | | | LABORATORY (Cont'd.) | | | | PROCEDURES | | |
| | Moderate Complex | 99203 | | | Wet Mount | 87210 | | | EKG  93000 | 93005 | |
| | Moderate/High Comp. | 99204 | | | Pap Smear | 88150 | | | Resp. Function Test | 94010 | |
| | High Complexity | 99205 | | | Handling | 99000 | | | Ear Lavage | 69210 | |
| | OFFICE VISITS | EST. PT | | | Hemoccult Stool | 82270 | | | Injection Inter. Jt.* | 20605 | |
| | Minimal | 99211 | | | Glucose | 82948 | | | Injection Major Jt.* | 20610 | |
| | Self Limited Comp. | 99212 | | | INJECTIONS | | | | Anoscopy | 46600 | |
| | Low/Moderate Comp. | 99213 | | | Vitamin B12/B Complex | J3420 | | | Sigmoidoscopy | 45355 | |
| | Moderate Complex | 99214 | | | ACTH | J0140 | | | I & D* | 10060 | |
| | High Complexity | 99215 | | | Depo-Estradiol | J1000 | | | Electrocautery* | 17200 | |
| | CONSULTATIONS | OFFICE | | | Depo Testosterone | J1070 | | | Thromb Hemor.* | 46320 | |
| | Moderate Complexity | 99243 | | | Imferon | J1760 | | | Inj. Tendon* | 20550 | |
| | Mod. to High Comp. | 99244 | | | Tetanus Toxoid | J3180 | | | | | |
| | HOME | EST. PT | | | Influenza Vaccine - Flu | 90724 | | | MISCELLANEOUS | | |
| | Moderate Complexity | 99352 | | | Pneumococcal Vaccine | 90732 | | | Drugs, Supplies, Materials | 99070 | |
| | ER | | | | TB Tine Test | 86585 | | | Special Reports | 99080 | |
| | Moderate Severity | 99283 | | | Aminophyllin | J0280 | | | Services After Hrs. | 99050 | |
| | High Severity | 99284 | | | Terbutaline Sulf. | J3105 | | | Services 10pm - 8am | 99052 | |
| | LABORATORY | | | | Demerol HCL | J0990 | | | Services Sun. & Holidays | 99054 | |
| | Urinalysis - Complete | 81000 | | | Compazine | J0780 | | | Counseling | 99403 | |
| | Hemoglobin | 85018 | | | Injection Therapeutic | 90782 | | | | | |
| | Culture, Strep/Monilia | 87081 | | | Estrone Susp. | J1410 | | | | | |

**DIAGNOSIS:**

| | | | | |
|---|---|---|---|---|
| □ Allergic Rhinitis ... 477.9 | □ Chronic Fatigue Synd. ... 300.5 | □ Hemorrhoids ... 455.6 | □ Peripheral Vascular Dis ... 443.9 | |
| □ Anemia ... 280.9 | □ COPD ... 496 | □ Hiatal Hernia ... 553.3 | □ Pharyngitis ... 462.0 | |
| □ Angina Pectoris ... 413 | □ Costochondritis ... 733.99 | □ Hiatal Hernia & Reflux ... 530.1 | □ Pneumonia, Bacterial ... 482.9 | |
| □ Anxiety ... 300.00 | □ CVA ... 431 | □ HVD ... 402.10 | □ Pneumonia, Viral ... 480.9 | |
| □ Aortic Stenosis ... 424.1 | □ Cystitis ... 595.9 | □ Hyperlipidemia ... 272.4 | □ Prostatitis, Chronic/Acute ... 601 | |
| □ ASCVD ... 429.2 | □ Deg. Disc. Disease, CX ... 722.4 | □ Hypoestrogenism ... 256.3 | □ Rectal Bleeding ... 569.3 | |
| □ ASHD ... 414.9 | □ Deg. Disc. Dis., Lumbar ... 722.52 | □ Hypothyroidism ... 244.9 | □ Renal Failure, Chronic ... 585 | |
| □ Asthma ... 493.9 | □ Depression, Endogenous ... 296.2 | □ Impacted Cerumen ... 380.4 | □ Rheumatoid Arthritis ... 714.0 | |
| □ Atrial Fibrillation ... 427.31 | □ Dermatitis ... 692.9 | □ Influenza, Viral ... 487.1 | □ Sinusitis ... 461.9 | |
| □ Bigeminy ... 427.89 | □ Diabetes Mellitus, Adult ... 250.0 | □ Irritable Bowel Syndrome ... 564.1 | □ Supraventr. Tachycardia ... 427.0 | |
| □ BPH ... 600 | □ Diarrhea ... 558.9 | □ Laryngitis ... 464.0 | □ T.I.A. ... 435.9 | |
| □ Bronchitis, Acute ... 466.1 | □ Diverticulitis ... 562.11 | □ Menopausal Syndrome ... 627.2 | □ Tachycardia ... 426.89 | |
| □ Bronchitis, Chronic ... 491.9 | □ Esophagitis ... 530.1 | □ Mitral Insufficiency ... 396.2 | □ Tendinitis ... 726.90 | |
| □ Bursitis ... 726 | □ Fibrocystic Breast Disease ... 610.11 | □ Moniliasis ... 112 | □ Tonsillitis ... 463 | |
| □ Cardiomyopathy ... 425.4 | □ Fissure in Ano ... 565.0 | □ Myocardial Infarction ... 410.9 | □ Ulcer Duodenal ... 532.9 | |
| □ Carotid Artery Disease ... 433.1 | □ Gastroenteritis ... 558.9 | □ Neuritis ... 729.2 | □ Ulcer Gastric ... 531.9 | |
| □ Cerebral Vascular Disease ... 437.9 | □ Gout ... 274.9 | □ Osteoarthritis ... 715.9 | □ URI ... 465.9 | |
| □ CHF ... 428.0 | □ HCVD ... 429.2 | □ Osteoporosis ... 733.0 | □ UTI ... 599.0 | |
| □ Cholecystitis ... 575.1 | □ Headache, Vascular ... 784.0 | □ Otitis Media ... 382.9 | □ Vaginitis ... 616.10 | |
| | □ Headache, Migraine ... 346.9 | □ Parkinsonism ... 332 | □ Vertigo ... 780.4 | |

DIAGNOSIS: (IF NOT CHECKED ABOVE)

REF. DR. & #

| DOCTOR'S SIGNATURE / DATE | NO SERVICES PURCHASED | SERVICE PERFORMED | ACCEPT ASSIGNMENT | TODAY'S FEE | |
|---|---|---|---|---|---|

**INSTRUCTIONS TO PATIENT FOR FILING INSURANCE CLAIMS**

1. MAIL THIS FORM DIRECTLY TO YOUR INSURANCE COMPANY.
   ATTACH YOUR OWN INSURANCE COMPANY'S FORM.

**PLEASE REMEMBER THAT PAYMENT IS YOUR OBLIGATION, REGARDLESS OF INSURANCE OR OTHER THIRD PARTY INVOLVEMENT.**

| | |
|---|---|
| OFFICE □ | YES □ |
| E.R. □ | NO □ |
| HOME □ | |

AMT. REC'D TODAY

TOTAL DUE

Charge form for question 10.

**ASSIGNMENT SHEET**

**Section 2: THE ADMINISTRATIVE ASSISTANT**

**Chapter 6: ORAL AND WRITTEN COMMUNICATIONS**

Review the objectives and text for each unit before completing the assignment sheet for that unit. When you have completed all sheets for the chapter, remove them from this Workbook and give them to the instructor for evaluation.

**Unit 1: TELEPHONE COMMUNICATIONS**

**A. Multiple Choice: Place the correct letter or letters on the blank line for each question.**

_____ 1. Desirable skills and qualities that the medical assistant who handles phone calls should have are
    a. courtesy                          c. active listening
    b. good grooming             d. great personality

_____ 2. When the phone rings in the office, it should be answered by the ____ ring.
    a. first                             c. third
    b. second                       d. fourth

_____ 3. When holding the phone to your ear, the receiver should be ____ inches in front of your mouth.
    a. 1–2 inches                  c. 4–5 inches
    b. 2–3 inches                  d. 6–8 inches

_____ 4. Patients who phone the office for an appointment should be given ____ choices.
    a. one                           c. three
    b. two                         d. four

_____ 5. You should _____ file a report that the physician has not seen.
    a. never                       c. always
    b. sometimes                d. immediately

**B. Fill in the Blank**

1. Essential items that should be next to each telephone in a medical facility are a _____ _____ and a _____

2. The _____ established by the medical assistant who answers the phone will contribute to successful communication with patients.

3. The responsibility of responding to phone calls in a medical office takes a great deal of _____ and _____

4. It is a sensible practice to have all _____ phone numbers listed by each phone in the office.

5. All telephone messages that are urgent should be given _____ and handled as soon as possible.

6. You should be _____ about your knowledge and experience with phone systems.

7. When answering a phone call of a patient, make sure you get the caller's _____ and _____ in case the call is an emergency and it is interrupted.

8. The appointment should be _____ by reading the appointment time back to the patient after it has been recorded in the appointment book.

9. Only patient information that has been _____ by the patient in writing, with the patient's signature, may be given to another party.

10. If you have made an error on a patient's bill, be sure to _____ it, _____ and offer to send a _____ statement.

11. When placing long-distance phone calls, it is advisable to consult a telephone directory for a _____ so you can establish the appropriate time to call.

12. Never tell anyone over the phone (or in person) that you are _____ as it may be an invitation for undesirable behavior.

13. If the physician requests that you monitor a phone call, it is important that the caller _____ to your listening and taking notes.

**C. True or False: Place a "T" for true or "F" for false in the space provided. For false statements, explain why they are false.**

_____ 1. A pleasant voice and good listening skills are essential in telephone communications.

_____ 2. When patients call for information about their condition or lab report results, it is not necessary to pull their chart.

_____ 3. All telephone calls, regardless of what you feel about their importance, should be documented.

_____ 4. The answering machine in the medical office should be turned on to leave a message to callers only on weekends when the physician is not in the office.

_____ 5. Telephone callers form a picture of you as they listen to your voice.

_____ 6. When you finish a conversation over the phone with a patient, you should hang up first to let the patient know you are finished talking.

_____ 7. When an attorney phones for information about a patient, you must provide the necessary information immediately.

_____ 8. Always be sure to make a copy of any correspondence mailed out so you have a copy for the patient's chart.

_____ 9. The physician usually does not wish to speak to unidentified phone callers during busy office hours.

_____ 10. When answering the medical office phone, and the physician is not there, you should always know where to reach him or her.

_____ 11. You should never leave a patient on hold for more than 10 minutes.

_____ 12. You should screen and complete as many calls as possible before adding names to the physician's call-back list.

**D. Brief Answer**

1. List the common types of calls that are received in a medical office. _____

_____

_____

_____

2. Explain why a telephone triage manual should be kept by the phone to manage telephone calls in a medical facility. _____

_____

_____

_____

3. List the important items of a telephone message. _____

_____

_____

_____

**E. Crossword Puzzle**

ACROSS

1. A number of sheets of paper fastened together
3. A given point of time
4. Relevant, applicable
5. To analyze by application of reagents—to prove knowledge
7. Induce to action
9. Mechanical device for recording sounds
10. An associate in an office, usually one of similar status
14. Person practicing medical profession
15. Writing instrument
17. A receptionist will answer telephone _____
20. Made known in words or actions
21. Conventional rules for correct behavior
24. A preliminary or indicating procedure
25. A helper or co-worker in a specific occupation
26. Tool or plan
27. Pertaining to medicine

DOWN

1. The personal or individual quality that makes one person different from another
2. The sound of a bell
3. A book containing lists of names and addresses
6. A chance of a life ____
8. Place for healing
10. Verified; ratified
11. Sympathetically trying to identify one's feelings with those of another
12. Pronouncing clearly
13. Sixty in each hour
16. Type of work or commerce
18. Prove to be true; supported by facts
19. Depend; trust
22. Coming next after second in a series
23. Sound produced through mouth

DIRECTIONS: Read the following situations out loud in class and role-play how you would handle them. Answers will vary. Your instructor may want to guide the situations.

**TELEPHONE WORKSHEET 1: "I HAVE TO SEE THE DOCTOR—TODAY!"**

Doctor's Identity:    (Use names of local physicians)

Solo or Group:    Two-physician partnership

Specialty:    Family practice

Time:    8:30 A.M.

Situation:    Both physicians are on hospital rounds and are not expected until 10:00 A.M.
The appointment book is full.

Patient:    (insert name of student or fictitious name), a patient since infancy

-------------------------------------------------------------------------------------------------

"I need an appointment today—right away. I'm leaving for college tomorrow, and the doctor just has to see me. Just for a minute. I need a quick physical and a form filled out. It's nothing really."
"I can't register for class unless the doctor sees me. I just have to have an appointment. I know this is last minute—but just this once, please. Certainly, you understand, you have to."

-------------------------------------------------------------------------------------------------

How did you handle this?
Instructor will need to evaluate each student answer. Answers will vary.

**TELEPHONE WORKSHEET 2:  MOTHER WHO WANTS TO MAKE AN APPOINTMENT FOR
HERSELF AND HER CHILD**

Doctor's Identity:            (Use name of local physician)

Solo or Group:              Solo practice

Specialty:                    OB/GYN

Time:                         10:00 A.M.

Situation:                  The physician is in an area where there are a number of pediatricians, and he does not
see pediatric patients.

Patient:                    (fictitious name) Mrs. _____

-------------------------------------------------------------------------------------------------------------------------

Mrs. _____ is new in the area and got the doctor's name from calling the county medical society. She has a
history of menstrual difficulty. She has no immediate problem, but wants to make an appointment with an
OB/GYN physician in this new location in order to establish a "regular" doctor.
She tells the medical assistant that she wants to bring (fill in name of child) with her, and wants to make an
appointment for _____ too, immediately following her appointment. _____ is her 4-year-old daughter.
Mrs. _____ does not want to accept the fact that Dr. _____ will not see _____. She argues that she has to bring
_____ with her, there is no one to take care of her, and this is not really an inconvenience to Dr. _____. It will
just take a 10-minute check for _____ , and Mrs. _____ is willing to make an appointment two or three weeks
in advance for the doctor's convenience.

-------------------------------------------------------------------------------------------------------------------------

How did you handle this?
Instructor will need to evaluate each student answer. Answers will vary.

**TELEPHONE WORKSHEET 3: PATIENT INSISTS ON APPOINTMENT**

Doctor's Identity:     (Use names of local physicians)

Solo or Group:     Two-physician partnership

Specialty:     Internal medicine

Time:     3:30 P.M.

Situation:     Dr. _____ is out of the office today.

Dr. _____ is in the examining room with a patient. The office is already behind schedule because Dr. _____ has had to work in a couple of emergency patients of Dr. _____.

Patient:     (fictitious name) Mrs. _____ is a regular patient (she has been to the office two or three times a year). The medical assistant knows her well enough to recognize the name and identify it with a 64-year-old widow living alone. Mrs. _____ has always been very nice, but is a little bit on the "dramatic" side.

--------------------------------------------------------------------------------

Mrs. _____ calls and says she is very ill and would like to see (Dr. who is out of the office) right away. She says she has had a headache since mid-morning and it is getting worse. She has had these headaches before, and Dr. _____ has always given her something to stop them. She doesn't have any more of the little pills and she feels just awful. She knows she will be sick all night if something isn't done right away. Although she feels real bad, she will get in a cab and come to the office right now.

She will see (Dr. in office) if necessary, but she prefers to see (Dr. who is out of the office) since he is her regular doctor. She thinks the doctor should see her now when she feels so bad. There is no use for the doctor to see her two or three days from now, when she may be feeling all right—if she lives through the night.

She doesn't threaten or get abusive, but is persistent and keeps repeating that she must see the doctor right now.

--------------------------------------------------------------------------------

How did you handle this?

Instructor will need to evaluate each student answer. Answers will vary.

**TELEPHONE WORKSHEET 4: "WE'RE ON VACATION"**

Doctor's Identity:        (Use name of local physician)

Solo or Group:        Solo practice

Specialty:        Internist

Time:        Late afternoon in July

Situation:        The doctor is in and he is seeing his last scheduled patient for the day.

Patient:        (fictitious name)

--------------------------------------------------------------------------------

The caller simply identifies herself as Mrs. _____. She has a thick southern accent. The medical assistant does not know her.

The woman is sniffling and is saying, "My baby, my baby, _____ is so sick. Is the doctor there? I just know my baby needs help. Is the doctor there? I'm just visiting here, my husband left me in the hotel here and has been out fishing and camping for two days. The baby has a high fever and just keeps crying. I'm all alone, I don't know what to do."

--------------------------------------------------------------------------------

How did you handle this?
Instructor will need to evaluate each student answer. Answers will vary.

**TELEPHONE WORKSHEET 5: THE ANGRY AND ABUSIVE PATIENT**

Doctor's Identity:        (Use name of local physician)

Solo or Group:        Solo practice

Specialty:        Family practice

Time:        1:30 P.M.

Situation:        The appointment book is completely filled and the only time for a regular office visit is 2½ weeks ahead, on Thursday at 2:00 P.M.

Patient:        (fictitious name) Mrs. _____ has been in the office two or three times during the past year, and has always been rather quiet and reserved. Mrs. _____ has high blood pressure, which is being handled very well with medication, but she is supposed to come into the office every three or four months for a checkup. This office does not schedule appointments that far in advance. The doctor has simply said, "Come back every two or three months." Mrs. _____ has never seemed unreasonable before, but today she is in a very bad mood.

--------------------------------------------------------------------------------

Mrs. _____ calls for an appointment and the medical assistant advises her that the first opening is 2½ weeks ahead. When the medical assistant gives her this information, her immediate response is that this is not at all convenient. She says that she planned to see the doctor in the next several days and that she has no idea where she will be in 2½ weeks. She thinks she might be taking a vacation trip somewhere, and she simply does not want to wait this long for an appointment.

As the conversation continues, Mrs. _____ gets more and more argumentative and points out that all she wants is a checkup, which will take the doctor only a few minutes, and that if it was anything more than that she would probably be dead before the doctor could get around to seeing her. She argues that she isn't demanding to see the doctor immediately, that an appointment in the next three or four days will be satisfactory, but that waiting 2½ weeks for a simple checkup is not reasonable.

Finally, Mrs. _____ gets nasty. She says she wants to talk to the doctor. She wants to know just who is running the medical practice. She doesn't think the doctor really knows what is going on. She mentions that she is running low on her pills and doesn't think that her medication will last for 2½ weeks more.

--------------------------------------------------------------------------------

How did you handle this?
Instructor will need to evaluate each student answer. Answers will vary.

**TELEPHONE WORKSHEET 6:  INSISTS ON TALKING TO THE DOCTOR**

Doctor's Identity:          (Use name of local physician)

Solo or Group:          Solo practice

Specialty:          Family practice

Time:          Early Monday morning

Situation:          The doctor is in the examining room with a patient. The appointment schedule is already overbooked, and this is going to be another day when all of the patients have a long wait in the reception room, and both the doctor and the medical assistant will be working overtime.

Patient:          (fictitious name) An elderly widower, a regular patient who makes an appointment to see the doctor almost every month most of the time for imagined ills.

------------------------------------------------------------------------------------------------------------------

Mr. _____ calls and says, "I need to talk with Dr. _____. I've had a splitting headache all weekend. I knew he would be out on the golf course or some such thing—so I waited until now to call. I just can't wait any longer. Put me through to him. I'll only take a minute.

The medical assistant replies that Dr. _____ is seeing a patient in the examining room and that he will call back. "That's what you always say," Mr. _____ replies. "If I was dying I would have to wait for a convenient time? All I want to do is talk to the doctor for just a minute."

The medical assistant repeats that the doctor is in the examining room and suggests a call-back.

Mr. _____, "I had to get out of bed to come to the phone, so I'll just hang on. That certainly isn't going to inconvenience him. You just tell him that I'm holding the phone. I don't like waiting—I waited all weekend and I don't want to be put off a moment longer than necessary. I pay my bills and I deserve to talk to the doctor when I need him."

------------------------------------------------------------------------------------------------------------------

How did you handle this?

Instructor will need to evaluate each student answer. Answers will vary.

**TELEPHONE WORKSHEET 7: CALL TO NOTIFY PATIENT**

| | |
|---|---|
| Doctor's Identity: | (Use names of local physicians) |
| Solo or Group: | Partnership |
| Specialty: | OB/GYN |
| Time: | 1:00 P.M. |

Situation: Both physicians have called in to say that they will be late in returning to the office. It seems all of the babies in town decided to be born today. Dr. _____ , anticipating a caesarean section, says he may not be in at all. Dr. _____ says that he will be at least one hour late, and maybe longer. Here office protocol is to notify patients, who have not as yet arrived, of the delay.

Patient: (fictitious name)

---

You call Mrs. _____ and tell her of the delay. She has an appointment for 3:00 P.M., which she made about three weeks ago. She is upset—you can tell this from the tone of her voice.

The medical assistant knows from past experience that the best thing to do would be to cancel Mrs. _____'s appointment and reschedule her. This can't be done. About the earliest time that Dr. _____ can see Mrs. _____ will be 5:00 to 5:30 P.M.

Mrs. _____ is not enthusiastic about either alternative.

---

How did you handle this?
Instructor will need to evaluate each student answer. Answers will vary.

**TELEPHONE WORKSHEET 8:  THE CASE OF THE HOLD BUTTON**

Doctor's Identity:       (Use name of local physician, female)

Solo or Group:       Solo practice

Specialty:       General surgery

Time:       10:00 A.M.

Situation:       Dr. _____ has advised the patient that if her incision continues to ooze, she is to call the doctor. The doctor has advised the medical assistant that if the patient calls, she will want to talk with her.

Patient:       (fictitious name)

----------------------------------------------------------------------------------------------------

Mrs. _____ calls; the doctor is in her consulting office and the medical assistant plans to transfer the call immediately to Dr. _____. Mrs. _____ is not upset, or doesn't seem to be, on the telephone. Dr. _____ is upset after talking with Mrs. _____ because she was having no trouble with her incision. All she needed was an appointment.

----------------------------------------------------------------------------------------------------

What did the medical assistant fail to do?
Instructor will need to evaluate each student answer. Answers will vary.

**TELEPHONE WORKSHEET 9:  THE PATIENT WHO HAS BEEN A NO-SHOW**

Doctor's Identity:          (Use name of local physician)

Solo or Group:          Solo practice

Specialty:          Family practice

Time:          11:30 A.M.

Situation:          The patient calls for an appointment. The patient had an appointment the previous week, but didn't show or call in. The patient simply says she was busy last Thursday and just couldn't make it. The appointment was only for a checkup, but she wants to make another appointment for now.

Patient:          (fictitious name)

-----------------------------------------------------------------------------------------------------------------

The medical assistant can make an appointment for approximately two weeks from today. Mrs. _____ is willing to accept that.

-----------------------------------------------------------------------------------------------------------------

What should the medical assistant say in regard to the previous "no-show"?
Instructor will need to evaluate each student answer. Answers will vary.

## TELEPHONE WORKSHEET 10: "I *MUST* SPEAK TO THE DOCTOR!"

Doctor's Identity:          (Use names of local physicians)

Solo or Group:           Two-physician partnership

Specialty:                    OB/GYN

Time:                           3:00 P.M.

Situation:                     Both physicians are in the office, and are busy seeing patients. They have a well-established practice and haven't been taking new patients unless they have been referred by associates.

Patient:                       (fictitious name)

--------------------------------------------------------------------------------------

A woman calls and identifies herself as _____. Mrs. _____ is obviously very upset. She says, "I need to talk with a doctor right away. My friend _____ told me that Dr. _____ was the best doctor in town." The medical assistant explains the doctor's policy.

Breathlessly, Mrs. _____ continues. "I need to talk to the doctor, really. I'm new in town. I don't know what to do. My sister in Omaha just called to say that she has found a lump on her breast and it has been identified as cancer. We lost our mother from cancer last year. I'm scared. I need to talk to the doctor. Please—can't you make an exception just this once?" Mrs. _____ then begins sobbing on the telephone.

--------------------------------------------------------------------------------------

How did you handle this?
Instructor will need to evaluate each student answer. Answers will vary.

**ASSIGNMENT SHEET**

**Chapter 6: ORAL AND WRITTEN COMMUNICATIONS**

**Unit 2: SCHEDULE APPOINTMENTS**

**A. Brief Answer**

1. What are the most important points in scheduling when a patient calls the office for an appointment?

   *mark off the hours when the doctor will be unable to see patients.*
   *(include hospitals round, lunch hr, vacation, etc)*
   *Attempt to give patients 2 choices of times for one appoint.*

2. Describe the best way to schedule a patient who is always late. _____

   _____

   _____

3. List the advantages of a computer scheduling system. _____

   _____

   _____

   _____

4. What information should be in the office procedure manual that would be helpful in making appointments outside the office? _____

   _____

   _____

**B. Multiple Choice: Place the correct letter or letters on the blank line for each question.**

_____ 1. Time blocked off in the schedule book that is not for patient appointments is called the

   a. schedule          c. manual
   b. matrix            d. cancelation

_____ 2. When patients cancel appointments, you should

   a. cross them off the schedule with one line through their name
   b. note C & C on the chart and the reason for canceling
   c. notify the physician
   d. a and b only

_____ 3. How long should medical office appointment books be kept in a secured area away from patient access and any unauthorized persons?

   a. indefinitely       c. five years
   b. three years        d. seven years

_____ 4. The preferred method of payment for services provided by the physician is/are

   a. cash              c. credit card
   b. check/money order  d. a and b

_____ 5. To keep medical records updated, how often should you ask patients about any changes in their personal data (insurance, phone number, address, etc,)?

   a. at each visit      c. once a year
   b. every six months   d. not necessary, patient will tell you

_____ 6. When do patients have to precertify services with their insurance company to ensure coverage?

   a. mental health counseling    c. emergency services where they live
   b. all office visits           d. substance abuse counseling

## C. Matching: MATCH the definition in column II with the correct term in column I.

COLUMN I

_____ 1. Wave
_____ 2. Open hours
_____ 3. Streaming
_____ 4. Clustering
_____ 5. Single-booking
_____ 6. Modified wave
_____ 7. Double-booking

COLUMN II

a. Appointments are made to accommodate specific needs of patients according to the amount of time that is generally adequate (for continuous patient flow)

b. This method is used for patients who will take a considerable amount of time-45 minutes to an hour

c. Appointment times are given to two or more patients for the same time

d. No appointments made; patients sign, in noting time of arrival

e. Appointments are made in the first 30 minutes of each hour—second half hour is for work-ins

f. A group of patients with the same complaint, diagnosis, or other commonality are scheduled sequentially every 10 minutes

g. Same as wave with additional scheduling of the second half of the hour in 10- to 20-minute intervals, according to the medical problem

## D. True or False: Place a "T" for true or "F" for false in the space provided. For false statements, explain why they are false.

_____ 1. Information regarding office hours should be placed in phone directories and wherever applicable.

_____ 2. Downtime refers to the time when the computer is not functional.

_____ 3. You should place an OUTguide in place of every chart that is pulled for the daily schedule.

_____ 4. The process of rescheduling involves calling each scheduled patient and offering an alternative appointment time as close to the original one as possible.

_____ 5. When scheduling an appointment for a patient, you should offer several choices of times for the appointment.

_____ 6. The term *precertification* means that certain procedures and treatments must be approved with the patient's insurance company for guaranteed payment of services before the patient receives the service.

_____ 7. Leaving the appointment book open for unauthorized persons to view breaks the laws of confidentiality.

_____ 8. Delays in the appointment schedule do not have to be made known to patients because it will upset them.

_____ 9. Appropriate printed information and instructions should be given to a patient for a referral appointment.

## E. Word Search: Find the following words hidden in the puzzle.

| | | |
|---|---|---|
| SERVICE | RAPPORT | WAVE |
| SEVERE | CODES | STAFF |
| TRIAGE | DOWNTIME | STYLE |
| GATEKEEPER | ROUTINE | FLEX |
| PERIODIC | CRITERION | PHONE |
| PRECERTIFICATION | PATIENT | REMOTE |
| APPOINTMENT | SCHEDULE | GUARANTOR |
| STREAMING | COMPLICATIONS | INFORMATION |
| SEQUENTIALLY | DELAY | STRESS |
| GOALS | | |

```
P E R I O D I C S O M R I S S S
G O A L S C L O S W A A N E E E
A P P O I N T M E N T P F Q V V
T R I A G E D P R S R P O U E C
E C O D E S H L T T I O R E R R
K D A I L Y J I S A X R M N E I
E M S E R V I C E F I T A T R T
E W S T Y L E A Z F L P T I O E
P A I D O W N T I M E H I A U R
E V E A P A T I E N T O O L T I
R E M O T E D O U B F N N L I O
S T R E A M I N G T L E K Y N N
D E L A Y F E S C H E D U L E Z
G U A R A N T O R A X P B C V O
P R E C E R T I F I C A T I O N
```

## F. Completion

Use the appointment schedule provided. Establish the matrix. Office hours are:

> Mondays: 8–5 P.M. (Lunch break 12:00–1:15 P.M.)
> Tuesdays: 8:30 A.M.–2:30 P.M. (Lunch break 12–12:30 P.M.)
> Wednesdays: 12:30–6:00 P.M.

Use the list of patients and list of abbreviations in Figure 6-14 of the textbook to fill in the appointment schedule. You should be able to find room for all on the schedule.

## INFORMATION SHEET FOR APPOINTMENTS

| | NAME | PHONE | COMPLAINT OR PROCEDURE | MINUTES | BEST TIME |
|---|---|---|---|---|---|
| 1. | Koch, Curtis | 555-0123 | Stepped on rusty nail | 15 | emergency |
| 2. | Harris, Dezzie | 555-1234 | Shortness of breath, dizziness | 14 | early p.m. |
| 3. | Hall, Pauline | 555-2345 | Smallpox vaccination for travel | 15 | any time |
| 4. | Graves, Connie | 555-3456 | Headache and sinus trouble | 15 | after work |
| 5. | Ford, Kenneth | 555-4567 | Cough and cold | 15 | any time |
| 6. | Edwards, Melvin | 555-5678 | Rectal examination and consultation | 15 | late p.m. |
| 7. | Dennis, Mrs. P.A. | 555-6789 | Annual physical exam; Pap test | 30 | a.m. |
| 8. | Daniels, Dave | 555-8910 | New patient | 30 | Monday |
| 9. | Carr, Bruce | 555-9102 | Company examination, new employee | 30 | Monday |
| 10. | Booth, Vivian | 555-1023 | Injury to ankle | 15 | Monday, p.m. |
| 11. | Block, Jimmy | 555-3457 | Check leg cast | 15 | a.m. |
| 12. | Bergstrom, Stephen | 555-4680 | Examination; complaint of pain in hands and knees | 15 | late Wednesday |
| 13. | Applegate, Elmo | 555-1357 | Follow-up exam and ECG | 15 | Monday, late p.m. |
| 14. | Anders, L.K. | 555-0987 | Treatment of leg ulcer | 15 | early a.m. |
| 15. | Appleby, Nathan | 555-1193 | Injection and consultation | 15 | Monday, late p.m. |
| 16. | Jefferson, Thomas | 555-7890 | Remove sutures and dressing, following hernia operation | 15 | any time |
| 17. | Benson, Mrs. C.L. | 555-5789 | Exam and consult regarding gallbladder surgery | 30 | Wednesday, after 4 |
| 18. | Hanning, Dianne | 555-6890 | Remove small growth by eye under local | 30 | a.m. |
| 19. | Blair, Robert | 555-7901 | Chest congestion | 15 | receive complaint today |
| 20. | Frost, Theresa | 555-8012 | IUD insertion | 30 | late p.m. |
| 21. | Booth, Earl | 555-9123 | Injury to ankle | 15 | Monday, p.m. |
| 22. | Ford, Anna | 555-0985 | Dressing to injured finger | 15 | Wednesday |
| 23. | Callahan, Barbara | 555-0984 | Remove wood splinter in leg | 30 | emergency |
| 24. | Dyer, Sandra | 555-0983 | Excise lesion on back | 30 | early p.m. |
| 25. | Carter, Gertrude | 555-0982 | Infection on face | 15 | Wednesday |
| 26. | Davis, Charles L. | 555-0981 | Examination, possible hernia | 15 | Tuesday |
| 27. | Guthrie, Mrs. June | 555-0980 | Desires weight reduction | 15 | a.m. |
| 28. | Underwood, Edgar | 555-0979 | Dog bite; left hand | 15 | emergency |
| 29. | Landers, Hubert | 555-0978 | Consultation regarding plastic surgery for facial scars from auto accident | 10 | near noon |
| 30. | Meyer, Thomas | 555-0977 | College examination, urinalysis, drug screen | 30 | any time |
| 31. | Thornton, Helen | 555-0976 | Weakness; patient thinks she is anemic | 15 | any time |
| 32. | Ochs, Glenn | 555-0975 | Preschool exam, booster injection | 15 | a.m. |
| 33. | Saunders, Mrs. G. | 555-0974 | Post-op dressing, breast surgery | 15 | early p.m. |
| 34. | Poff, Richard | 555-0973 | Crushed finger in car door | 15 | emergenc |
| 35. | Rambo, Clyde | 555-0963 | Complete physical exam | 30 | early p.m |
| 36. | Quinn, Mrs. Mary J. | 555-0953 | Influenza vaccine injection | 5 | any time |
| 37. | Owens, Russell | 555-0954 | Aspirate left elbow | 15 | late a.m |
| 38. | Stone, Ann | 555-0843 | Prolonged menstrual periods | 15 | after w |
| 39. | Lee, Felix | 555-0732 | Dressing to toe injury | 15 | noon |
| 40. | Nye, Peter | 555-0132 | Check blood pressure, weight, urine | 15 | a.m. |

Monday August 30 (242)

Tuesday August 31 (243)

Wednesday September 1 (244)

| | 00 |
| | 15 |
| 8 | 30 |
| | 45 |
| | 00 |
| 9 | 15 |
| | 30 |
| | 45 |
| | 00 |
| 10 | 15 |
| | 30 |
| | 45 |
| | 00 |
| 11 | 15 |
| | 30 |
| | 45 |
| | 00 |
| 12 | 15 |
| | 30 |
| | 45 |
| | 00 |
| 1 | 15 |
| | 30 |
| | 45 |
| | 00 |
| 2 | 15 |
| | 30 |
| | 45 |
| | 00 |
| 3 | 15 |
| | 30 |
| | 45 |
| | 00 |
| 4 | 15 |
| | 30 |
| | 45 |
| | 00 |
| 5 | 15 |
| | 30 |
| | 45 |

Appointment Schedule

6. Following information in the textbook on punctuation, capitalization, and mailable standards, type Letters 1, 2, and 3 following the instruction for each letter; letterheads are provided. Final copy should meet mailable standards. _____

7. List the problem areas to watch when proofreading. _____

_____

_____

8. Prepare corrected Letter 4 by interpreting proofreader's marks.

9. Given a dictating machine tape, produce a mailable letter according to Procedure 6-7, Compose a Business Letter. _____

10. Refer to the CAAHEP Standards in Appendix B of the textbook. Within the area of *Communication,* which three curriculum standards are discussed in this unit? _____

_____

## LETTER 1

The first letter is to Robert Jones, M.D., 5000 N. High Street, Yourtown, US 43200. The name of the patient is Juan Gomez. Use full block style seen in Figure 6-20(B) and proper capitalization, punctuation, and placement on the paper.

Dear dr jones

your patient juan gomez was first seen October 7, complaining of severe tinnitus in both ears.

On physical examination his hearing was 15/20 right ear 13/20 left ear audiogram was made which showed considerable loss of high tones Mr. gomez's complaints of tinnitus and decreased hearing are in accordance with the audiometric and clinical findings of beginning degeneration of his nerve of hearing. In all probability this condition has been caused by loud noises which he has encountered in his work.

despite treatment his hearing has not increased and tinnitus persists.

thank you for referring mr gomez.

very truly yours

## LETTER 2

Type the second letter using modified block style seen in Figure 6-20(C). Use current date for the letter. Address the letter to John Jones, M.D., 3530 Main Street, Cold Springs, KY 41076. The name of the patient is Mrs. Patty Segal. The dictating physician is Samuel E. Matthews, M.D.

I saw _____ on _____ for X-ray examination.

AP and lateral roentgenograms of the cervical spine show an aberration of the normal cervical curve. The curve is convexed posteriorly at the level of the fifth, sixth, and seventh cervical vertebrae. Normally, the posterior curve should be concave. There are no significant hypertrophic changes, but there are minimal true arthritic changes involving the articular facets in the lower cervical region.

A roentgenogram of the right shoulder shows no evidence of intrinsic bone disease. There is no periarticular soft tissue calcification in the region of the bruise.

Thank you for your referral

Very truly yours,

## LETTER 3

Type the following letter using modified block with indented paragraphs as seen in Figure 6-20(D). The letter is to Robert Jones, M.D., 5000 N. High Street, Yourtown, US 98765. The patient is Patricia Moriarty. The letter is from Kerry Smith, M.D.

Dear Dr. Jones:

I saw _____ in the office today. You will recall that she has suffered from menstrual discomfort and intermenstrual pain for the past 6 months.

On examination, the breasts are well developed and free of masses. On pelvic examination, the hymen is intact; and vaginal examination was not performed. On rectal examination, the uterus was anterior and freely movable. The right adnexa were normal. The left ovary was enlarged to the size of a walnut or slightly larger and was cystic. Compression of this ovary reproduced the patient's pain.

Patricia was asked to return in three weeks for re-examination to determine the need for treatment of ovarian enlargement.

Thank you for referring this patient.

Sincerely,

**LETTERHEAD 1**

**SAMUEL E. MATTHEWS, M.D.**

**SUITE 120  100 E. MAIN STREET**

**YOURTOWN, US  98765-4321**

**LETTERHEAD 2**

SAMUEL E. MATTHEWS, M.D.

SUITE 120  100 E. MAIN STREET

YOURTOWN, US  98765-4321

**LETTERHEAD 3**

**KERRY SMITH, M.D.**

**101 LANE AVENUE**

**YOURTOWN, US 12345**

**LETTER 4:  Letter to Be Corrected**

Kerry Smith, M.D.
101 Lane Avenue
Yourtown, US  12345


*e*
Robrt Jones, M.D.
5000 N. High Street
Yourtown, US  98765


Dear Dr. Jones:


I saw Patricia Moriarty in the office today.  You will recall that she has suffered from menstrual dis comfort and intermenstrual pain since July.


On examination, the breasts are well develloped and free of masses.  on pelvic examination, the hymen is intact;  and vaginal examination was not performed.  On Rectal examination, the uterus was anterior and freely movable.  The right adnexa were normal.  The left ovary was enlarged to the size of a walnut or slightly larger and was cystic. Compression of this ovary reproduced the patient's pain. Patricia was asked to return in three weeks for re-examination to determine the need for treatment of ovarian enlargement.


Thank you for referring this patient.


Sincerely,




Kerry Smith, M.D.

**LETTER 4**

**KERRY SMITH, M.D.**

**101 LANE AVENUE**

**YOURTOWN, US  12345**

**B. Word Puzzle:** Use the definitions below to spell out these terms.

1.        _ _ _ T _ _ _
2.        _ _ _ _ R _ _ _ _ _ _
3.        _ _ A _ _ _
4.        _ _ _ N _ _ _
5.  _ _ _ _ S _ _
6.        C _ _ _ _ _ _
7.        _ R _ _ _ _ _ _ _
8.        _ _ I _ _ _ _ _
9.        P _ _ _ _ _ _ _ _ _
10.      _ _ T _ _ _ _ _
11.      _ I _ _ _ _ _ _
12.      _ O _ _ _ _ _
13.      _ _ N _ _ _
14. _ _ _ _ I _ _ _ _ _
15. _ _ _ _ _ S _
16.      T _ _ _ _ _ _ _

1. The part of a written or spoken statement that surrounds a particular word or passage and can clarify its meaning
2. A shortened word or words formed by omitting or combining some of the letters or sounds
3. A section of a sentence
4. A noun substitute
5. A mark or series of marks used in writing or printing to indicate an omission, especially of letters or words
6. A critical examination of a thing or situation
7. Carefully read material for errors
8. An item suitable for mailing
9. An addition to a letter written after the writer's name
10. A mark imprinted on paper that is visible when it is held up to the light, usually a sign of quality
11. The name of a person as written by himself or herself
12. To qualify or limit the meaning
13. To indicate, to mean
14. Paper used for letters
15. To write, to form by combination of units or parts
16. A reference book containing words and their synonyms

**ASSIGNMENT SHEET**

**Chapter 6: ORAL AND WRITTEN COMMUNICATIONS**

**Unit 4: RECEIVING AND SENDING OFFICE COMMUNICATIONS**

**A. Brief Answer**

1. What supplies and equipment are needed to open the mail? _____

   _____

2. What information may be different on the envelope than on the contents of the letter? _____

   _____

3. The U.S. Postal Service has identified certain features of a letter that might be suspicious. List the three that would be the most inappropriate for a physician's office. _____

   _____

4. What should you do with a suspicious letter or package? _____

   _____

5. What incoming mail may be handled by the medical assistant alone? _____

   _____

6. How should unwanted drug samples be disposed of? _____

7. Using the following information, address the envelope below so it can be read by the OCR and sorted by the BCS. Send to: Medical Records, University Hospital, 100 E. First Street, Ourtown, US 12345-6789 (You may print your answer in lieu of typing.) Use Elizabeth R. Evans, M.D., Suite 205, 100 E. Main St., Yourtown, US 98765-4321 as the return address.

_Elizabeth R. Evans, M.D.,_
_Suite 205, 100 E_
_Main St, yourtown US_
_98765-4321_

_Medical Records university Hospital_
_100 E First st. ourtown US_
_12345-6789_

**Fill in the Blank:**

8. Below are some abbreviations pertaining to mail; spell out the words they stand for.

   A. USPS _____

   B. OCR _____

   C. BCS _____

   D. APT _____

E.  ATTN    _____  _____
F.  AVE     _____
G.  BLVD    _____
H.  HTS     _____
I.  HOSP    _____
J.  INST    _____
K.  LN      _____
L.  PKY     _____
M.  PL      _____
N.  PO      _____
O.  RR      _____

9.  What do the numbers in the following zip code 43221-4940 stand for?

4- _____

32- _____

21- _____

49- _____

40- _____

10. Name four things to remember in processing metered mail. _____

_____

_____

11. Where can current postal information be obtained? _____

12. List the six classifications of mail. _____

_____

13. What special sending or receiving features are associated with the following types of mailings?

A. Express— _____

B. Certificate of mailing— _____

C. Certified mail— _____

D. Registered— _____

E. Restricted delivery— _____

14. Refer to the Role Delineation Chart in Appendix A of the textbook. Within the area of *Operational Functions,*
what role relates to the content of this unit? _____

## B.  Matching:  MATCH the definition in column II with the correct term in column I.

COLUMN I

_____    1.  Fax
_____    2.  Pager
_____    3.  Voice mail
_____    4.  Cellular

_____    5.  Conference call
_____    6.  Teleconference
_____    7.  Telemedicine
_____    8.  E-mail
_____    9.  Internet

COLUMN II

a.  Involves phones, cameras, and television
b.  Portable telephone
c.  Needs computer, electronic address, and phone to receive messages
d.  Requires appropriate software, a modem, a service provider, and a search engine
e.  Sends written material electronically over phone lines
f.  Long-distance physical assessment
g.  Small receiver of electronic messages by phone signal
h.  Multi-phone call
i.  Receives messages in a "mailbox"

2. Use a calculator to determine the balance due o\n the following patient account. Total each appointment and payment, list monthly balances and final balance due. (Insurance filing charge not reimbursable.)

| | | Charges | Receipts | Balance |
|---|---|---|---|---|
| 6/1/97 | Office consult—extensive | 105.00 | | |
| | Diagnostic X-ray testing | 67.00 | | |
| | Laboratory | 35.00 | | _____ |
| 6/10/97 | Office, follow-up, extensive | 85.00 | | |
| | ECG | 65.00 | | |
| | Culture | 40.00 | | |
| | Injection, antibiotic | 30.00 | | _____ |
| 7/1/97 | Office, intermediate | 65.00 | | _____ |
| 7/21/97 | Office intermediate | 65.00 | | _____ |
| 8/1/97 | Insurance filed (Medicare, Travelers) | 10.00 | | _____ |
| 9/15/97 | Medicare payment | | 272.16 | |
| | Medicare write off | | 226.80 | _____ |
| 9/25/97 | Travelers payment | | 58.04 | _____ |

## B. Brief Answer

1. List the nine examples of items frequently copied. _____

_____

_____

2. What is microfilming? _____

_____

_____

3. How can microfilmed material be read? _____

_____

_____

4. You are having difficulty transcribing dictation due to the following possible reasons. What could you say to the physician to improve the quality of the content?

   a. You are not sure what type of dictation is to be transcribed or when it was recorded. _____

   _____

   _____

   b. The message is clear, but you do not know to whom it goes or where to send it. _____

   _____

   _____

   c. You can't tell if a pause is the end of the sentence or a break in dictation. _____

   _____

   _____

   d. The dictation seems to be muffled and slurred at times and often barely audible because of background noise. _____

   _____

   _____

   e. You are never sure if the dictation is finished or if it's a break in the message. _____

   _____

   _____

5. List four features of a word processor. _____

_____

_____

6. What is a computer? _____

_____

_____

_____

7. Name three types of printers _____

_____

8. Give 10 examples of medical management software uses. _____

_____

_____

_____

9. Refer to the ABHES Course Content Requirements in Appendix C of the textbook. Within the area of *Basic Keyboarding,* which content requirement relates to the content in this unit? _____

_____

**C. Matching: MATCH the definition in column II with the correct term in column I.**

COLUMN I

_____ 1. Batch
_____ 2. Bug
_____ 3. Cursor
_____ 4. Data
_____ 5. Disk
_____ 6. File
_____ 7. Font
_____ 8. Hard copy
_____ 9. Initialize
_____ 10. Memory
_____ 11. Modem
_____ 12. Monitor
_____ 13. Peripheral
_____ 14. Program
_____ 15. Scroll
_____ 16. Write-protect

COLUMN II

a. A readable paper copy or printout
b. Information that can be processed or produced by a computer
c. A single stored unit of information that is named
d. Formatting
e. Video display unit with a screen
f. To move the cursor up, down, right, or left
g. An error in a program
h. Anything plugged into a computer
i. A set of instructions written in computer language
j. An accumulation of data to be processed
k. Data held in storage
l. Process or code that prevents overwriting data or a program on a disk
m. A marker on the screen showing where the next character will be placed
n. An assortment of characters of a given size and style
o. A magnetic storage device made of plastic
p. A peripheral device that enables a computer to communicate over phone lines

**D. Word Search: Find the following words hidden in the puzzle.**

ACRONYM
CALCULATOR
COMPUTER
DICTATION
ELECTRONIC
HARDWARE
MENU
MICROFICHE

MICROFILM
PAYEE
PROCESSOR
PROGRAM
SOFTWARE
TECHNOLOGY
TRANSCRIPTION

```
E C P G T O U R A D W Y C M I B
X T R A C Q S P R O G R A M C T
U D O D B W C M I C R O F I L M
H R C D I C T A T I O N L C G E
A V E T O M E N U R P C S R Q Y
R X S A D L C U Z F G O O O H K
D J S L M Z H T S P C M F F W F
W B O T R A N S C R I P T I O N
A K R A C R O N Y M G U W C H J
R C A L C U L A T O R T A H K L
E L E C T R O N I C M E R E N P
S V A D C O G G H F C R E T R O
D G V K P A Y E E R H P Z W C A
```

**ACHIEVING SKILL COMPETENCY**

Reread the performance objective for each procedure and then practice the skills listed below, following the procedure in your textbook.

Procedure 6-1:   Answer the Office Phone
Procedure 6-2:   Process Phone Message
Procedure 6-3:   Record Telephone Mesage on Recording Device
Procedure 6-4:   Obtain Telephone Message from Phone Recording Device
Procedure 6-5:   Schedule Appointments
Procedure 6-6:   Arrange Referral Appointment
Procedure 6-7:   Compose a Business Letter
Procedure 6-8:   Total Charges on Calculator
Procedure 6-9:   Operate Copy Machine
Procedure 6-10:  Operate Transcriber
Procedure 6-11:  Operate Office Computer

When you feel you have mastered performance of a skill, sign your name on the appropriate evaluation sheet and give it to your instructor to indicate you are prepared to perform the procedure for evaluation.

After your instructor has returned your work to you, make all necessary corrections and place in a three-ring notebook for future reference.

**ASSIGNMENT SHEET**

**Chapter 7: RECORDS MANAGEMENT**

   Review the objectives and text for each unit before completing the assignment sheet for that unit. When you have completed all sheets for the chapter, remove them from this Workbook and give them to the instructor for evaluation.

**Unit 1: THE PATIENT'S MEDICAL RECORD**

**A. Brief Answer**

1. Define *subjective information.* _____

_____

2. Define *objective information.* _____

_____

_____

3. What is a progress note? _____

_____

4. Describe methods of recording progress notes. _____

_____

5. Describe the correct procedure for making corrections on progress notes. _____

_____

_____

_____

6. List the differences between a traditional record and the Problem Oriented Medical Record (POMR).

_____

_____

_____

_____

_____

7. What is a procrastinator? In terms of the medical office, what effect would this have on patients' records?

_____

_____

_____

## B. Word Scramble

1. _ _ _ _ _ _ _ _        DIFIGNSN
2. _ _ _ _ _ _ _ _        PSEFICCI
3. _ _ _ _ _ _            RDOCRE
4. _ _ _ _ _ _ _ _ _ _    CEJEVTIBSU
5. _ _ _ _ _ _ _ _        SPGESRRO
6. _ _ _ _ _ _ _          ACEDITT
7. _ _ _ _ _ _ _ _ _ _ _ _ _  NFOICTTYLIDAEIN
8. _ _ _ _ _ _ _ _ _ _ _ _    TANECIVOONNL
9. _ _ _ _ _ _ _ _ _        CEBTJIOVE
10. _ _ _ _ _ _ _ _ _       MDDCEUONTE
11. _ _ _ _ _ _ _          RTSHYIO
12. _ _ _ _ _ _ _ _ _       ENIOMRIPSS

## B. Write a sentence with each unscrambled word regarding the patient's medical record.

1. _____
2. _____
3. _____
4. _____
5. _____
6. _____
7. _____
8. _____
9. _____
10. _____
11. _____
12. _____

## C. Multiple Choice: Place the correct letter or letters on the blank line for each question.

_____ 1. What information in a medical record makes it a useful legal document?

a. progress notes          c. dates of injuries

b. dates of treatments     d. all of these

_____ 2. Which of the symptoms listed below are objective?

a. headache                c. swelling

b. rash                    d. bleeding

_____ 3. Which of the symptoms listed below are subjective?

a. red throat              c. bruise

b. nausea                  d. abdominal pain

_____ 4. Besides the clinical visit findings, what additional information is recorded on progress notes?

a. phone messages          c. phone/fax refills

b. marital status          d. cancelations

_____ 5. What color of ink should be used in recording patient information?

a. blue                    c. red

b. black                   d. any color

**C. True or False: Place a "T" for true or "F" for false in the space provided. For false statements, explain why they are false.**

_____ 1. The confidentiality of the patient's medical record must be maintained by careful management as it is used.

_____ 2. Only parts of the patient's record are necessary when the patient wishes the physician to testify in an injury case.

_____ 3. The patient must always sign an authorization form before any information can be released.

_____ 4. All patient information contained in the medical record is considered subjective information.

_____ 5. Progress notes should be arranged in chronological order with the most recent date on top.

_____ 6. The date and time should be recorded on the page for progress notes each time the patient is seen.

_____ 7. Using correction fluid is recommended to completely eliminate an error made on a patient's record.

_____ 8. Using black ink on the patient's record is important for making good copies.

_____ 9. The POMR record begins with the standard database.

After your instructor has returned your work to you, make all necessary corrections and place it in a three-ring notebook for future reference.

**ASSIGNMENT SHEET**

**Chapter 7: RECORDS MANAGEMENT**

**Unit 2: FILING**

**SUGGESTED RESPONSES TO CRITICAL THINKING CHALLENGE IN TEXTBOOK**

1. What did Judy's apparent haste cause to happen? _____
   _____

2. Do you think Judy had good intentions? _____

3. What do you think needs to be done to Mr. Jeffries' chart? _____
   _____

4. What do you think Francene said to Judy about this error? _____
   _____

5. Who should record the data on Mr. Stephens' chart? _____

6. What would you have done in this situation? _____
   _____
   _____

7. Would you call the temporary service to report Judy's error? _____
   _____

8. What do you think of the temporary service? _____
   _____

9. Would you call the temporary service again? _____

**A. Brief Answer**

1. What is meant by *indexing*? _____
   _____
   _____

2. Name and define the four basic filing methods.
   a. _____
   b. _____
   c. _____
   d. _____

3. Name and define the five steps in filing.
   a. _____
   _____
   b. _____
   c. _____
   d. _____
   e. _____

4. Describe the proper method of placing material in a file folder. _____
   _____

5. Describe the most efficient method of removing and replacing patient files. _____
   _____
   _____
   _____

6. List the storage media used for "paperless" filing systems. _____

_____

7. Describe ways to help find a missing chart. _____

_____

_____

_____

_____

## B. Indexing Practice

1. Index each name below on a 3 × 5 card or paper cut to that size. Start each name ½ inch from the top and ½ inch from the left margin. Arrange the cards in alphabetical order.

   a.  Curtis Koch
   b.  Dianne Hanning
   c.  Dezzie Harris
   d.  Connie Graves
   e.  Anna Epstein
   f.  Melvin Edwards
   g.  Charles L. Davis
   h.  Gertrude Carter
   i.  Barbara Cahill
   j.  Earl Block

   k.  Robert Blair
   l.  C.L. Benson
   m.  L.K. Ander
   n.  Elmo Applegate
   o.  Nathan Appleby
   p.  Bruce Carr
   q.  Sandra Dyer
   r.  Pauline Hall
   s.  P.A. Dennis
   t.  Dave Daniels

2. Index each name below on a 3 × 5 card or paper cut to that size. Start each name ½ inch from the top and ½ inch in from the left margin. Arrange the cards in alphabetical order.

   a.  Edgar Underwood
   b.  Richard Poff
   c.  Thomas Meyer
   d.  Felix Lee
   e.  Helen Thornton
   f.  Hubert Landers
   g.  Ann Stone
   h.  Mary June Quinn
   i.  Peter Nye
   j.  G. Saunders

   k.  Glen Ochs
   l.  Clyde Rambo
   m.  Russel Owens
   n.  Thomas Jefferson
   o.  June Guthrie
   p.  Theresa Frost
   q.  Kenneth Ford
   r.  Vivian Booth
   s.  Jimmy Block
   t.  Stephen Bergstrom

3. Code the names listed below by underlining the first unit and place 2, 3, 4 above other units in correct filing order. Then arrange the names in correct alphabetic and indexing order on the form provided.

Ex: L$\overset{2}{\text{i}}$sa / A$\overset{3}{\text{nn}}$ / Hale

a. Steve Van Meter
b. Victor Li-Lelaez
c. Min Kwang-Shik
d. Joan Vanmatre
e. Judy Kavang
f. Esther Corbie-Bender
g. Marila Corbitt
h. Asad Al-Alowi
i. Louise Gage
j. Frances Buntyn
k. Letticia Galindo
l. Don Durflinger
m. Anna Gunton

n. Louie Gage
o. Alfred D'Ambrosio
p. A./M. FitzHugh
q. Kelly LaBarba
r. Sylvia D'Ambrogi
s. Bill Fitz
t. Bryan LaBeff
u. C. W. McBrayer
v. Dr. Larry Mathis
w. Mrs. M.W. Smith (Mary)
x. Rev. Joan Sanders
y. Mrs. Carol Long (Mrs. William)
   Carol Long (Mrs.) William

## WORKSHEET FOR FILING ASSIGNMENTS

| 1st Unit | 2nd Unit | 3rd Unit | 4th Unit |
|---|---|---|---|
| a. | | | |
| b. | | | |
| c. | | | |
| d. | | | |
| e. | | | |
| f. | | | |
| g. | | | |
| h. | | | |
| i. | | | |
| j. | | | |
| k. | | | |
| l. | | | |
| m. | | | |
| n. | | | |
| o. | | | |
| p. | | | |
| q. | | | |
| r. | | | |
| s. | | | |
| t. | | | |
| u. | | | |
| v. | | | |
| w. | | | |
| x. | | | |
| y. | | | |

4. Code the names listed below by underlining the first unit and place 2, 3, 4 above other units in correct filing order. Then arrange the names in correct alphabetic and indexing order on the form provided.

   Ex: Abbott-Coltman. / Inc.

   a. Neu-Mor/Corp.
   b. Mt./Vernon/Mobile/Homes
   c. Richard's/Antiques
   d. Robt./Moriconi, (Jr.)
   e. Japan/Air Lines
   f. Aus-/Tex/Garden/Supply
   g. A./Ingram
   h. Northwest/Airlines
   i. Bill/New/Law/Office
   j. San/Antonio/Tours,/Inc.
   k. So-Lo/Diet/Center
   l. M/N/Insurance/Agency
   m. McFarland/Down Town/Motor/Co.
   n. Vivian/Richards, (M.D.)
   o. St./Paul/Printing/Co.

# WORKSHEET FOR FILING ASSIGNMENTS

| 1st Unit | 2nd Unit | 3rd Unit | 4th Unit |
|----------|----------|----------|----------|

a. _____

b. _____

c. _____

d. _____

e. _____

f. _____

g. _____

h. _____

i. _____

j. _____

k. _____

l. _____

m. _____

n. _____

o. _____

5. Use the 25 cards prepared in question 3. Write the following registry numbers in the upper-right-hand corner of the cards. Arrange the cards in numerical order and list the 25 names in the order in which they now appear.

a. _____    j. _____    r. _____

b. _____    k. _____    s. _____

c. _____    l. _____    t. _____

d. _____    m. _____    u. _____

e. _____    n. _____    v. _____

f. _____    o. _____    w. _____

g. _____    p. _____    x. _____

h. _____    q. _____    y. _____

i. _____

| | | |
|---|---|---|
| Van Meter 19-2-10 | Kavang 10-11-65 | Gage, Louise 12-70-45 |
| Li-Lelaez 22-12-65 | Corbie-Bender 50-30-25 | Buntyn 60-20-15 |
| Kwang-Shik 13-11-65 | Corbitt 13-30-25 | Galindo 12-70-45 |
| Vanmatre 10-22-10 | Al-Alowi 10-10-15 | Durflinger 40-40-25 |
| Gunton 10-70-45 | D'Ambrogi 19-40-25 | Mathis 40-12-75 |
| Gage, Louise 12-70-45 | Fitz 20-60-35 | Smith 13-23-95 |
| D'Ambrosio 10-10-25 | LaBeff 20-12-65 | Sanders 18-10-95 |
| FitzHugh 10-13-35 | McBrayer 30-23-75 | Long 13-30-65 |
| LaBarba 11-12-65 | | |

**C. Word Search: Find the following words hidden in the puzzle.**

ACCUMULATED

ALPHABETICAL

CODING

DATA

EXPEDITE

FILING

GEOGRAPHIC

ILLUMINATING

INDEXING

INSPECT

NUMERICAL

SEQUENCE

SORT

STORE

SUBSEQUENT

SUPPLEMENTED

SYSTEMATICALLY

UNIT

UNPRODUCTIVE

```
P O I U L K J H M N B V O I U Y L L A C I T A M E T S Y S
Q W E R F D S A Z X C V K J H N B U N P R O D U C T I V E
H J K F G H D F H S T O R E S D A W Q E T R E F O C N M Q
B V C X Z G F D S O M D E T A L U M U C C A I U D O S N U
L K J M N B T Y U R I O T M N B H G F A P O I U I K P L E
S U B S E Q U E N T X P I W A B M Y I P O U J H N B E M N
L O J Y F E D S W G Z Q D B Y N T M I T T R E W G D C X C
O P U I T Y T R E N A S E W E R I P F I L I N G Y N T G E
L K J M N B H G F I P L P D E X N V B O M I Y R E D D L K
A S D W E Q R T B X N H X I L L U M I N A T I N G C A B N
P O K I J M N B F E D T E H G F D S A Q W E R T Y O T L K
F D S A E R T W C D B N M J H L A C I T E B A H P L A K J
L O I K J M N H Y N P O M N U M E R I C A L J N B M L O P
E R W D S F B V C I M J H K I U O C I H P A R G O E G I N
P O I N T S U P P L E M E N T E D P O K E R D C S Q N T L
```

**D. Multiple Choice: Place the correct letter on the blank line for each question.**

_____ 1. Bar code files eliminate the need for

    a. data entry

    b. OUTguides

    c. progress notes

    d. all of these

_____ 2. Placing all documents in a patient's chart in _____ order makes it easier to obtain information.

    a. color-coded

    b. alphabetical

    c. chronological

    d. categorical

_____ 3. The method of filing that provides the most patient privacy is

    a. alphabetical

    b. numeric

    c. categorical

    d. chronological

_____ 4. In a miscellaneous file, when there are more than ____ papers on one subject or person, you should remove them and make a separate folder.

    a. two

    b. three

    c. four

    d. five

_____ 5. _____ make it easy to obtain phone numbers and addresses.

    a. bar code files

    b. desktop files

    c. tickler files

    d. numeric files

_____ 6. Removing the files of patients who are no longer being seen by the physician is called
   a. processing                          c. sorting
   b. indexing                            d. purging

_____ 7. When there is a signature on a patient's chart, J. Williams (CL), whose initials are in the parentheses?
   a. patient's                           c. medical assistant's
   b. physician's                         d. office manager's

## ACHIEVING SKILL COMPETENCY

Reread the performance objective for each procedure and then practice the skills listed below, following the procedure in your textbook.

Procedure 7-1: File Item(s) Alphabetically
Procedure 7-2: Pull File Folder from Alphabetic files
Procedure 7-3: File Item(s) Numerically
Procedure 7-4: Pull file Folder from Numeric Files

When you have mastered the performances of a skill, sign your name on the appropriate evaluation sheet and give it to your instructor to indicate you are prepared to perform the procedure for evaluation.

After your instructor has returned your work to you, make all necessary corrections and place in a three-ring notebook for future reference.

**ASSIGNMENT SHEET**

## Chapter 8: COLLECTING FEES

Review the objectives and text for each unit before completing the assignment sheet for that unit. When you have completed all sheets for the chapter, remove them from this Workbook and give them to the instructor for evaluation.

### Unit 1: MEDICAL CARE EXPENSES

**A. Brief Answers**

1. What are the factors to consider in determining fees for patient care?

_____

_____

_____

2. When insurance companies and government agencies establish a fee profile for physicians, how does it affect payment for patients?

_____

_____

_____

3. Explain what you should do if an indigent patient wants an appointment in your facility and your physician cannot accept another indigent patient at this time.

_____

_____

_____

_____

4. List the information that should be obtained on the personal data sheet of each patient.

a. _____

b. _____

c. _____

d. _____

e. _____

f. _____

g. _____

h. _____

i. _____

j. _____

**B. True or False: Place a "T" for true or "F" for false in the space provided. For false statements, explain why they are false.**

_____ 1. Physicians are the ones who discuss fees with patients.

_____ 2. Insurance companies and government agencies establish a fee profile for physicians based on charges averaged over a period of time.

_____ 3. Physicians should never be told when a patient is unhappy with the cost of treatment.

_____ 4. Indigent patients should receive the same care as paying patients.

_____ 5. Two copies of the reduced fee agreement, with the words "without prejudice" stated, should be witnessed as they are signed for those with limited income.

_____ 6. Each time the patient comes in for an appointment, you should verify the personal data sheet information.

_____ 7. The personal data sheet should ask for additional insurance coverage.

_____ 8. It is not necessary for the records release form to have a witness sign it.

_____ 9. On the third-party liability statement, the name of the patient and the name of the responsible party are always one and the same person.

**C. Word Puzzle:** **For each word listed below, provide another word that has the same meaning (or is similar in meaning) to fill in the blank spaces.**

1. Complicated      1. _ _ _ _ _ _ _ _ _ _ _

2. Poor             2. _ _ _ _ _ _ _ _

3. Inexpensive      3. _ _ _ _ _ _ _ _

4. Succeeding       4. _ _ _ _ _ _ _ _ _ _

5. Confirm          5. _ _ _ _ _ _

**D. Multiple Choice:** **Place the correct letter on the blank line for each question.**

_____ 1. Completed annually, this form provides a "signature on file" for your records.
  a. personal/patient data sheet          c. medication list
  b. medical history form                 d. charges statement

_____ 2. Fees should be discussed with patients
  a. in the reception area                c. in a private area
  b. in the exam room                     d. in groups

_____ 3. At each office visit you should ask patients for their insurance card so that you can
  a. read it                              c. release information
  b. copy it                              d. check their birth date

_____ 4. If a third party is responsible for a patient's charges, that person should sign a
  a. liability statement                  c. records release form
  b. data sheet                           d. estimate form

_____ 5. You should obtain a release of information form
  a. as needed                            c. at the first visit
  b. when patients are moving             d. at each visit

After your instructor has returned your work to you, make all necessary corrections and place in a three-ring notebook for future reference.

**ASSIGNMENT SHEET**

**Chapter 8: COLLECTING FEES**

**Unit 2: CREDIT ARRANGEMENTS**

**A. Brief Answers**

1. Explain when you should discuss payment planning and health insurance coverage with patients and give examples.

   _____

   _____

   _____

   _____

2. What is specified in the Truth in Lending Act?

   _____

   _____

   _____

3. How are physicians required under the AMA Code of Ethics to allow patients to use credit cards for services?

   _____

   _____

   _____

4. Why are credit card payments advantageous if there is a 1% to 3% assessment charged to the physician?

   _____

   _____

   _____

5. What is the purpose of the Bureau of Medical Economics?

   _____

6. If a request is received from a credit bureau regarding a patient, what information are you to disclose in your answer?

   _____

   _____

   _____

**B. Multiple Choice: Place the correct letter or letters on the blank line for each question.**

_____ 1. Assisting patients with a plan for payment of costly medical expenses is the responsibility of the
   a. physician                          c. medical assistant
   b. interpreter                         d. physician assistant

_____ 2. How long must the (signed) Truth in Lending form be kept on file?
   a. two years                          c. 10 years
   b. six years                          d. indefinitely

_____ 3. Patients should be reminded to check with their _____ for the amount that they are responsible for (co-pay), if their insurance does not pay the total cost.
   a. bank                               c. insurance company
   b. financial planner                  d. loan company

_____ 4. In large cities it is wise to check ____ before extending credit for a large medical expense.
    a. marital status          c. credit references
    b. medical history         d. insurance

_____ 5. It is a violation of the law if you disclose ____ in requests from creditors regarding patients.
    a. opening date of account         c. character of patient
    b. paying habits          d. largest amount of account

## C. Word Search: Find the following words hidden in the puzzle.

```
I A D V A N C E A C T
A D D I S C L O S E H
D E L I N Q U E N T C
V C L O E T H I C S O
T R U T H   C A R D S
I N S T A L L M E N T
C P A Y M E N T D E S
I A F I N A N C I N G
L T E S T I M A T E F
O I N C H A R G E S A
S U B S T A N T I A L
```

CARDS
INSTALLMENT
CHARGES
FINANCING
ETHICS
COSTS
DISCLOSE
PAYMENT
TRUTH
ESTIMATE
DELINQUENT
ADVANCE
ACT
CREDIT
SOLICIT
SUBSTANTIAL

## D. True or False: Place a "T" for true or "F" for false in the space provided. For false statements, explain why they are false.

_____ 1. A cost estimate sheet for surgery should include cost of the surgery and the approximate cost of the anesthesia, consultants, and hospital costs.

_____ 2. The Truth in Lending Act is enforced by the International Trade Commission.

_____ 3. Physicians may increase charges for services to patients who wish to use credit cards for medical services.

_____ 4. It is not only lawful but good practice to disclose information to referring offices regarding paying habits of patients.

_____ 5. The Truth in Lending form must be signed by the patient in your presence.

After your instructor has returned your work to you, make all necessary corrections and place in a three-ring notebook for future reference.

## ASSIGNMENT SHEET

**Chapter 8:  COLLECTING FEES**

**Unit 3:  BOOKKEEPING PROCEDURES**

**A. Multiple Choice:  Place the correct letter or letters on the blank line for each question.**

_____  1. A patient account shows the

      a. balance due              c. payments

      b. charges                d. a and b only

_____  2. Besides the appointment schedule, the ___ will reflect the names of all patients seen each day.

      a. patient's ledger         c. itemized statement

      b. daily log sheet          d. all receipts

_____  3. Patients should be ____ from sending cash payments through the mail.

      a. encouraged           c. discouraged

      b. stopped              d. restrained

_____  4. Dividing account cards into groups to correspond to the number of times billing is done is called

      a. bookkeeping         c. business transactions

      b. cycle billing          d. balancing

_____  5. Patients who have filed bankruptcy may continue to see the physician, but must pay with

      a. cash               c. insurance

      b. credit card           d. check

**B. Matching:  Match the definition in column II with the correct term in column I.**

COLUMN I

_____  1. Posted

_____  2. Trial balance

_____  3. Cash payment

_____  4. Petition

_____  5. Proprietorship

_____  6. Bankruptcy

_____  7. Bookkeeper

_____  8. Journalizing

COLUMN II

a. Owner-manager of a business

b. Formal written application seeking specific judicial action

c. Legal petition to the courts if one is unable to pay creditors

d. One who records transactions/accounts of a business

e. To record bookkeeping transactions in a journal

f. Total owed/record of accounts receivable

g. Transfer of information from one record to another

h. Write-it-once bookkeeping system

i. Must be given a receipt

**C. Brief Answer**

1. Use half sheets of paper and type the invoice shown in Figure 8-7. Type itemized statements from the five families who still owe money. _____

_____

2. Describe the exceptions to the usual billing procedures. _____

_____

_____

_____

_____

_____

_____

Name _____

3. Describe the advantages of a write-it-once bookkeeping system. _____

_____

_____

_____

_____

**D.** 1. Use the following information to fill in a daily log for each of the three days indicated. Be careful to calculate charges when more than one is listed and put only the total in the charge column. Be sure to itemize in column listing description. Be careful to list payments in payment column and break down each in either cash or check payment column.

December 27, XX_____

    Juan Gomez - paid $17.00 ck

    Sue Schmidt - O.C. limited $27.00; Inj. B 12 $15.00

    Susan Segal - O.C. New intermediate $48.00

    Sue Schmidt - paid $62.00 ck

    Carol Sue Kostrevski - O.C. Comprehensive $70.00; paid $50.00 cash

    LaChar Holley - (NP) Comprehensive $85.00

January 5, XX_____

    Geoff Segal - paid $48.00 cash for Susan

    Juan Gomez - Extended exam $46.00

    June Kostrevski - Allergy testing $100.00

    Carol Sue Kostrevski - Inj. Penicillin $12.00

    Joan Moriarty - O.C. Intermediate $30.00; x-ray left knee $76.00; paid $50.00 ck

    Carol Schmidt - O.C. Extended $46.00

    Boris Kostrevski - Paid $150.00 ck

January 8, XX_____

    Boris Kostrevski - CPE comprehensive New $85.00; chest x-ray $79.00;

      ECG $50.00; Lab Physical Profile $113.00;

      Draw blood $5.00; Urinalysis $10.00

    Patrick Moriarty - O.C. Intermediate $30.00; paid $38.00 ck

    Tina Schmidt - cast removal $35.00

    Juan Gomez- O.C. Limited $27.00

    Geoff Segal - N.C.

    June Kostrevski - Ck. Aetna Ins. $100.00

    LaChar Holley - Hospital 12/29 thru 1/6

      Initial visit $85.00

      6 days at $25.00

      Total charges $235.00

    Boris Kostrevski - Medicare pd. ck $40.00

    Juan Gomez - Medical pd. ck $12.50

    After your instructor has returned your work to you, make all necessary corrections and place in a three-ring notebook for future reference.

| DATE | NAME | DESCRIPTION | CHARGES | CREDITS | | CASH | CHK |
|------|------|-------------|---------|---------|---------|------|-----|
| | | | | PAYMENTS | ADJ. | | |
| | | | | | | | |
| | | | | | | | |
| | | | | | | | |
| | | | | | | | |
| | | | | | | | |
| | | | | | | | |
| | | | | | | | |
| | | | | | | | |
| | | | | | | | |
| | | | | | | | |
| | | | | | | | |
| | | | | | | | |
| | | | | | | | |

| DATE | NAME | DESCRIPTION | CHARGES | √ | CREDITS | | CASH | CHK |
| | | | | | PAYMENTS | ADJ. | | |
|---|---|---|---|---|---|---|---|---|
| | | | | | | | | |
| | | | | | | | | |
| | | | | | | | | |
| | | | | | | | | |
| | | | | | | | | |
| | | | | | | | | |
| | | | | | | | | |
| | | | | | | | | |
| | | | | | | | | |
| | | | | | | | | |
| | | | | | | | | |
| | | | | | | | | |
| | | | | | | | | |
| | | | | | | | | |

| DATE | NAME | DESCRIPTION | CHARGES | √ | CREDITS | | | CASH | CHK |
|------|------|-------------|---------|---|---------|---|---|------|-----|
| | | | | | PAYMENTS | ADJ. | | | |
| | | | | | | | | | |
| | | | | | | | | | |
| | | | | | | | | | |
| | | | | | | | | | |
| | | | | | | | | | |
| | | | | | | | | | |
| | | | | | | | | | |
| | | | | | | | | | |
| | | | | | | | | | |
| | | | | | | | | | |
| | | | | | | | | | |

2. Prepare ledger cards for the patients listed below. The additional names are of family members who would be listed on the separate account cards. After the account cards are prepared, post the three daily log days to the account cards. Be sure to itemize all charges under description column. Your instructor may provide you with account cards, or you may use the blank cards printed in this Workbook for completion of this assignment. If you use separate cards, they should always be in alphabetical order. _____

---

Boris Kostrevski - Mrs. June; Carol Sue
1493 S. James Road
(Your city and ZIP code)
$55.00 Balance brought forward

Patrick Moriarty - Mrs. Joan
397 North Tony Road
(Your city and ZIP code)
$38.00 Balance brought forward

George Schmidt - Mrs. Sue; Tina; Carol Susan
2349 E. Remington Road
(Your city and ZIP code)
$75.00 Balance brought forward

Juan Gomez
293 West High Street
(Your city and ZIP code)
$25.00 Balance brought forward

Patty and Geoff Segal - Susan
410 North Tony Road
(Your city and ZIP code)

LaChar Holley
4567 Charcoal Lane
(Your city and ZIP code)

If you would like more practice experience in completion of day sheets and account cards, your instructor has additional assignments in the Instructor's Manual.

## Form 1 (Segal, Patty)

Samuel E Matthews, M D
Suite 120
100 E Main Street
Yourtown  US  98765-4321
(654) 789-0123

Segal, Patty
410 North Tony Road
Anywhere, USA  00000

| DATE | DESCRIPTION | CHARGE | CREDITS | | CURRENT BALANCE |
|------|-------------|--------|---------|-----|-----------------|
| | | | PAYMENTS | ADL. | |
| | BALANCE FORWARD → | | | | |

PLEASE PAY LAST AMOUNT IN THIS COLUMN ←

276L

## Form 2 (Gomez, Juan)

Samuel E Matthews, M D
Suite 120
100 E Main Street
Yourtown  US  98765-4321
(654) 789-0123

Gomez, Juan
293 West High Street
Anywhere, USA  00000

| DATE | DESCRIPTION | CHARGE | CREDITS | | CURRENT BALANCE |
|------|-------------|--------|---------|-----|-----------------|
| | | | PAYMENTS | ADL. | |
| | BALANCE FORWARD → | | | | |

PLEASE PAY LAST AMOUNT IN THIS COLUMN ←

276L

**Samuel E Matthews, M D**
Suite 120
100 E Main Street
Yourtown US 98765-4321
(654) 789-0123

Moriarty, Joan
397 Tony Road
Anywhere, USA 00000

| DATE | DESCRIPTION | CHARGE | CREDITS | | CURRENT BALANCE |
| --- | --- | --- | --- | --- | --- |
| | | | PAYMENTS | ADJ. | |
| | BALANCE FORWARD → | | | | |
| | | | | | |

PLEASE PAY LAST AMOUNT IN THIS COLUMN ◄

276L

**Samuel E Matthews, M D**
Suite 120
100 E Main Street
Yourtown US 98765-4321
(654) 789-0123

Holley, LaChar
4567 Charcoal Lane
Anywhere, USA 00000

| DATE | DESCRIPTION | CHARGE | CREDITS | | CURRENT BALANCE |
| --- | --- | --- | --- | --- | --- |
| | | | PAYMENTS | ADJ. | |
| | BALANCE FORWARD → | | | | |
| | | | | | |

PLEASE PAY LAST AMOUNT IN THIS COLUMN ◄

276L

## Form 1 (Kostrevski)

Samuel E Matthews, M D
Suite 120
100 E Main Street
Yourtown  US  98765-4321
(654) 789-0123

Kostrevski, Carol Sue
1493 S. James Road
Anywhere, USA  00000

| DATE | DESCRIPTION | CHARGE | CREDITS | | CURRENT |
| | | | PAYMENTS | ADJ. | BALANCE |
|---|---|---|---|---|---|
| | BALANCE FORWARD | | | | |
| | | | | | |

PLEASE PAY LAST AMOUNT IN THIS COLUMN

276L

## Form 2 (Moriarty)

Samuel E Matthews, M D
Suite 120
100 E Main Street
Yourtown  US  98765-4321
(654) 789-0123

Moriarty, Patrick
397 North Tony Road
Anywhere, USA  00000

| DATE | DESCRIPTION | CHARGE | CREDITS | | CURRENT |
| | | | PAYMENTS | ADJ. | BALANCE |
|---|---|---|---|---|---|
| | BALANCE FORWARD | | | | |
| | | | | | |

PLEASE PAY LAST AMOUNT IN THIS COLUMN

276L

## Statement 1

Samuel E Matthews, M D
Suite 120
100 E Main Street
Yourtown US 98765-4321
(654) 789-0123

Kostrevski, June
1493 S. James Road
Anywhere, USA 00000

| DATE | DESCRIPTION | CHARGE | CREDITS |  | CURRENT BALANCE |
|------|-------------|--------|---------|---------|-----------------|
|      |             |        | PAYMENTS | ADL. |                 |
|      | BALANCE FORWARD | | | | |
|      |             |        |         |         |                 |
|      |             |        |         |         |                 |
|      |             |        |         |         |                 |
|      |             |        |         |         |                 |
|      |             |        |         |         |                 |
|      |             |        |         |         |                 |
|      |             |        |         |         |                 |
|      |             |        |         |         |                 |
|      |             |        |         |         |                 |
|      |             |        |         |         |                 |
|      |             |        |         |         |                 |
|      |             |        |         |         |                 |

PLEASE PAY LAST AMOUNT IN THIS COLUMN

276L.

## Statement 2

Samuel E Matthews, M D
Suite 120
100 E Main Street
Yourtown US 98765-4321
(654) 789-0123

Kostrevski, Boris
1493 S. James Road
Anywhere, USA 00000

| DATE | DESCRIPTION | CHARGE | CREDITS |  | CURRENT BALANCE |
|------|-------------|--------|---------|---------|-----------------|
|      |             |        | PAYMENTS | ADL. |                 |
|      | BALANCE FORWARD | | | | |
|      |             |        |         |         |                 |
|      |             |        |         |         |                 |
|      |             |        |         |         |                 |
|      |             |        |         |         |                 |
|      |             |        |         |         |                 |
|      |             |        |         |         |                 |
|      |             |        |         |         |                 |
|      |             |        |         |         |                 |
|      |             |        |         |         |                 |
|      |             |        |         |         |                 |
|      |             |        |         |         |                 |
|      |             |        |         |         |                 |

PLEASE PAY LAST AMOUNT IN THIS COLUMN

276L.

Samuel E Matthews, M D
Suite 120
100 E Main Street
Yourtown  US  98765-4321
(654) 789-0123

Schmidt, Sue
2349 E. Remington Road
Anywhere, USA  00000

| DATE | DESCRIPTION | CHARGE | CREDITS | | CURRENT |
| | | | PAYMENTS | ADL. | BALANCE |
|---|---|---|---|---|---|
| | BALANCE FORWARD ➡ | | | | |
| | | | | | |
| | | | | | |
| | | | | | |
| | | | | | |
| | | | | | |
| | | | | | |
| | | | | | |
| | | | | | |
| | | | | | |
| | | | | | |
| | | | | | |
| | | | | | |
| | | | | | |
| | | | | | |

PLEASE PAY LAST AMOUNT IN THIS COLUMN ⬅

276L.

---

Samuel E Matthews, M D
Suite 120
100 E Main Street
Yourtown  US  98765-4321
(654) 789-0123

Schmidt, George
2349 E. Remington Road
Anywhere, USA  00000

| DATE | DESCRIPTION | CHARGE | CREDITS | | CURRENT |
| | | | PAYMENTS | ADL. | BALANCE |
|---|---|---|---|---|---|
| | BALANCE FORWARD ➡ | | | | |
| | | | | | |
| | | | | | |
| | | | | | |
| | | | | | |
| | | | | | |
| | | | | | |
| | | | | | |
| | | | | | |
| | | | | | |
| | | | | | |
| | | | | | |
| | | | | | |
| | | | | | |
| | | | | | |

PLEASE PAY LAST AMOUNT IN THIS COLUMN ⬅

276L.

## Statement 1

**Samuel E Matthews, M D**
Suite 120
100 E Main Street
Yourtown US 98765-4321
(654) 789-0123

Schmidt, Tina
2349 E. Remington Road
Anywhere, USA 00000

| DATE | DESCRIPTION | CHARGE | CREDITS | | CURRENT BALANCE |
|------|-------------|--------|---------|-----|-----------------|
| | | | PAYMENTS | ADJ. | |
| | BALANCE FORWARD → | | | | |
| | | | | | |
| | | | | | |
| | | | | | |
| | | | | | |
| | | | | | |
| | | | | | |
| | | | | | |
| | | | | | |
| | | | | | |
| | | | | | |
| | | | | | |

276L
PLEASE PAY LAST AMOUNT IN THIS COLUMN ←

## Statement 2

**Samuel E Matthews, M D**
Suite 120
100 E Main Street
Yourtown US 98765-4321
(654) 789-0123

Schmidt, Carol Susan
2349 E. Remington Road
Anywhere, USA 00000

| DATE | DESCRIPTION | CHARGE | CREDITS | | CURRENT BALANCE |
|------|-------------|--------|---------|-----|-----------------|
| | | | PAYMENTS | ADL. | |
| | BALANCE FORWARD → | | | | |
| | | | | | |
| | | | | | |
| | | | | | |
| | | | | | |
| | | | | | |
| | | | | | |
| | | | | | |
| | | | | | |
| | | | | | |
| | | | | | |
| | | | | | |

276L
PLEASE PAY LAST AMOUNT IN THIS COLUMN ←

**Samuel E Matthews, M D**
Suite 120
100 E Main Street
Yourtown US 98765-4321
(654) 789-0123

Segal, Susan
410 North Tony Road
Anywhere, USA 00000

| DATE | DESCRIPTION | CHARGE | CREDITS PAYMENTS | CREDITS ADL. | CURRENT BALANCE |
|------|-------------|--------|----------|-----|------------------|
| | | BALANCE FORWARD → | | | |
| | | | | | |

PLEASE PAY LAST AMOUNT IN THIS COLUMN ←

276L

---

**Samuel E Matthews, M D**
Suite 120
100 E Main Street
Yourtown US 98765-4321
(654) 789-0123

Segal, Geoff
410 North Tony Road
Anywhere, USA 00000

| DATE | DESCRIPTION | CHARGE | CREDITS PAYMENTS | CREDITS ADL. | CURRENT BALANCE |
|------|-------------|--------|----------|-----|------------------|
| | | BALANCE FORWARD → | | | |
| | | | | | |

PLEASE PAY LAST AMOUNT IN THIS COLUMN ←

276L

**ASSIGNMENT SHEET**

**Chapter 8: COLLECTING FEES**

**Unit 4: COMPUTER BILLING**

**A. Brief Answer**

1. Describe the advantages of computerized billing. _____

_____

_____

_____

_____

_____

2. Describe different ways to locate an account in a computer system. _____

_____

_____

3. List reasons why billing statements would/should be withheld. _____

_____

_____

_____

4. Define *alpha search*. _____

_____

_____

**B. Multiple Choice: Place the correct letter on the blank line for each question.**

_____  1. A patient's account history is also referred to as a
      a. family history                 c. fee statement
      b. monthly summary          d. patient ledger

_____  2. A back-up file disk of all transactions ___ is necessary to keep billing records secure.
      a. often                    c. weekly
      b. daily                    d. monthly

_____  3. In computer terminology, a record of the information obtained for every patient is a(n)
      a. account history          c. charge slip
      b. insurance form          d. journal report

_____  4. _____ should be programmed into the computer along with their descriptions and the fees to be charged for each.
      a. ICD codes             c. CPT codes
      b. account numbers      d. insurance numbers

_____  5. A computer statement should show the portion of the amount due that is current,
      a. over 30 days          c. over 90 days
      b. over 60 days          d. all of these

**B. True or False:  Place a "T" for true or "F" for false in the space provided. For false statements, explain why they are false.**

_____  1. So that you don't have to ask patients to sign insurance forms each time they are seen, you can have them sign a form initially and keep it as a "signature on file."

_____  2. When the computer system accepts a number only, you must maintain a cross-reference file of an alphabetical listing of patients along with their account numbers.

_____  3. For an alpha search, the account number is entered in the computer to find the patient's ledger card.

After your instructor has returned your work to you, make all necessary corrections and place in a three-ring notebook for future reference.

**ASSIGNMENT SHEET**

**Chapter 8: COLLECTING FEES**

**Unit 5: COLLECTING OVERDUE PAYMENTS**

**SUGGESTED RESPONSES TO CRITICAL THINKING CHALLENGE IN TEXTBOOK**

1. Does there seem to be a lack of continuity and communication among the office personnel? _____

2. What should have been done about this? Whose fault was it? _____

   . _____

3. What should Clara have done when she realized the patient couldn't understand her? _____

   _____

4. Should the person who took care of the cash payment have alerted someone about having very little information about this lady? _____

   _____

5. What happens if the patient has a reaction to the medication? _____

   _____

6. Do you think this is a critical issue that should be discussed at a staff meeting? _____

7. What would you have done in this situation? _____

   _____

**A. Brief Answer**

1. Define *aging of accounts.* _____

   _____

2. How long are accounts ordinarily carried before being referred to a collection agency? _____

   _____

3. Should accounts automatically be referred to collection after the prescribed period of time? Why? _____

   _____

4. List the advantages of the use of telephone calls for account collection. _____

   _____

5. List conditions necessary when using the telephone for account collection.

   a. _____
   b. _____
   c. _____
   d. _____
   e. _____
   f. _____
   g. _____
   h. _____
   i. _____
   j. _____

6. Compose and type collection letters for the accounts of LaChar Holley, Juan Gomez, George Schmidt, and Boris Kostrevski. Use the examples in Figure 8-11 as a guide. If you use dates, be sure they compatible with the account cards you are using for a reference. Use a different form for each letter. Read typed letters.

7. Define *statute of limitations.* _____

   _____

   _____

**B. True or False: Place a "T" for true or "F" for false in the space provided. For false statements, explain why they are false.**

_____ 1. Making idle threats can encourage patients to pay their bill.

_____ 2. The process of computer analysis of accounts receivable is known as aging of accounts.

_____ 3. If you make collection calls early in the morning or late at night, you can be held liable for harassment.

_____ 4. You should have a reminder file to help you follow up on promises to pay.

**SAMUEL E. MATTHEWS, MD**
**SUITE 120**
**100 E. MAIN STREET**
**YOURTOWN, US 98765-4321**
**(654) 789-0123**

**SAMUEL E. MATTHEWS, MD**
**SUITE 120**
**100 E. MAIN STREET**
**YOURTOWN, US 98765-4321**
**(654) 789-0123**

**SAMUEL E. MATTHEWS, MD**
**SUITE 120**
**100 E. MAIN STREET**
**YOURTOWN, US 98765-4321**
**(654) 789-0123**

**SAMUEL E. MATTHEWS, MD**
**SUITE 120**
**100 E. MAIN STREET**
**YOURTOWN, US 98765-4321**
**(654) 789-0123**

## ACHIEVING SKILL COMPETENCY

Reread the performance objective for each procedure and then practice the skills listed below, following the procedure in your textbook.

Procedure 8-1: Prepare Patient Ledger Card
Procedure 8-2: Record Charges and Credits
Procedure 8-3: Generate Itemized Statement
Procedure 8-4: Compose Collection Letter

When you feel you have mastered the performance of the skill, sign your name on the appropriate evaluation sheet and give it to your instructor to indicate you are prepared to perform the procedure for evaluation.

After your instructor has returned your work to you, make all necessary corrections and place in a three-ring notebook for future reference.

**ASSIGNMENT SHEET**

**Chapter 9: HEALTH CARE COVERAGE**

   Review the objectives and text for each unit before completing the assignment sheet for that unit. When you have completed all sheets for the chapter, remove them from this Workbook and give them to the instructor for evaluation.

**Unit 1: FUNDAMENTALS OF MANAGED CARE**

**A. Brief Answer**

   1. What type of medical insurance has created competition in the insurance industry? _____

   2. Why are HMOs so popular? _____

   3. How did the phrase *managed care* originate? _____

   4. What is generally the cost of health care to employees whose employer offers an HMO as part of their benefit package? _____

   5. Describe managed care today. _____

   6. What is the initial purpose of the HMO? _____

   7. What are the two major types of health insurance? _____

   8. In regard to health insurance coverage, how can the medical assistant be helpful to patients? _____

   9. Where can patients find the names of physicians who participate in their HMO? _____

   10. Describe a helpful practice that should be performed at the beginning of each office visit regarding the patient's insurance card. _____

   11. List the four conditions of the birthday rule in regard to insurance coverage. _____

   12. What is critical to ensure successful reimbursement for medical services rendered to patients? _____

Name _____

13. List the subject areas the medical assistant must be knowledgeable about to process medical claims forms and explain why they are important. _____

_____

14. Refer to the CAAHEP Standards in Appendix B of the textbook. Within the area of *Medical Assisting Administrative Procedures,* which curriculum standard is discussed in this unit? _____

_____

## B. Matching: Match the definition in column II with the correct term in column I.

COLUMN I

_____ 1. Attending physician
_____ 2. Signed authorization
_____ 3. Advance directives
_____ 4. Admitting physician
_____ 5. Capitation
_____ 6. Balance billing
_____ 7. Assignment of benefits
_____ 8. Accounts receivable
_____ 9. Claim

COLUMN II

a. Fixed amount paid to physician per month
b. Physician who admits patient to hospital
c. Total charges that have not been paid
d. Patient authorizes payment directly to the physician
e. Physician who cares for patient in hospital
f. Authorization to release medical information
g. Also known as a living will
h. Charges insurance did not pay
i. Request for insurance company payment

## C. Fill in the Blank

1. _____ was established to aid personnel and dependents of the armed services with medical expenses.

2. _____ was established for disabled veterans, their spouses, and their dependents to aid with medical expenses.

3. A predetermined amount that the insured must pay before the insurance company pays is called the _____

4. A printed description of the benefits provided by the insurer to the beneficiary is known as the _____

5. _____ is the term given to the primary care physician for coordinating the patient's care to specialists, hospital admissions, and so on.

6. A specific amount that the insured must pay toward the charge for professional services rendered is called

7. The _____ is the one who writes his or her signature on the back of a check that is made out to him or her.

8. A list of approved professional services for which the insurance company will pay along with the maximum fee is called a _____

9. A _____ is a printed form that has patient information and a listing of the services and code numbers with the total charges.

10. A program that provides complete health care for children and encourages early detection of health problems is known as _____

11. _____ is a system of medical team members organized into groups to provide quality and cost-effective care that encompasses both the delivery of health care and the payment of services

**D. Word Search:** **Provide the term for each definition below. Then find the terms and the words in italics hidden in the puzzle. (Abbreviations may be used.)**

1. Standard claims *form* of the *Health* Care Finance Administration to submit for third-*party* payment. _____

2. A joint funding program by the federal and by state governments (but not Arizona) for those on public assistance for medical *care.* _____

3. Private *insurance* to supplement Medicare benefits for non-covered services. _____

4. A *group* of physicians who continue to practice independently in their own offices. _____

5. Coding system used to *document* diseases, injuries, illnesses, and modalities. _____

6. Non-profit organization created to improve patient care *quality* and health plan performance. _____

7. Another name for *encounter* form. _____

8. Transferring words into numbers to facilitate use of *computers* in claims processing. _____

9. Moneys paid for an insurance *contract.* _____

10. *Fee* schedule based on relative *value* of resources that physicians spend to provide services to Medicare patients. _____

11. The person who has been insured; insurance *policy* holder. _____

12. Prior authorization must be obtained before the patient is admitted to the hospital or receives some specified outpatient or in-office *procedures.* _____

```
V A L U E R M I N S U R A N C E
E R A C I D E M N C Z A U C O D
R A M I F I D A C O A T I E N T
B O C A R E I D Q D H E A L T H
R W O R A H C F A I 5 0 0 L R D
V S M M C H A J P N S W X L A T
S U P E R B I L L G Y B P F C J
P B U D I C D 9 C M F O R M T Q
O S T I F E N C O U N T E R E U
L C E F E E G P R T F A M I P A
I R R I P A R T Y S X D I K U L
C I S L N C O G J X K O U Z M I
Y B M L B T U X D O C U M E N T
M E D I G A P R O C E D U R E Y
P R E C E R T I F I C A T I O N
```

**E. True or False:** **Place a "T" for true or "F" for false in the space provided. For false statements, explain why they are false.**

_____ 1. An indemnity plan is a company that bills the physician for medical services.

_____ 2. The Medicare fee schedule is a list of approved professional services that includes the maximum fee that Medicare will pay for each service.

_____ 3. A preexisting condition is a condition that existed before the insured's policy was issued.

_____ 4. A contract is an agreement between two or more parties for certain services or obligations to be discussed.

_____ 5. For patients who are minors or who are incompetent, a guardian must sign for any release of information and for any services to be completed.

_____ 6. Utilization management refers to a panel that keeps track of what services were ordered and checks if medical care was completed.

_____ 7. The usual fee is the charge that physicians make for services for their private patients.

_____ 8. A skilled nursing facility is a medical facility licensed primarily to provide skilled nursing care to patients ordered by workers' compensation.

After your instructor has returned your work to you, make all necessary corrections and place in a three-ring notebook for future reference.

## ASSIGNMENT SHEET

**Chapter 9: HEALTH CARE COVERAGE**

**Unit 2: HEALTH CARE PLANS**

### A. Brief Answer

1. What is significant regarding premiums and benefits of private commercial insurance companies?

   _____

2. Why was Blue Cross health insurance originally set up?

   _____

3. What coverage does Blue Cross now include besides hospital expenses?

   _____

4. Name the additional plans Blue Cross Blue Shield offer today.

   _____

5. What do indemnity plans require of the patient regarding payments?

   _____

6. What is the usual co-payment required of patients who have an HMO plan?

   _____

7. List the available types of HMOs and briefly describe each of them.

   a. _____
   b. _____
   c. _____
   d. _____

   _____

8. What are the responsibilities of the NCQA?

   _____

9. Refer to the CAAHEP Standards in Appendix B of the textbook. Within the area of *Medical Assisting Administrative Procedures,* which role relates to the content of this unit? _____

10. In October 2001, what four changes were made to help inform Medicare recipients? _____

    _____

    _____

### B. Fill in the Blank: For each plan below, identify if it is considered private or government by placing a "P" or "G" in the space provided.

_____ 1. Foundations for medical care

_____ 2. Medicare

_____ 3. Blue Shield

_____ 4. TRICARE (CHAMPUS)

_____ 5. Workers' compensation

_____ 6. Blue Cross

_____ 7. Easter Seal Rehabilitation Centers

_____ 8. Medicaid

_____ 9. Commercial health insurance

_____ 10. Health maintenance organizations

## C. Fill in the Blank

1. To qualify as a(n) _____ an organization must present proof of its ability to provide comprehensive health care.

2. One of the four levels of NCQA accreditation is full accreditation given for _____ indicating excellent performance.

3. The primary care physician is also referred to as _____

4. HMOs mail _____ to the provider's office to keep the office apprised of policy changes between representatives' visits.

5. Besides the four principal types of state benefits, workers' compensation also includes _____ _____ for severely disabled employees.

6. Patients who have had an industrial injury should have a _____ and a separate account card for that injury.

7. One common reason for delay in payment of claims is that they are _____

8. Medicare B is the coverage that pays for _____

9. Physicians who choose not to be participating providers must collect _____ _____ for the services rendered.

10. If the physician provides a non-covered service for a Medicare patient, an _____ must be signed by the patient.

11. There is a special _____ on the HCFA-1500 form that allows the claims processor to assign a unique identification number to the claim during microfilming.

12. In processing Medicare forms, use ICDA codes for _____ CPT codes for _____ and HCPCS codes for _____

## D. True or False: Place a "T" for true or "F" for false in the space provided. For false statements, explain why they are false.

_____ 1. TRICARE (CHAMPUS) covers all military personnel.

_____ 2. Medicare encourages all providers to file claims electronically.

_____ 3. The NPI (National Provider Identification) is used in blocks 24k and 33 of the HCFA-1500 to identify the location of the service.

_____ 4. Ideally, all insurance forms should be signed and dated by the patient.

_____ 5. The only time a patient's signature is not necessary is when you have been given verbal permission from that patient to release information.

_____ 6. Claims will be returned to the provider if the NPI number is missing from the HCFA form.

_____ 7. Medicare Part B patients usually are responsible for the first $100 of covered services.

_____ 8. For Medicaid patients, a general rule is that prior authorization is necessary to provide medical treatment except in an emergency.

_____ 9. Workers' compensation requires that a patient have reevaluations at intervals with her or his physician, who must promptly give a supplemental report regarding the patient's condition.

After your instructor has returned your work to you, make all necessary corrections and place in a three-ring notebook for future reference.

**ASSIGNMENT SHEET**

**Chapter 9: HEALTH CARE COVERAGE**

**Unit 3: PREPARING CLAIMS**

**SUGGESTED RESPONSES TO CRITICAL THINKING CHALLENGE IN TEXTBOOK**

1. What should Maria do? _____

_____

_____

_____

2. Is she liable for filing fraudulent insurance claims when in reality she just enters what the physician has
   indicated? _____

   _____

3. There is a phone number to report Medicare fraud (800-447-8477). Should she call and report her suspicion?

   _____

4. What do you think would be the ramifications if she approaches the physician with her observations? _____

   _____

   _____

5. Because this position is so perfect for her and she is paid well, should she just overlook the occasional
   irregularities? After all, physicians are only allowed to charge so much for services, and they need to add a
   little to help make up the difference. _____

   _____

6. Do you think it is possible that the physician realizes her personal situation and might take advantage of her
   loyalty? _____

   _____

   _____

**ANSWERS TO WORKBOOK ASSIGNMENT**

**Mixed Quiz**

1. What does the phrase *third-party reimbursement* mean? _____

   _____

2. Why were claim forms developed? _____

   _____

3. When did the first attempt at classifying the causes of deaths occur? _____

4. What significant event occurred in 1938? _____

   _____

   _____

5. Fill in the blank

   Coding is, in reality, the _____ of _____ or _____ of

   _____ or _____ into _____ to _____

   _____ which can be _____ into _____ and _____

   _____

6. List three reasons why coding is beneficial.

   a. _____
   _____
   _____

   b. _____

   c. _____
   _____

7. What change occurred with the Catastrophic Coverage Act of 1988? _____

8. What does *sequencing* mean? _____

9. What is the main rule to remember when coding, and what does it mean? _____

10. Look at a copy of an approved HCFA-1500 insurance form. Where would you enter the following information?

   _____ A. Health care coverage being billed
   _____ B. Patient's name
   _____ C. Insured's name
   _____ D. Patient's condition is result of employment
   _____ E. Name of insured's employer
   _____ F. Indicate there is another health plan
   _____ G. Have patient sign
   _____ H. Dates patient unable to work
   _____ I. Diagnosis codes
   _____ J. Procedure codes
   _____ K. Physician's tax ID number
   _____ L. Assignment acceptance
   _____ M. Physician's signature

11. Complete the five insurance forms provided using the following information: Code 11, office, for places of service: (24B) The physician is Samuel E. Matthews, MD, Suite 120, 100 E. Main Street, Yourtown, US 98765-4321. His SS# is 987654321. Phone 654-789-0123. PIN 7654321. The patients all live in Yourtown, US.

   a. Juan Gomez, 293 West High Street 98765

      Medicare. Phone 263-5538. BD 2/17/21. Male. SS# 291166966-A. Patient is insured person. Other insurance BC, BS #2911669660; signature on file. Abdominal pain and diabetes mellitus. (Consult this unit for code numbers. Consult code book for code numbers needed for procedures.) Seen in office.

      5/18/___   Office visit, intermediate 30.00
                    Test feces for blood     15.00
                    Automated hemogram   10.00
                    Blood drawing   5.00

   b. LaChar Holley, 4567 Charcoal Lane 98765

      Travelers Insurance. Phone 122-7768. BD 10/7/60. Female. SS# 505209821. Patient is insured person. No other insurance. Not related to employment or accident. Signature on file. Arthritis, acute back pain. Seen in office.

      6/15/___   Office visit, intermediate 30.00
                    X ray lumbar spine, AP & lateral  118.00
                    Blood drawing   5.00
                    Automated hemogram   10.00

c.  Tina Schmidt, daughter. BD 12/27/90. Phone 891-7145. Insured George Schmidt, 1249 E. Remington Road 98769. Self-employed. BC and BS Insurance. SS# of insured 888207777. BD 10/6/49. No other insurance. Phone 441-0050. Signature on file. Impetigo. Seen in office.

6/20/__    Office visit, limited          27.00

d.  Joan Moriarty, wife. BD 12/19/62. Insured Patrick Moriarty, 397-½ North Tony Road 98768. Self-employed. Metropolitan-Insurance. SS# of insured 887105566. BD 11/14/60. Phone 431-6943. No other insurance. Signature on file. Cervicitis, cystitis, acute edema. Patient seen in office.

9/20/__    Office visit, extended        46.00
            Catheterization, urethra  20.00
            Endometrial biopsy        125.00
            Urinalysis          10.00

e.  Boris Kostrevski, 1493 S. James Road 98765. Medicare and Aetna Insurance. SS# of insured 505208800-A. BD 7/14/22. Phone 298-6483. Signature on file. Diabetes mellitus, coronary atherosclerosis. Seen in office.

6/20/__    Office visit, intermediate 30.00
            Assay blood fluid, glucose        10.00
            Blood drawing    5.00

12. Refer to ABHES Course Content Requirements in Appendix C of the textbook. Within the area of *Medical Office Business Procedures/Management,* which content requirement is discussed in this unit?

_____

# HEALTH INSURANCE CLAIM FORM

APPROVED OMB-0938-0008

PICA                                                                 PICA

| 1. ☐ MEDICARE (Medicare #) ☐ MEDICAID (Medicaid #) ☐ CHAMPUS (Sponsor's SSN) ☐ CHAMPVA (VA File #) ☐ GROUP HEALTH PLAN (SSN or ID) ☐ FECA BLK LUNG (SSN) ☐ OTHER (ID) | 1a. INSURED'S I.D. NUMBER (FOR PROGRAM IN ITEM 1) |

| 2. PATIENT'S NAME (Last Name, First Name, Middle Initial) | 3. PATIENT'S BIRTH DATE MM ¦ DD ¦ YY   SEX M☐ F☐ | 4. INSURED'S NAME (Last Name, Firts Name, Middle Initial) |

| 5. PATIENT'S ADDRESS (No., Street) | 6. PATIENT RELATIONSHIP TO INSURED ☐Self ☐Spouse ☐Child ☐Other | 7. INSURED'S ADDRESS (No., Street) |

| CITY | STATE | 8. PATIENT STATUS ☐Single ☐Married ☐Other | CITY | STATE |

| ZIP CODE | TELEPHONE (Include Area Code) ( ) | Employed ☐ Full-Time Student ☐ Part-Time Student ☐ | ZIP CODE | TELEPHONE (Include Area Code) ( ) |

| 9. OTHER INSURED'S NAME (Last Name, First Name, Middle Initial) | 10. IS PATIENT'S CONDITION RELATED TO: | 11. INSURED'S POLICY GROUP OR FECA NUMBER |

| a. OTHER INSURED'S POLICY OR GROUP NUMBER | a. EMPLOYMENT? (CURRENT OR PREVIOUS) ☐YES ☐NO | a. INSURED'S DATE OF BIRTH MM ¦ DD ¦ YY   SEX M☐ F☐ |

| b. OTHER INSURED'S DATE OF BIRTH MM ¦ DD ¦ YY   SEX M☐ F☐ | b. AUTO ACCIDENT?   PLACE (State) ☐YES ☐NO | b. EMPLOYER'S NAME OR SCHOOL NAME |

| c. EMPLOYER'S NAME OR SCHOOL NAME | c. OTHER ACCIDENT? ☐YES ☐NO | c. INSURANCE PLAN NAME OR PROGRAM NAME |

| d. INSURANCE PLAN NAME OR PROGRAM NAME | d. RESERVED FOR LOCAL USE | d. IS THERE ANOTHER HEALTH BENEFIT PLAN? ☐YES ☐NO If yes, return to and complete item 9 a-d. |

**READ BACK OF FORM BEFORE COMPLETING & SIGNING THIS FORM.**

12. PATIENT'S OR AUTHORIZED PERSON'S SIGNATURE I authorize the release of any medical or other information necessary to process this claim. I also request payment of government benefits either to myself or to the party who accepts assignments below.

SIGNED_____  DATE_____

13. INSURED'S OR AUTHORIZED PERSON'S SIGNATURE I authorize payment of medical benefits to the undersigned physician or supplier for services described below.

SIGNED_____

| 14. DATE OF CURRENT: MM ¦ DD ¦ YY  ILLNESS (First sympton) OR INJURY (Accident)OR PREGNANCY (LMP) | 15. IF PATIENT HAS HAD SAME OR SIMILAR ILLNESS. GIVE FIRST DATE MM ¦ DD ¦ YY | 16. DATES PATIENT UNABLE TO WORK IN CURRENT OCCUPATION MM ¦ DD ¦ YY    MM ¦ DD ¦ YY FROM          TO |

| 17. NAME OR REFERRING PHYSICIAN OR OTHER SOURCE | 17a. I.D. NUMBER OF REFERRING PHYSICIAN | 18. HOSPITALIZATION DATES RELATED TO CURRENT SERVICES MM ¦ DD ¦ YY    MM ¦ DD ¦ YY FROM          TO |

| 19. RESERVED FOR LOCAL USE | 20. OUTSIDE LAB? ☐YES ☐NO   $ CHARGES |

| 21. DIAGNOSIS OR NATURE OF ILLNESS OR INJURY. (RELATE ITEMS 1,2,3 OR 4 TO ITEM 24E BY LINE) 1.|_____.____   3.|_____.____   2.|_____.____   4.|_____.____ | 22. MEDICAID RESUBMISSION CODE    ORIGINAL REF. NO. 23. PRIOR AUTHORIZATION NUMBER |

| 24. | A | | | | B | C | D | | E | F | G | H | I | J | K |
|---|---|---|---|---|---|---|---|---|---|---|---|---|---|---|---|
| | DATE(S) OF SERVICE From | | | To | Place of Service | Type of Service | PROCEDURES, SERVICES, OR SUPPLIES (Explain Unusual Circumstances) | | DIAGNOSIS CODE | $ CHARGES | DAYS OR UNITS | EPSDT Family Plan | EMG | COB | RESERVED FOR LOCAL USE |
| | MM DD YY | | MM | DD YY | | | CPT/HCPCS | MODIFIER | | | | | | | |
| 1 | | | | | | | | | | | | | | | |
| 2 | | | | | | | | | | | | | | | |
| 3 | | | | | | | | | | | | | | | |
| 4 | | | | | | | | | | | | | | | |
| 5 | | | | | | | | | | | | | | | |
| 6 | | | | | | | | | | | | | | | |

| 25. FEDERAL TAX I.D. NUMBER   SSN EIN ☐ ☐ | 26. PATIENT'S ACCOUNT NO. | 27. ACCEPT ASSIGNMENT? (For govt. claims, see back) ☐YES ☐NO | 28. TOTAL CHARGE $ | 29. AMOUNT PAID $ | 30. BALANCE DUE $ |

| 31. SIGNATURE OF PHYSICIAN OR SUPPLIER INCLUDING DEGREES OR CREDENTIALS (I certify that the statements on the reverse apply to this bill and are made a part thereof.) SIGNED _____ DATE _____ | 32. NAME AND ADDRESS OF FACULTY WHERE SERVICES WERE RENDERED (If other than home or office) | 33. PHYSICIAN'S, SUPPLIER'S BILLING NAME, ADDRESS, ZIP CODE & PHONE# PIN #              GRP # |

(APPROVED BY AMA COUNCIL ON MEDICAL SERVICE 8/88)   *PLEASE PRINT OR TYPE*

FORM HCFA-1500 (U2) (12-90)
FORM OWCP -1500        FORM RRB-1500

CARRIER
PATIENT AND INSURED INFORMATION
PHYSICIAN OR SUPPLIER INFORMATION

PLEASE
DO NOT
STAPLE
IN THIS
AREA

APPROVED OMB-0938-0008

**HEALTH INSURANCE CLAIM FORM**

PICA                                               PICA

1. MEDICARE   MEDICAID   CHAMPUS   CHAMPVA   GROUP HEALTH PLAN   FECA BLK LUNG   OTHER     1a. INSURED'S I.D. NUMBER   (FOR PROGRAM IN ITEM 1)

☐ (Medicare #)  ☐ (Medicaid #)  ☐ (Sponsor's SSN)  ☐ (VA File #)  ☐ (SSN or ID)  ☐ (SSN)  ☐ (ID)

2. PATIENT'S NAME (Last Name, First Name, Middle Initial)

3. PATIENT'S BIRTH DATE   SEX   MM  DD  YY   M ☐  F ☐

4. INSURED'S NAME (Last Name, Firts Name, Middle Initial)

5. PATIENT'S ADDRESS (No., Street)

6. PATIENT RELATIONSHIP TO INSURED   ☐ Self  ☐ Spouse  ☐ Child  ☐ Other

7. INSURED'S ADDRESS (No., Street)

CITY     STATE

8. PATIENT STATUS   ☐ Single  ☐ Married  ☐ Other

CITY     STATE

ZIP CODE   TELEPHONE (Include Area Code)  ( )

Employed ☐  Full-Time Student ☐  Part-Time Student ☐

ZIP CODE   TELEPHONE (Include Area Code)  ( )

9. OTHER INSURED'S NAME (Last Name, First Name, Middle Initial)

10. IS PATIENT'S CONDITION RELATED TO:

11. INSURED'S POLICY GROUP OR FECA NUMBER

a. OTHER INSURED'S POLICY OR GROUP NUMBER

a. EMPLOYMENT? (CURRENT OR PREVIOUS)  ☐ YES  ☐ NO

a. INSURED'S DATE OF BIRTH   SEX   MM  DD  YY   M ☐  F ☐

b. OTHER INSURED'S DATE OF BIRTH   SEX   MM  DD  YY   M ☐  F ☐

b. AUTO ACCIDENT?   PLACE (State)  ☐ YES  ☐ NO

b. EMPLOYER'S NAME OR SCHOOL NAME

c. EMPLOYER'S NAME OR SCHOOL NAME

c. OTHER ACCIDENT?  ☐ YES  ☐ NO

c. INSURANCE PLAN NAME OR PROGRAM NAME

d. INSURANCE PLAN NAME OR PROGRAM NAME

d. RESERVED FOR LOCAL USE

d. IS THERE ANOTHER HEALTH BENEFIT PLAN?  ☐ YES  ☐ NO  If yes, return to and complete item 9 a-d.

**READ BACK OF FORM BEFORE COMPLETING & SIGNING THIS FORM.**

12. PATIENT'S OR AUTHORIZED PERSON'S SIGNATURE I authorize the release of any medical or other information necessary to process this claim. I also request payment of government benefits either to myself or to the party who accepts assignments below.

13. INSURED'S OR AUTHORIZED PERSON'S SIGNATURE I authorize payment of medical benefits to the undersigned physician or supplier for services described below.

SIGNED_____   DATE_____

SIGNED_____

14. DATE OF CURRENT:  MM  DD  YY   ◄ ILLNESS (First sympton) OR INJURY (Accident)OR PREGNANCY (LMP)

15. IF PATIENT HAS HAD SAME OR SIMILAR ILLNESS. GIVE FIRST DATE  MM  DD  YY

16. DATES PATIENT UNABLE TO WORK IN CURRENT OCCUPATION  MM  DD  YY   MM  DD  YY   FROM   TO

17. NAME OR REFERRING PHYSICIAN OR OTHER SOURCE

17a. I.D. NUMBER OF REFERRING PHYSICIAN

18. HOSPITALIZATION DATES RELATED TO CURRENT SERVICES  MM  DD  YY   MM  DD  YY   FROM   TO

19. RESERVED FOR LOCAL USE

20. OUTSIDE LAB?  ☐ YES  ☐ NO   $ CHARGES

21. DIAGNOSIS OR NATURE OF ILLNESS OR INJURY. (RELATE ITEMS 1,2,3 OR 4 TO ITEM 24E BY LINE)

1.l_____.___     3. l_____.___

2.l_____.___     4. l_____.___

22. MEDICAID RESUBMISSION CODE   ORIGINAL REF. NO.

23. PRIOR AUTHORIZATION NUMBER

| 24. A DATE(S) OF SERVICE | | | | | B Place of Service | C Type of Service | D PROCEDURES, SERVICES, OR SUPPLIES (Explain Unusual Circumstances) | | E DIAGNOSIS CODE | F $ CHARGES | G DAYS OR UNITS | H EPSDT Family Plan | I EMG | J COB | K RESERVED FOR LOCAL USE |
|---|---|---|---|---|---|---|---|---|---|---|---|---|---|---|---|
| From MM | DD | YY | To MM | DD YY | | | CPT/HCPCS | MODIFIER | | | | | | | |
| 1 | | | | | | | | | | | | | | | |
| 2 | | | | | | | | | | | | | | | |
| 3 | | | | | | | | | | | | | | | |
| 4 | | | | | | | | | | | | | | | |
| 5 | | | | | | | | | | | | | | | |
| 6 | | | | | | | | | | | | | | | |

25. FEDERAL TAX I.D. NUMBER   SSN ☐ EIN ☐

26. PATIENT'S ACCOUNT NO.

27. ACCEPT ASSIGNMENT? (For govt. claims, see back)  ☐ YES  ☐ NO

28. TOTAL CHARGE  $

29. AMOUNT PAID  $

30. BALANCE DUE  $

31. SIGNATURE OF PHYSICIAN OR SUPPLIER INCLUDING DEGREES OR CREDENTIALS (I certify that the statements on the reverse apply to this bill and are made a part thereof.)

SIGNED _____ DATE _____

32. NAME AND ADDRESS OF FACULTY WHERE SERVICES WERE RENDERED (If other than home or office)

33. PHYSICIAN'S, SUPPLIER'S BILLING NAME, ADDRESS, ZIP CODE & PHONE#

PIN #     GRP #

(APPROVED BY AMA COUNCIL ON MEDICAL SERVICE 8/88)   *PLEASE PRINT OR TYPE*   FORM HCFA-1500 (U2) (12-90)   FORM OWCP -1500   FORM RRB-1500

CARRIER ►   PATIENT AND INSURED INFORMATION   PHYSICIAN OR SUPPLIER INFORMATION

PLEASE
DO NOT
STAPLE
IN THIS
AREA

APPROVED OMB-0938-0008

PICA

# HEALTH INSURANCE CLAIM FORM

PICA

1. MEDICARE     MEDICAID     CHAMPUS     CHAMPVA     GROUP          FECA          OTHER
                                                     HEALTH PLAN    BLK LUNG
   ☐(Medicare #) ☐(Medicaid #) ☐(Sponsor's SSN) ☐(VA File #) ☐(SSN or ID) ☐(SSN) ☐(ID)

1a. INSURED'S I.D. NUMBER          (FOR PROGRAM IN ITEM 1)

2. PATIENT'S NAME (Last Name, First Name, Middle Initial)

3. PATIENT'S BIRTH DATE          SEX
   MM    DD    YY          M ☐    F ☐

4. INSURED'S NAME (Last Name, Firts Name, Middle Initial)

5. PATIENT'S ADDRESS (No., Street)

6. PATIENT RELATIONSHIP TO INSURED
   ☐ Self  ☐ Spouse  ☐ Child  ☐ Other

7. INSURED'S ADDRESS (No., Street)

CITY                          STATE

8. PATIENT STATUS
   ☐ Single    ☐ Married    ☐ Other

CITY                          STATE

ZIP CODE          TELEPHONE (Include Area Code)
                  (    )

Employed ☐  Full-Time ☐  Part-Time ☐
            Student      Student

ZIP CODE          TELEPHONE (Include Area Code)
                  (    )

9. OTHER INSURED'S NAME (Last Name, First Name, Middle Initial)

10. IS PATIENT'S CONDITION RELATED TO:

11. INSURED'S POLICY GROUP OR FECA NUMBER

a. OTHER INSURED'S POLICY OR GROUP NUMBER

a. EMPLOYMENT? (CURRENT OR PREVIOUS)
   ☐ YES          ☐ NO

a. INSURED'S DATE OF BIRTH          SEX
   MM    DD    YY          M ☐    F ☐

b. OTHER INSURED'S DATE OF BIRTH          SEX
   MM    DD    YY          M ☐    F ☐

b. AUTO ACCIDENT?          PLACE (State)
   ☐ YES          ☐ NO

b. EMPLOYER'S NAME OR SCHOOL NAME

c. EMPLOYER'S NAME OR SCHOOL NAME

c. OTHER ACCIDENT?
   ☐ YES          ☐ NO

c. INSURANCE PLAN NAME OR PROGRAM NAME

d. INSURANCE PLAN NAME OR PROGRAM NAME

d. RESERVED FOR LOCAL USE

d. IS THERE ANOTHER HEALTH BENEFIT PLAN?
   ☐ YES          ☐ NO  If yes, return to and complete item 9 a-d.

**READ BACK OF FORM BEFORE COMPLETING & SIGNING THIS FORM.**

12. PATIENT'S OR AUTHORIZED PERSON'S SIGNATURE I authorize the release of any medical or other information necessary to process this claim. I also request payment of government benefits either to myself or to the party who accepts assignments below.

13. INSURED'S OR AUTHORIZED PERSON'S SIGNATURE I authorize payment of medical benefits to the undersigned physician or supplier for services described below.

SIGNED_____     DATE_____

SIGNED_____

14. DATE OF CURRENT:          ILLNESS (First sympton) OR
    MM    DD    YY            INJURY (Accident)OR
                             PREGNANCY (LMP)

15. IF PATIENT HAS HAD SAME OR SIMILAR ILLNESS.
    GIVE FIRST DATE     MM    DD    YY

16. DATES PATIENT UNABLE TO WORK IN CURRENT OCCUPATION
    MM    DD    YY          MM    DD    YY
    FROM                TO

17. NAME OR REFERRING PHYSICIAN OR OTHER SOURCE

17a. I.D. NUMBER OF REFERRING PHYSICIAN

18. HOSPITALIZATION DATES RELATED TO CURRENT SERVICES
    MM    DD    YY          MM    DD    YY
    FROM                TO

19. RESERVED FOR LOCAL USE

20. OUTSIDE LAB?          $ CHARGES
    ☐ YES  ☐ NO

21. DIAGNOSIS OR NATURE OF ILLNESS OR INJURY. (RELATE ITEMS 1,2,3 OR 4 TO ITEM 24E BY LINE)

1.I_____.____          3. I_____.____

2.I_____.____          4. I_____.____

22. MEDICAID RESUBMISSION
    CODE          ORIGINAL REF. NO.

23. PRIOR AUTHORIZATION NUMBER

| 24. | A | | | | | B | C | D | | | E | F | G | H | I | J | K |
|---|---|---|---|---|---|---|---|---|---|---|---|---|---|---|---|---|---|
| | DATE(S) OF SERVICE | | | | | Place | Type | PROCEDURES, SERVICES, OR SUPPLIES | | | | | DAYS | EPSDT | | | RESERVED FOR |
| | From | | | To | | of | of | (Explain Unusual Circumstances) | | | DIAGNOSIS | | OR | Family | | | LOCAL USE |
| | MM | DD | YY | MM | DD | YY | Service | Service | CPT/HCPCS | | MODIFIER | CODE | $ CHARGES | UNITS | Plan | EMG | COB | |
| 1 | | | | | | | | | | | | | | | | | | |
| 2 | | | | | | | | | | | | | | | | | | |
| 3 | | | | | | | | | | | | | | | | | | |
| 4 | | | | | | | | | | | | | | | | | | |
| 5 | | | | | | | | | | | | | | | | | | |
| 6 | | | | | | | | | | | | | | | | | | |

25. FEDERAL TAX I.D. NUMBER     SSN EIN
                                ☐     ☐

26. PATIENT'S ACCOUNT NO.

27. ACCEPT ASSIGNMENT?
    (For govt. claims, see back)
    ☐ YES  ☐ NO

28. TOTAL CHARGE
    $

29. AMOUNT PAID
    $

30. BALANCE DUE
    $

31. SIGNATURE OF PHYSICIAN OR SUPPLIER INCLUDING DEGREES OR CREDENTIALS
(I certify that the statements on the reverse apply to this bill and are made a part thereof.)

32. NAME AND ADDRESS OF FACULTY WHERE SERVICES WERE RENDERED (If other than home or office)

33. PHYSICIAN'S, SUPPLIER'S BILLING NAME, ADDRESS, ZIP CODE & PHONE#

SIGNED _____ DATE ____

PIN #          GRP #

(APPROVED BY AMA COUNCIL ON MEDICAL SERVICE 8/88)          ***PLEASE PRINT OR TYPE***

FORM HCFA-1500 (U2) (12-90)
FORM OWCP -1500          FORM RRB-1500

**PLEASE DO NOT STAPLE IN THIS AREA**

APPROVED OMB-0938-0008

PICA

# HEALTH INSURANCE CLAIM FORM

PICA

| 1. MEDICARE | MEDICAID | CHAMPUS | CHAMPVA | GROUP HEALTH PLAN | FECA BLK LUNG | OTHER | 1a. INSURED'S I.D. NUMBER | (FOR PROGRAM IN ITEM 1) |
|---|---|---|---|---|---|---|---|---|
| ☐ (Medicare #) | ☐ (Medicaid #) | ☐ (Sponsor's SSN) | ☐ (VA File #) | ☐ (SSN or ID) | ☐ (SSN) | ☐ (ID) | | |

2. PATIENT'S NAME (Last Name, First Name, Middle Initial)

3. PATIENT'S BIRTH DATE   MM | DD | YY   SEX   M ☐  F ☐

4. INSURED'S NAME (Last Name, Firts Name, Middle Initial)

5. PATIENT'S ADDRESS (No., Street)

6. PATIENT RELATIONSHIP TO INSURED   ☐ Self ☐ Spouse ☐ Child ☐ Other

7. INSURED'S ADDRESS (No., Street)

CITY          STATE

8. PATIENT STATUS   ☐ Single   ☐ Married   ☐ Other

CITY          STATE

ZIP CODE   TELEPHONE (Include Area Code)   (   )

Employed ☐   Full-Time ☐ Student   Part-Time ☐ Student

ZIP CODE   TELEPHONE (Include Area Code)   (   )

9. OTHER INSURED'S NAME (Last Name, First Name, Middle Initial)

10. IS PATIENT'S CONDITION RELATED TO:

11. INSURED'S POLICY GROUP OR FECA NUMBER

a. OTHER INSURED'S POLICY OR GROUP NUMBER

a. EMPLOYMENT? (CURRENT OR PREVIOUS)   ☐ YES   ☐ NO

a. INSURED'S DATE OF BIRTH   MM | DD | YY   SEX   M ☐  F ☐

b. OTHER INSURED'S DATE OF BIRTH   MM | DD | YY   SEX   M ☐  F ☐

b. AUTO ACCIDENT?   PLACE (State)   ☐ YES   ☐ NO

b. EMPLOYER'S NAME OR SCHOOL NAME

c. EMPLOYER'S NAME OR SCHOOL NAME

c. OTHER ACCIDENT?   ☐ YES   ☐ NO

c. INSURANCE PLAN NAME OR PROGRAM NAME

d. INSURANCE PLAN NAME OR PROGRAM NAME

d. RESERVED FOR LOCAL USE

d. IS THERE ANOTHER HEALTH BENEFIT PLAN?   ☐ YES   ☐ NO   If yes, return to and complete item 9 a-d.

**READ BACK OF FORM BEFORE COMPLETING & SIGNING THIS FORM.**

12. PATIENT'S OR AUTHORIZED PERSON'S SIGNATURE I authorize the release of any medical or other information necessary to process this claim. I also request payment of government benefits either to myself or to the party who accepts assignments below.

SIGNED_____   DATE_____

13. INSURED'S OR AUTHORIZED PERSON'S SIGNATURE I authorize payment of medical benefits to the undersigned physician or supplier for services described below.

SIGNED_____

14. DATE OF CURRENT:   MM | DD | YY   ILLNESS (First sympton) OR INJURY (Accident)OR PREGNANCY (LMP)

15. IF PATIENT HAS HAD SAME OR SIMILAR ILLNESS. GIVE FIRST DATE   MM | DD | YY

16. DATES PATIENT UNABLE TO WORK IN CURRENT OCCUPATION   MM | DD | YY   MM | DD | YY   FROM          TO

17. NAME OR REFERRING PHYSICIAN OR OTHER SOURCE

17a. I.D. NUMBER OF REFERRING PHYSICIAN

18. HOSPITALIZATION DATES RELATED TO CURRENT SERVICES   MM | DD | YY   MM | DD | YY   FROM          TO

19. RESERVED FOR LOCAL USE

20. OUTSIDE LAB?   ☐ YES   ☐ NO   $ CHARGES

21. DIAGNOSIS OR NATURE OF ILLNESS OR INJURY. (RELATE ITEMS 1,2,3 OR 4 TO ITEM 24E BY LINE)

1. I_____.____   3. I_____.____

2. I_____.____   4. I_____.____

22. MEDICAID RESUBMISSION   CODE   ORIGINAL REF. NO.

23. PRIOR AUTHORIZATION NUMBER

| 24. A | | | | | B | C | D | | E | F | G | H | I | J | K |
|---|---|---|---|---|---|---|---|---|---|---|---|---|---|---|---|
| DATE(S) OF SERVICE | | | | | Place of Service | Type of Service | PROCEDURES, SERVICES, OR SUPPLIES (Explain Unusual Circumstances) | | DIAGNOSIS CODE | $ CHARGES | DAYS OR UNITS | EPSDT Family Plan | EMG | COB | RESERVED FOR LOCAL USE |
| From | | | To | | | | CPT/HCPCS | MODIFIER | | | | | | | |
| MM | DD | YY | MM | DD | YY | | | | | | | | | | |
| 1 | | | | | | | | | | | | | | | |
| 2 | | | | | | | | | | | | | | | |
| 3 | | | | | | | | | | | | | | | |
| 4 | | | | | | | | | | | | | | | |
| 5 | | | | | | | | | | | | | | | |
| 6 | | | | | | | | | | | | | | | |

25. FEDERAL TAX I.D. NUMBER   SSN ☐ EIN ☐

26. PATIENT'S ACCOUNT NO.

27. ACCEPT ASSIGNMENT? (For govt. claims, see back)   ☐ YES   ☐ NO

28. TOTAL CHARGE   $

29. AMOUNT PAID   $

30. BALANCE DUE   $

31. SIGNATURE OF PHYSICIAN OR SUPPLIER INCLUDING DEGREES OR CREDENTIALS (I certify that the statements on the reverse apply to this bill and are made a part thereof.)

SIGNED _____ DATE _____

32. NAME AND ADDRESS OF FACULTY WHERE SERVICES WERE RENDERED (If other than home or office)

33. PHYSICIAN'S, SUPPLIER'S BILLING NAME, ADDRESS, ZIP CODE & PHONE#

PIN #          GRP #

(APPROVED BY AMA COUNCIL ON MEDICAL SERVICE 8/88)

**PLEASE PRINT OR TYPE**

FORM HCFA-1500 (U2) (12-90)
FORM OWCP -1500   FORM RRB-1500

*Side labels:* CARRIER — PATIENT AND INSURED INFORMATION — PHYSICIAN OR SUPPLIER INFORMATION

135

PLEASE
DO NOT
STAPLE
IN THIS
AREA

APPROVED OMB-0938-0008

PICA

# HEALTH INSURANCE CLAIM FORM

PICA

1. MEDICARE    MEDICAID    CHAMPUS    CHAMPVA    GROUP HEALTH PLAN    FECA BLK LUNG    OTHER    1a. INSURED'S I.D. NUMBER    (FOR PROGRAM IN ITEM 1)

☐ (Medicare #)  ☐ (Medicaid #)  ☐ (Sponsor's SSN)  ☐ (VA File #)  ☐ (SSN or ID)  ☐ (SSN)  ☐ (ID)

2. PATIENT'S NAME (Last Name, First Name, Middle Initial)

3. PATIENT'S BIRTH DATE    SEX
MM   DD   YY    M ☐   F ☐

4. INSURED'S NAME (Last Name, Firts Name, Middle Initial)

5. PATIENT'S ADDRESS (No., Street)

6. PATIENT RELATIONSHIP TO INSURED
☐ Self  ☐ Spouse  ☐ Child  ☐ Other

7. INSURED'S ADDRESS (No., Street)

CITY    STATE

8. PATIENT STATUS
☐ Single  ☐ Married  ☐ Other

CITY    STATE

ZIP CODE    TELEPHONE (Include Area Code)
(    )

Employed ☐  Full-Time Student ☐  Part-Time Student ☐

ZIP CODE    TELEPHONE (Include Area Code)
(    )

9. OTHER INSURED'S NAME (Last Name, First Name, Middle Initial)

10. IS PATIENT'S CONDITION RELATED TO:

11. INSURED'S POLICY GROUP OR FECA NUMBER

a. OTHER INSURED'S POLICY OR GROUP NUMBER

a. EMPLOYMENT? (CURRENT OR PREVIOUS)
☐ YES  ☐ NO

a. INSURED'S DATE OF BIRTH    SEX
MM   DD   YY    M ☐   F ☐

b. OTHER INSURED'S DATE OF BIRTH    SEX
MM   DD   YY    M ☐   F ☐

b. AUTO ACCIDENT?    PLACE (State)
☐ YES  ☐ NO

b. EMPLOYER'S NAME OR SCHOOL NAME

c. EMPLOYER'S NAME OR SCHOOL NAME

c. OTHER ACCIDENT?
☐ YES  ☐ NO

c. INSURANCE PLAN NAME OR PROGRAM NAME

d. INSURANCE PLAN NAME OR PROGRAM NAME

d. RESERVED FOR LOCAL USE

d. IS THERE ANOTHER HEALTH BENEFIT PLAN?
☐ YES  ☐ NO  If yes, return to and complete item 9 a-d.

**READ BACK OF FORM BEFORE COMPLETING & SIGNING THIS FORM.**
12. PATIENT'S OR AUTHORIZED PERSON'S SIGNATURE I authorize the release of any medical or other information necessary to process this claim. I also request payment of government benefits either to myself or to the party who accepts assignments below.

SIGNED_____    DATE_____

13. INSURED'S OR AUTHORIZED PERSON'S SIGNATURE I authorize payment of medical benefits to the undersigned physician or supplier for services described below.

SIGNED_____

14. DATE OF CURRENT:
MM   DD   YY
◄ ILLNESS (First sympton) OR
INJURY (Accident)OR
PREGNANCY (LMP)

15. IF PATIENT HAS HAD SAME OR SIMILAR ILLNESS.
GIVE FIRST DATE    MM   DD   YY

16. DATES PATIENT UNABLE TO WORK IN CURRENT OCCUPATION
MM   DD   YY    MM   DD   YY
FROM    TO

17. NAME OR REFERRING PHYSICIAN OR OTHER SOURCE

17a. I.D. NUMBER OF REFERRING PHYSICIAN

18. HOSPITALIZATION DATES RELATED TO CURRENT SERVICES
MM   DD   YY    MM   DD   YY
FROM    TO

19. RESERVED FOR LOCAL USE

20. OUTSIDE LAB?    $ CHARGES
☐ YES  ☐ NO

21. DIAGNOSIS OR NATURE OF ILLNESS OR INJURY. (RELATE ITEMS 1,2,3 OR 4 TO ITEM 24E BY LINE)

1. I____.___    3. I____.___

2. I____.___    4. I____.___

22. MEDICAID RESUBMISSION CODE    ORIGINAL REF. NO.

23. PRIOR AUTHORIZATION NUMBER

| 24. | A | | | | | B | C | D | | E | F | G | H | I | J | K |
|---|---|---|---|---|---|---|---|---|---|---|---|---|---|---|---|---|
| | DATE(S) OF SERVICE | | | | | Place of Service | Type of Service | PROCEDURES, SERVICES, OR SUPPLIES (Explain Unusual Circumstances) | | DIAGNOSIS CODE | $ CHARGES | DAYS OR UNITS | EPSDT Family Plan | EMG | COB | RESERVED FOR LOCAL USE |
| | From | | | To | | | | CPT/HCPCS | MODIFIER | | | | | | | |
| | MM | DD | YY | MM | DD | YY | | | | | | | | | | | |
| 1 | | | | | | | | | | | | | | | | |
| 2 | | | | | | | | | | | | | | | | |
| 3 | | | | | | | | | | | | | | | | |
| 4 | | | | | | | | | | | | | | | | |
| 5 | | | | | | | | | | | | | | | | |
| 6 | | | | | | | | | | | | | | | | |

25. FEDERAL TAX I.D. NUMBER    SSN ☐ EIN ☐

26. PATIENT'S ACCOUNT NO.

27. ACCEPT ASSIGNMENT? (For govt. claims, see back)
☐ YES  ☐ NO

28. TOTAL CHARGE    $

29. AMOUNT PAID    $

30. BALANCE DUE    $

31. SIGNATURE OF PHYSICIAN OR SUPPLIER INCLUDING DEGREES OR CREDENTIALS (I certify that the statements on the reverse apply to this bill and are made a part thereof.)

SIGNED _____ DATE _____

32. NAME AND ADDRESS OF FACULTY WHERE SERVICES WERE RENDERED (If other than home or office)

33. PHYSICIAN'S, SUPPLIER'S BILLING NAME, ADDRESS, ZIP CODE & PHONE#

PIN #    GRP #

(APPROVED BY AMA COUNCIL ON MEDICAL SERVICE 8/88)    **PLEASE PRINT OR TYPE**

FORM HCFA-1500 (U2) (12-90)
FORM OWCP -1500    FORM RRB-1500

CARRIER
PATIENT AND INSURED INFORMATION
PHYSICIAN OR SUPPLIER INFORMATION

## ACHIEVING SKILL COMPETENCY

Reread the performance objective for the procedure and then practice the skill listed below, following the procedure in your textbook.

Procedure 9-1:  Complete a Claim Form

When you have mastered the performance of the skill, sign your name on the appropriate evaluation sheet and give it to your instructor to indicate you are prepared to perform the procedure for evaluation.

After your instructor has returned your work to you, make all necessary corrections and place in a three-ring notebook for future reference.

**ASSIGNMENT SHEET**

## Chapter 10: MEDICAL OFFICE MANAGEMENT

Review the objectives and text for each unit before completing the assignment sheet for that unit. When you have completed all sheets for the chapter, remove them from this Workbook and give them to the instructor for evaluation.

## Unit 1: THE LANGUAGE OF BANKING

**Mixed Quiz**

1. Matching: Match the definition in column II with the correct term in column I.

| COLUMN I | COLUMN II |
|---|---|
| _____ 1. Agent | a. Record of deposit given to customer by bank |
| _____ 2. Bankbook | b. A person authorized to act for another |
| _____ 3. Bank statement | c. A bank account against which checks are written |
| _____ 4. Cashier's check | d. Record of deposits, withdrawals, and interest earned |
| _____ 5. Check register | e. An itemized list of cash and checks deposited |
| _____ 6. Certified check | f. Check stub |
| _____ 7. Checking account | g. Purchaser pays full amount of check issued by bank |
| _____ 8. Currency | h. Paper money issued by government |
| _____ 9. Deposit | i. A record sent to customer showing all banking activity for a set period of time |
| _____ 10. Debit | j. Money being placed in a bank account |
| _____ 11. Deposit record | k. Bank stamps customer's own check and holds funds aside to cover check |
| _____ 12. Deposit slip | l. An entry of an amount owed that has been charged to the account |

2. Matching: Match the definition in column II with the correct term in column I.

| COLUMN I | COLUMN II |
|---|---|
| _____ 1. Endorsement | a. Negotiable instrument purchased for a fee to be used instead of a check |
| _____ 2. Endorser | b. Check made out for a future date |
| _____ 3. Insufficient funds | c. Person to whom check is written |
| _____ 4. Limited check | d. Payee's signature on back of check |
| _____ 5. Maker | e. A bank term used to indicate that writer of check did not have enough money in account to cover check |
| _____ 6. Money order | f. Person who signs check |
| _____ 7. Note | g. An amount sent electronically toa savings or checking account |
| _____ 8. Payee | h. Legal evidence of debt |
| _____ 9. Payer | i. Same as payee on check |
| _____ 10. Postdated check | j. Check that will be void if written over designated amount or kept beyond time limit of when it should be cashed |
| _____ 11. Direct deposit | k. Individual who signs a check |

3. Matching:  Match the definition in column II with the correct term in column I.

COLUMN I

_____ 1. Power of attorney
_____ 2. Savings account
_____ 3. Service charge
_____ 4. Stale check

_____ 5. Negotiable

_____ 6. Stop payment
_____ 7. Teller
_____ 8. Traveler's check

_____ 9. Voucher check

_____ 10. Warrant

_____ 11. Withdrawal

COLUMN II

a. Bank employee who is main contact between customer and bank
b. Fees charged by bank for services rendered
c. Removal of funds from depositor's account
d. Method by which maker of check may change his mind about making payment
e. Check with detachable form used to state purpose for which check was written
f. A bank account upon which depositor earns interest
g. Evidence of a debt due but is not negotiable
h. Special check issued by bank in exchange for cash that must be signed when purchased and again when used
i. A check presented for payment after date specified when would be honored
j. A legal procedure that authorizes one person to act as agent for another
k. Something that is able to be transferred or exchanged

4. Explain the bank code on a check.
   a. What is an ABA number? _____
   b. Who originated the number concept? _____
   c. What is its purpose? _____
   _____

5. Spell out the acronym MICR. _____
   a. Explain what each series of numbers means.
      1. _____
      2. _____
      3. _____
   b. What does a bank add to the check? _____
   c. Why is MICR used? _____
   _____

6. Label the ABA and MICR codes on the check. Refer to Figure 10-1 in the textbook.

Labeling:

**JAMES C. MORRISON**      **101**
1765 SHERIDAN DRIVE
YOUR CITY, STATE, 12345

_____, 19_____    00–6789/0000    — A

PAY TO THE
ORDER OF _____ | $ _____

_____ DOLLARS

DELUXE CHECK PRINTERS
YOUR CITY, U.S.A. 12345

MEMO _____

|:00006  7894|:  12345678;'  0101  ;0000039158;

B      C      D      E

a. _____

b. _____

c. _____

d. _____

e. _____

7. Explain the difference between overdraft and overdrawn. _____

_____

_____

8. a. List five pieces of information the bank requires to stop payment on a check.

1. _____

2. _____

3. _____

4. _____

5. _____

b. For what reasons may payment be stopped?

1. _____

2. _____

9. Define the term *postdated check* and explain what you must do with such a check. _____

_____

_____

10. What is an electronic fund transfer system? _____

_____

11. Describe the one-write check writing system. _____

_____

12. What would you do in the event a bank deposit is not credited? _____

_____

_____

13. Refer to the Role Delineation Chart in Appendix A of the textbook. Within the area of *Practice Finances,* which two roles relate to the content of this unit?

    a. _____

    b. _____

After your instructor has returned your work to you, make all necessary corrections and place in a 3-ring notebook for future reference.

**ASSIGNMENT SHEET**

**Chapter 10: MEDICAL OFFICE MANAGEMENT**

**Unit 2: CURRENCY, CHECKS, AND PETTY CASH**

**Mixed Quiz**

1. Explain why comparing shipments to packing lists or invoices is important. _____
   _____
   _____
   _____

2. Using the following information, write four checks to suppliers of goods and services. Use the current date
   and sign the checks with the physician's name with your name below the line. Complete the stub end,
   subtracting each subsequent check. (Two extra checks are provided in case you make an error.)
   a. Physician's Supply, Inc.   $125.50
   b. Clinical Laboratory Services      $987.45
   c. Brown Office Equipment  $535.99
   d. Jones Building Maintenance      $1,248.75

3. Fill in the Blanks
   Currency is the name given to _____ It can be made up of _____ and
   _____ When receiving cash from a patient, always _____ the money while the patient is
   watching. When the amount is entered on the ledger card or other form, always indicate the payment is in
   _____ All cash in an offfice should be kept _____ Daily proceeds are usually
   _____ or _____ at the close of the day.

4. List the seven features you must examine to be sure the check is valid. _____
   _____
   _____

5. Why should you refuse a third-party check? _____

6. Why should you not accept a check for more than the amount due? _____
   _____

7. Why may a check marked "payment in full" be a problem? _____
   _____

8. Name the two kinds of endorsements, explaining the meaning of each one.
   a. _____
   _____
   b. _____

9. How do you process a check when the name of the payee is misspelled? _____
   _____

10. Where should a check be endorsed? _____

## Check 1490

| 1490 | BAL. BRO'T FOR'D | | |
|---|---|---|---|
| _____ 19___ | | | |
| TO _____ | DEPOSITS | | |
| FOR _____ | TOTAL | | |
| | THIS CHECK | | |
| | BALANCE | | |

ELIZABETH R. EVANS, M.D.
SUITE 205 100 E. MAIN ST.
YOURTOWN, US 98765-4321

1490

_____ 19____   25-64/440

PAY TO THE ORDER OF _____ $ _____

_____ DOLLARS

THE NEVER FAIL BANK
ANYWHERE, U.S.A 00000

7-88-25

FOR _____

|:00006 7894|: 12345678;' 01490 ;0000039158;

## Check 1491

| 1491 | BAL. BRO'T FOR'D | | |
|---|---|---|---|
| _____ 19___ | | | |
| TO _____ | DEPOSITS | | |
| FOR _____ | TOTAL | | |
| | THIS CHECK | | |
| | BALANCE | | |

ELIZABETH R. EVANS, M.D.
SUITE 205 100 E. MAIN ST.
YOURTOWN, US 98765-4321

1491

_____ 19____   25-64/440

PAY TO THE ORDER OF _____ $ _____

_____ DOLLARS

THE NEVER FAIL BANK
ANYWHERE, U.S.A 00000

7-88-25

FOR _____

|:00006 7894|: 12345678;' 01491 ;0000039158;

## Check 1492

| 1492 | BAL. BRO'T FOR'D | | |
|---|---|---|---|
| _____ 19___ | | | |
| TO _____ | DEPOSITS | | |
| FOR _____ | TOTAL | | |
| | THIS CHECK | | |
| | BALANCE | | |

ELIZABETH R. EVANS, M.D.
SUITE 205 100 E. MAIN ST.
YOURTOWN, US 98765-4321

1492

_____ 19____   25-64/440

PAY TO THE ORDER OF _____ $ _____

_____ DOLLARS

THE NEVER FAIL BANK
ANYWHERE, U.S.A 00000

7-88-25

FOR _____

|:00006 7894|: 12345678;' 01492 ;0000039158;

## Check 1493

| 1493 | BAL. BRO'T FOR'D | | |
|---|---|---|---|
| _____ 19___ | | | |
| TO _____ | DEPOSITS | | |
| FOR _____ | TOTAL | | |
| | THIS CHECK | | |
| | BALANCE | | |

ELIZABETH R. EVANS, M.D.
SUITE 205 100 E. MAIN ST.
YOURTOWN, US 98765-4321

1493

_____ 19____   25-64/440

PAY TO THE ORDER OF _____ $ _____

_____ DOLLARS

THE NEVER FAIL BANK
ANYWHERE, U.S.A 00000

7-88-25

FOR _____

|:00006 7894|: 12345678;' 01493 ;0000039158;

## Check 1494

| 1494 | BAL. BRO'T FOR'D | | |
|---|---|---|---|
| _____ 19___ | | | |
| TO _____ | DEPOSITS | | |
| FOR _____ | TOTAL | | |
| | THIS CHECK | | |
| | BALANCE | | |

ELIZABETH R. EVANS, M.D.
SUITE 205 100 E. MAIN ST.
YOURTOWN, US 98765-4321

1494

_____ 19____   25-64/440

PAY TO THE ORDER OF _____ $ _____

_____ DOLLARS

THE NEVER FAIL BANK
ANYWHERE, U.S.A 00000

7-88-25

FOR _____

|:00006 7894|: 12345678;' 01494 ;0000039158;

## Check 1495

| 1495 | BAL. BRO'T FOR'D | | |
|---|---|---|---|
| _____ 19___ | | | |
| TO _____ | DEPOSITS | | |
| FOR _____ | TOTAL | | |
| | THIS CHECK | | |
| | BALANCE | | |

ELIZABETH R. EVANS, M.D.
SUITE 205 100 E. MAIN ST.
YOURTOWN, US 98765-4321

1495

_____ 19____   25-64/440

PAY TO THE ORDER OF _____ $ _____

_____ DOLLARS

THE NEVER FAIL BANK
ANYWHERE, U.S.A 00000

7-88-25

FOR _____

|:00006 7894|: 12345678;' 01495 ;0000039158;

11. Prepare a bank deposit using the following list of cash and check payments.

Currency/coin:  $35.50, $40.00, $50.75, $25.00, $15.75

Checks:  Holley, check #134—$40.00

Segal, check #285—$25.00

Gomez, check #596—$55.00

Schmidt, check #436—$32.00

Moriarty, check #1073—$38.00

Kostrevski, check #735—$47.00

Kendrix, check #489—$150.00

Cartloano, check #634—$45.00

Money orders:  Chin, $45.00; Jackson, $55.00

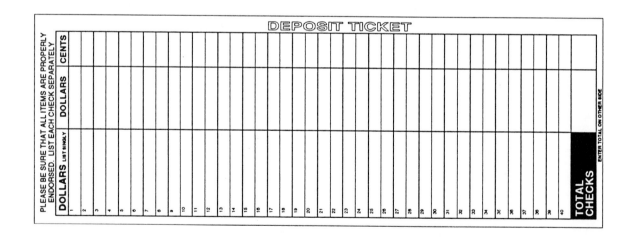

12. What must you do if a mail deposit is lost? _____

_____

13. Use the following figures to reconcile the bank account on the form provided. You may assume the opening balance agrees with the previous statement.

STATEMENT OF ACCOUNT

THE NEVER FAIL BANK • ANYWHERE, USA 00000

For the month of _____, _____(year)

Checks written during the month

| #101 | 25.00 | 111 | 500.00 | 122 | 35.00 |
|------|-------|-----|--------|-----|-------|
| 102 | 600.00 | 112 | 18.22 | 123 | 95.94 |
| 103 | 75.00 | 113 | 133.28 | 124 | 19.00 |
| 104 | 37.54 | 114 | 57.50 | 125 | 75.00 |
| 105 | 30.00 | 115 | 38.60 | 126 | 400.00 |
| 106 | 95.94 | 116 | 500.00 | 127 | 78.37 |
| 107 | 73.87 | 117 | 785.00 | 128 | 95.94 |
| 108 | 44.00 | 118 | 28.37 | 129 | 200.00 |
| 109 | 130.00 | 119 | 60.00 | 130 | 33.60 |
| 110 | 95.94 | 120 | 36.30 | 131 | 1200.00 |
|  |  | 121 | 115.45 | 132 | 100.00 |

Checkbook balance end of last month $3173.71

Deposit mailed but not appearing on statement $191.00

| Checks Paid Out | | Deposits | Balance |
|--------|--------|----------|---------|
| **Balance Brought Forward** | | | 1840.57 |
| 25.00 | 95.94 | 500.00 | 1815.57 |
| 600.00 | 44.00 | 750.00 | 1715.57 |
| 30.00 | 500.00 | 350.00 | 2339.63 |
| 73.87 | 38.60 | 700.00 | 2441.76 |
| 95.94 | 115.45 | 335.00 | 2394.32 |
| 57.50 | 95.94 | 500.00 | 2133.22 |
| 28.37 | 75.00 | 440.50 | 2604.85 |
| 60.00 | 78.37 | 180.00 | 2985.35 |
| 36.30 | 33.60 | 175.00 | 3013.60 |
| 35.00 | 130.00 | 520.00 | 3057.66 |
| 19.00 | 18.22 | 522.50 | 3483.66 |
| 400.00 | 500.00 | 720.00 | 3431.85 |
| 200.00 | 95.94 | 600.00 | 3918.25 |
| 100.00 | 133.28 | 662.00 | 4414.98 |
| | 3.27 SC | | 5076.98 |

No. checks 28

No. deposits 14

Service charge 3.27

Ending balance 5076.98

## RECONCILE THE BANK STATEMENT

Bank statement balance          _____

Outstanding checks

_____

_____

_____

_____

Subtract total outstanding checks     _____

Adjusted balance     _____

Add deposits not credited     _____

Corrected bank statement balance     _____

Checkbook balance     _____

Subtract bank charges     _____

Corrected checkbook balance     _____

14. For what purpose is a petty cash fund used? _____

_____

15. Word Puzzle: Use the clues below to spell out these terms.

```
1.                    _ E _ _ _ _ _ _
2.            _ _ _ _ N _ _ _ _
3.            _ _ _ _ D _ _ _ _ _
4.                    _ O _ _
5.              _ _ _ R _ _ _ _
6.            _ _ _ _ S _ _ _
7                     _ E _ _ _ _ _
8.              _ _ _ M _ _ _
9.            _ _ _ _ _ E _
10.            _ _ _ N _ _ _ _ _ _ _
11. _ _ _ _ _ _ _ _ _ T _ _ _
```

1. All consumed, none left
2. Make agree
3. Payee other than patient
4. Cancel, make invalid
5. Cash
6. A record
7. To place in an account
8. A sum paid toward a balance
9. A paper designating payment
10. Action occurring
11. Power given, permission granted

16. Refer to the Role Delineation Chart in Appendix A of the textbook. Within the area of *Practice Finances,* which three roles relate to the content of this unit? _____

_____

After your instructor has returned your work to you, make all necessary corrections and place in a three-ring notebook for future reference.

**ASSIGNMENT SHEET**

**Chapter 10: MEDICAL OFFICE MANAGEMENT**

**Unit 3: SALARY, BENEFITS, AND TAX RECORDS**

**Mixed Quiz**

1. Fill in the Blanks

   All employees in a physician's office must have a _____ Forms to apply for the number can be obtained from local _____ _____ and _____ Each employee must also complete an _____ indicating the number of exemptions claimed. In addition, recent federal legislation requires the completion of an _____ This form is issued by the _____ _____ Its purpose is to ensure all persons employed are either _____ or _____ In addition to these federal requirements, forms must also be processed for _____ and _____ tax records.

2. What information should be listed on payroll record keeping forms?

   a. _____
   b. _____
   c. _____
   d. _____
   e. _____
   f. _____
   g. _____
   h. _____
   i. _____
   j. _____
   k. _____
   l. _____
   m. _____

3. a. What determines the amount of federal tax withheld?

      1. _____
      2. _____
      3. _____
      4. _____

   b. How are state and local taxes determined? _____

   c. What is net pay? _____

4. What is the physician's responsibility in relation to state and federal regulations?

   a. _____
   b. _____
   c. _____
   d. _____

5. List twelve examples of fringe benefits.

a. _____   g. _____
b. _____   h. _____
c. _____   i. _____
d. _____   j. _____
e. _____   k. _____
f. _____   l. _____

6. What does the term *vested* mean? _____
_____

7. Spelling: Each line contains three different spellings of a word. Underline the correctly spelled word.

| accountent | accontant | accountant |
| disability | disibility | disebility |
| longevity | lonjevity | longitevy |
| egemption | exeption | exemption |
| deducktions | deductions | deductshuns |

8. Refer to the Role Delineation Chart in Appendix A of the textbook. Within the area of *Practice Finances,* which role relates specifically to the content of this unit? _____

9. Word Puzzle: Use the clues below to spell out these terms.

1.        _ _ _     _ _ _ _ _ _
2.     _ _ _ _ _    _ _ _ _
3.          _     _ _ _ _ _ _
4.       _ _ _     _ _ _ _ _ _ _ _ _
5.      _ _ _ _     _ _ _ _
6.   _ _ _ _ _ _     _ _ _
7          _ _     _ _
8. _ _ _ _ _ _ _ _
9.          _     _ _ _ _ _ _
10.         _     _ _ _ _
11.             _ _
12.     _ _ _ _ _     _ _ _ _ _ _ _

1. Eligible credits to reduce tax
2. One who examines fiscal matters
3. Additional to salary
4. Without work
5. To excuse
6. Lack of ability
7. Total earnings
8. Length of time
9. One hired for a job
10. Eligible to receive
11. Remaining
12. Participation in distribution of earnings

After your instructor has returned your work to you, make all necessary corrections and place in a three-ring notebook for future reference.

Name _____

Date _____ Score _____

**ASSIGNMENT SHEET**

**Chapter 10: MEDICAL OFFICE MANAGEMENT**

**Unit 4: GENERAL MANAGEMENT DUTIES**

**SUGGESTED RESPONSES TO CRITICAL THINKING CHALLENGE IN TEXTBOOK**

1. What are some options open to Michelle? _____

_____

2. What do you think about establishing a different job description with perhaps a little more responsibility in order to justify a salary increase? _____

_____

_____

3. Could additional fringe benefits be established for employees such as Rosie, who have been employed for five years? _____

_____

4. Is there any guarantee that Rosie would stay even if Michelle did manage to arrange a salary increase? _____

_____

_____

_____

5. What really is important for job satisfaction? _____

_____

_____

6. How would being given more responsibility, a *title,* and a sense of control over some portion of the operation provide any incentive? _____

_____

_____

_____

_____

_____

_____

**A. Mixed Quiz**

1. Why is it necessary to maintain a sense of fiscal status? _____

_____

2. What kinds of information are supplied to the practice monthly by an accountant?

   a. _____

   b. _____

   c. _____

3. What are three consequences of a missed appointment?

a. _____

b. _____

c. _____

4. List eight topics that should be covered by the office policy manual: _____

_____

_____

5. What is the purpose of an office procedure manual? _____

_____

6. What kind of information should be indicated on an inventory card?

a. _____

b. _____

c. _____

d. _____

7. When might a patient's account be overpaid? _____

What must you check before refunding any amount? _____

8. All items must be stored properly. Identify the following correct storage places.

a. Medications in _____

b. Narcotics in _____

c. Some laboratory supplies in _____

d. Supplies _____

9. List an office manager's responsibility to the support staff.

a. _____

b. _____

c. _____

d. _____

e. _____

f. _____

g. _____

10. List an office manager's responsibilities to physicians.

a. _____

b. _____

c. _____

_____

d. _____

e. _____

11. List six organizations that might conduct an on-site visit. _____

12. Refer to the ABHES Course Content Requirements in Appendix C of the textbook. Within the area of *Medical Office Business Procedures/Management,* which three content requirements are discussed in this unit?

_____

_____

13. Unscramble

```
A P R E M I U M S D B C D
M E E S F G E D H E M A I
A C I T F I X R J L A C N
N A M A I N T E N A N C E
A L B T S C E C K G U O G
G I U U C O N O L A A U L
E B R S A M S R M T L N I
M R S N L E I D O I P T G
E A E Q R S V S T O U V E
N T M W X R E F U N D Y N
T I E X P E D I T U R E T
Z O N I N V E N T O R Y A
B N T C P O L I C Y D E F
```

| | |
|---|---|
| ACCOUNT | MANAGEMENT |
| CALIBRATION | MANUAL |
| DELEGATION | NEGLIGENT |
| EXPENDITURE | POLICY |
| EXTENSIVE | PREMIUMS |
| FISCAL | RECORDS |
| INCOME | REFUND |
| INVENTORY | REIMBURSEMENT |
| MAINTENANCE | STATUS |

## ACHIEVING SKILL COMPETENCY

Reread the performance objective for each procedure and practice the skills listed below, following the procedures in your textbook.

        Procedure 10-1: Prepare a Check

        Procedure 10-2: Prepare a Deposit Slip

        Procedure 10-3: Reconcile a Bank Statement

When you feel you have mastered the performance of the skill, sign your name on the appropriate evaluation sheet and give it to your instructor to indicate you are prepared to perform the procedure for evaluation.

After your instructor has returned your work to you, make all necessary corrections and place in a three-ring notebook for future reference.

**ASSIGNMENT SHEET**

**Section 3: STRUCTURE AND FUNCTION OF THE BODY**

**Chapter 11: ANATOMY AND PHYSIOLOGY OF THE HUMAN BODY**

Review the objectives and text for each unit before completing the assignment sheet for that unit. When you have completed all sheets for the chapter, remove them from this Workbook and give them to the instructor for evaluation.

**Unit 1: ANATOMICAL DESCRIPTORS AND FUNDAMENTAL BODY STRUCTURES**

**A. Mixed Quiz**

1. Define *anatomy*. _Is the study of the physical structure of the body and it's organs_

2. Name and define the two subdivisions of anatomy. _gross anatomy= study of those features_

3. Define *physiology*. _the science of function cells, tissues & organs of the body._

4. Describe the meaning of the phrase *anatomical position*. _Standing erect, with arms down at the sides. and the palms of the hands facing foward_

5. Fill in the Blank

   In anatomical position, the patient's right side is across from your _left_ side. Something toward the midline is said to be _medical_ if it is away from the midline it is _lateral_ Arms and legs are known as _extremities_ The front of the body is called the _Anterior_ or _Ventrial_ section. The back section is called the _Dorsal_ or _Posterior_ side. The body has two main cavities. The anterior cavity is further divided into an upper _thoracic_ and a lower _abdominal_ cavity. The posterior body section has a _cranial_ cavity and a _spinal_ cavity.

6. List the organs within each body cavity.

   a. Thoracic: _thorax_
   b. Abdominal: _abdomel_
   c. Pelvic: _pelvis_
   d. Cranial: _cranium or skull_
   e. Spinal: _spinal colum, canal or cord_

7. Refer to CAAHEP Standards in Appendix B of the textbook. Within the area of *Medical Terminology*, which curriculum standard addresses the appropriate use of medical terms in this unit? _____

_____

8. Labeling: Label the directional reference terms on the illustrations of anatomical position. Refer to Figures 11-1 and 11-2 in the textbook.

Median (Sagital) Plane

Proximal
(nearest point
of attachment)

Distal
(farthest
from point of
attachment)

Medial
(toward the
median)

Lateral
(away from
the median)

Midline

Right          Left

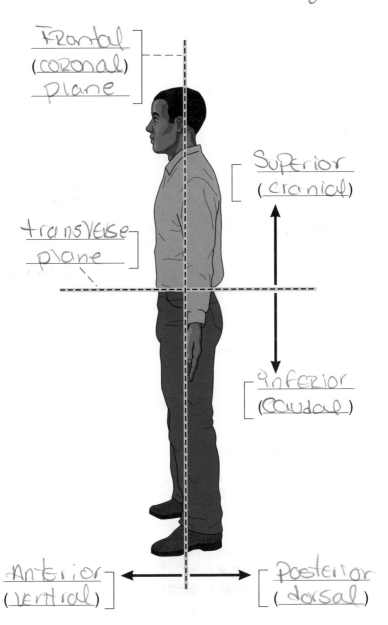

Frontal (coronal) plane

transverse plane

Superior (cranial)

inferior (caudal)

Anterior (ventral)

Posterior (dorsal)

9. Labeling: Label the eight body cavities on the following illustration. Refer to Figure 11-3 in the textbook.

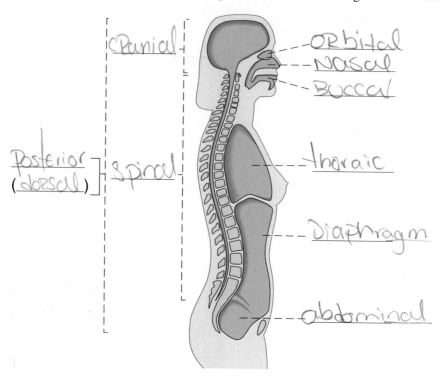

Cranial

Orbital
Nasal
Buccal

Posterior
(dorsal)

spinal

thoraic

Diaphragm

abdominal

10. Labeling: Label the thoracic and abdominal organs. Refer to Figure 11-4 in the textbook.

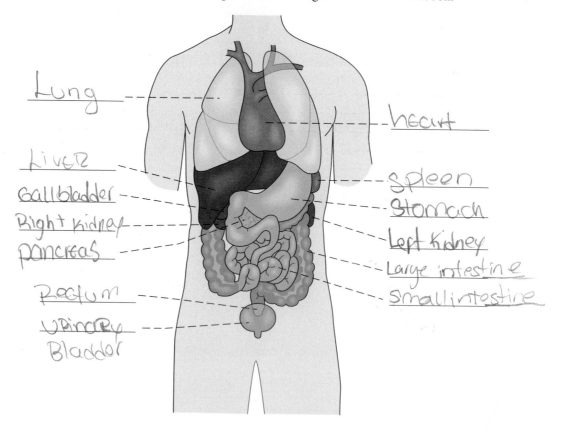

Lung

heart

Liver
Gallbladder
Right kidney
pancreas

spleen
Stomach
Left kidney
Large intestine
Small intestine

Rectum
Urinary
Bladder

11. The abdomen can be divided into four sections for reference purposes. Name the sections.
   a. _Right upper Quadrant_
   b. _Left Upper "_
   c. _Right Lower "_
   d. _Left Lower "_

12. Labeling: Label the nine anatomical divisions and one reference point of the abdomen on the following illustration. Refer to Figure 11-6 in the textbook.

Epigastric

Right hypochondriac
umbilicos
Right lumbar, lateral
Right iliac, inguinal

Left hypochondriac
umbilical
Left lumbar lateral
Left iliac, inguinal
Hypogastric pubic

13. List the structures of a cell.
   a. _organelles_
   b. _nucleus_
   c. _mitochondria_
   d. _Ribosomes_
   e. _centriole_
   f. _endoplastic Reticulum_
   g. _golgi apparatus_
   h. _lysosomes_
   i. _mitosis_
   j. _chromosomes._

14. List three things that may cause a mutation to occur. _____

15. Name three types of inheritance patterns and explain how they affect an individual's inherited traits.
   a. _dominant_
   b. _recessive_
   c. _X-linked_

16. List the six processes by which materials pass through cell membranes.
   a. _diffusion_
   b. _osmosis_
   c. _filtration_
   d. _phagocytosis_
   e. _Active_
   f. _transport_

17. Fill in the Blank

The osmotic characteristics of solutions are classified by their effect on *red blood cells* If the solution is the same osmotic pressure as blood serum, it is known as an *isotonic* solution. When osmolality is lower, the solution is called *hypotonic* If it is higher, it is called *hypertonic* A salt solution with the same salt content as that of a red blood cell is called *normal saline*

18. Matching: Match the acid or base in column I with its possible location in column II.

COLUMN I

___d___ Acetic acid
___f___ Boric acid
___e___ Hydrochloric acid
___a___ Sulfuric acid
___b___ Ammonium hydroxide
___g___ Magnesium hydroxide
___c___ Sodium hydroxide

COLUMN II

a. Found in batteries
b. Household liquid cleaners
c. Lye
d. Found in vinegar
e. Found in the stomach
f. Weak eyewash
g. Milk of Magnesia

19. Indicate whether the following pH value is acidic or alkaline and which body fluid has a similar value.

| pH Value | Acidic/Alkaline | Body Fluid |
| --- | --- | --- |
| a. 8.0 | Sodium bicarbonate | pancreatic juice |
| b. 7.4 | Blood | Pure water Neutral |
| c. 6.0 | Urine | |
| d. 7.3 | tears | water neutral |
| e. 1.5 | | |

20. Matching: Match the following genetic conditions have visible abnormal characteristics that make them readily recognized. Match the condition in column I to its visible sign in column II.

COLUMN I

___c___ Cleft lip
___e___ Cleft palate
___f___ Down syndrome
___g___ Spina bifida
___a___ Klinefelter's syndrome
___b___ Talipes
___d___ Turner's syndrome

COLUMN II

a. Male with long legs with short, obese trunk
b. Malformation of one or both feet
c. Verticle split in upper lip
d. Female with webbing of the neck
e. Opening in the top of mouth
f. Small head and slanting eyes
g. A malformation of the back

21. What is the name of the project that sequenced genes? _____ DNA

22. Explain the term *DNA fingerprinting* and how it can be used. is a detection
Identification
barcode

23. List the four types of tissues. Identify three places in the body where the tissue can be found.

a. Epithreal
  1. intestinal
  2. Respiratory
  3. urinal tract
b. connective
  1. tendons
  2. ligaments
  3. organs capsule

c. Nerve
  1. eye
  2. ear
  3. Brain
d. _____
  1. _____
  2. _____
  3. _____

Name ___Angela Plave___

24. List the 10 systems of the body.

a. _____muscular system_____
b. _____skeletal_____
c. _____Nervous_____
d. _____endocrine_____
e. _____circulatory_____
f. _____lymphatic_____
g. _____Respirator_____
h. _____digestive_____
i. _____Urinary_____
j. _____reproductive_____

25. Word Search: Find the following words hidden in the puzzle.

| | | |
|---|---|---|
| ANATOMY | EPITHELIAL | ORGAN |
| ANTERIOR | FEET | PELVIC |
| CAVITY | GENE | PKU |
| CLEFT | GENETIC | POSTERIOR |
| CONNECTIVE | ILIAC | SKIN |
| CRANIAL | LATERAL | SMOOTH |
| DNA | LIP | SPINA |
| DORSAL | LUMBAR | TISSUE |
| DOWN | MIDLINE | VENTRAL |
| EDEMA | MUSCLE | |
| EPIGASTRIC | NERVE | |

```
S P I N A G E N E T I C W P
S P L N C L E F T D O W N C
P K U I A F E N M T I C T V
S P I E P I T H E L I A L E
S P A N T E R I O R G A N K
S M I N A G P N S T I C E P
S U I N A G E E S I C R O
S S V E N T R A L T U C V S
S C I N A G O N I V F E E T
S L R N E D E M A L I C T E
S E I A A G E N Y T I C T R
S C O N N E C T I V E A T I
S P I E P I G A S T R I C O
S P D O R S A L U M B A R R
S L A T E R A L S M O O T H
S M I D L I N E C A V I T Y
```

26. Matching: Match the meaning in column II with the correct term in column I.

COLUMN I

| Answer | Term |
|---|---|
| D | 1. Cardiac |
| N | 2. Cranial |
| P | 3. Cytoplasm |
| S | 4. Diaphragm |
| Y | 5. Dorsal |
| W | 6. Epigastric |
| R | 7. Homeostasis |
| CC | 8. Hypochondriac |
| A | 9. Inguinal |
|  | 10. Lateral |
| e | 11. Medial |
| C | 12. Myelin |
| b | 13. Neuron |
| g | 14. Proximal |
| J | 15. Smooth |
| N | 16. Striated |
| X | 17. Thoracic |
| M | 18. Tissue |
| K | 19. Umbilical |
| V | 20. Ventral |
| F | 21. Mutation |
| LL | 22. Chromosome |
| U | 23. X-linked gene |
| I | 24. PKU |
| O | 25. Down syndrome |

COLUMN II

a. Groin area
b. A nerve cell
c. A covering on a nerve
d. Heart tissue
e. Toward the midline
f. Change in the genetic code
g. Part of extremity nearest the body
h. Cavity that holds the brain
i. Lack of liver enzyme to act upon phenylalanine
j. Muscle tissue in organs
k. Abdominal area around navel
l. Stores hereditary material of the cell
m. Consists of like cells
n. Skeletal muscle tissue
o. A genetic condition due to improper chromosome 21 division
p. Cellular fluid
q. Part of extremity farthest away from body
r. State of normal functioning
s. Muscle that divides anterior cavity
t. Away from the midline
u. Carried by X chromosome
v. The anterior section
w. Abdominal area above umbilical
x. Chest area
y. The posterior section
z. The abdominal area below the umbilical
aa. The cell nucleus
bb. Swelling in the tissues
cc. Abdominal area below ribs

**CRITICAL THINKING SCENARIOS: What would your responses be in the following situations?**

1. Your friend, Nancy Martin, shares with you that she is trying to become pregnant. You know she is 37 years old and has a younger brother with Down syndrome. _____

_____

_____

2. A neighbor confides in you that her 15-year-old son has not shown any signs of sexual maturity, even though he is very tall. You know he has also had some difficulty with school. _____

_____

_____

_____

_____

After your instructor has returned your work to you, make all necessary corrections and place in a three-ring notebook for future reference.

**ASSIGNMENT SHEET**

**Chapter 11: ANATOMY AND PHYSIOLOGY OF THE HUMAN BODY**

**Unit 2: THE NERVOUS SYSTEM**

**A. Mixed Quiz**

1. List the two main divisions of the nervous system.

    a. _____

    b. _____

2. What is a *synapse?* _____

    _____

3. Identify two types of peripheral nerves.

    a. _____

    b. _____

4. List the two types of spinal nerves and describe their functions.

    a. _____

    b. _____

5. Fill in the Blank

    Simple reflex actions involve an impulse traveling along a nerve to the _____ and _____ A common test used to illustrate this action is called the _____ Complex reflex actions involve an impulse traveling from its source through _____ to the _____ and up to the _____ The message is interpreted and the _____ carry the response message back to the _____ and out the appropriate nerve.

6. What is the purpose or function of the autonomic nervous system? _____

    _____

7. Name the two divisions of the autonomic nervous system, explaining their actions.

    a. _____

    b. _____

8. List the five divisions of the brain and identify what function each division provides.

    a. _____

    _____

    b. _____

    c. _____

    d. _____

    e. _____

9. List the lobes of the cerebrum and their associated functions.

    a. _____

    _____

    b. _____

    c. _____

    _____

    d. _____

10. List the two structures between the cerebrum and the midbrain, describing their functions.

   a. _____

      1. _____

   b. _____

      1. _____

      2. _____

      3. _____

      4. _____

      5. _____

      6. _____

      7. _____

      8. _____

11. List the three meninges, describing their location and function as given in the text.

   a. _____

   b. _____

   c. _____

12. What are the spaces called between the (a) dura mater and the arachnoid and (b) the arachnoid and the pia?

   a. _____

   b. _____

13. Name the fluid within the cavities of the CNS and describe its function. _____

   _____

14. Matching: Match the diagnostic tests in column I with their purpose in column II.

   COLUMN I                              COLUMN II

   _____  1. Arteriography            a. Detects abnormal electrical impulses in the brain

   _____  2. Brain scan               b. To detect tumors, bleeding, clots, brain size, and
                                           edema

   _____  3. Glasgow Coma Scale       c. Measure cerebrospinal fluid pressure or obtain a
                                           sample of fluid

   _____  4. CAT scan                 d. Images enhanced with color

   _____  5. E.E.G.                   e. To detect cranial fractures or dense cerebral areas

   _____  6. Electromyography         f. Instill a dye or air to show irregularities in the CNS

   _____  7. Lumbar puncture          g. Detects cerebral hemorrhage, aneurysm, or CVA

   _____  8. Myelography              h. To detect neuromuscular disorders or nerve damage

   _____  9. Skull X ray              i. Radioisotopes measured to detect abnormal masses or
                                           blood vessel lesions

   _____  10. Position Emission Tomography    j. To describe the level of consciousness

15. Label the illustration with the following terms. Refer to Figure 11-35 the textbook.

Brainstem     Medulla     Sulci

Cerebellum     Midbrain     Temporal lobe

Cerebrum     Occipital lobe

Convolutions     Parietal lobe

Frontal lobe     Pons

**Lateral View**

16. Matching:  Match the letter of the disease or disorder with the symptoms given.

1. _____ Sudden, acute onset of fever, headache, and vomiting, which progresses to a stiff neck and back, drowsiness, and eventual coma.

2. _____ Blurred or double vision with sensations of tingling or numbness; periods of attacks and remission characterized by tremor, muscular weakness, and paralysis.

3. _____ Severe muscle rigidity, drooling, tremor, and a characteristic bent forward position when walking.

4. _____ Temporary double vision, slurred speech, dizziness, staggering, and falling.

5. _____ Loss of sensation with paralysis of one side of the body.

6. _____ Sharp, piercing pain in the back of the thigh extending down the side of the leg.

7. _____ Weakness and paralysis on one side of the face causing drooping mouth, drooling, and inability to close the affected eye.

8. _____ Fluid-filled vesicles on the skin associated with fever, severe deep pain, itching, and abnormal skin sensations.

9. _____ Seizures of varying duration, possible loss of consciousness, loss of body function control, and convulsions.

10. _____ Abnormally large head, distended scalp veins, shiny scalp skin, irritability, vomiting.

11. _____ Hyperactive tendon reflexes, underdeveloped affected extremities, muscular contractions; may also have seizures, mental retardation, and impaired speech.

12. _____ High fever, chills, headache, positive Brudzinski's and Kernig's signs.

13. _____ Severe pain along the course of a nerve anywhere in the body.

14. _____ Excruciating facial pain upon stimulation of a trigger zone.

15. _____ Paralysis with loss of sensation and reflexes in lower extremities.

16. _____ Muscular weakness and atrophy; problems with speech, chewing, and swallowing; respirations may be affected; choking and drooling.

17. _____ Prodromal symptoms of fatigue, visual disturbances, tingling of face and lips, sensitivity to light, nausea, and vomiting.

18. _____ Incomplete closure of one or more vertebra, bladder and bowel control problems, hydrocephalus, weakness or paralysis of legs, often mental retardation.

19. _____ Vomiting, lethargy, liver dysfunction, hyperventilation, delirium and coma, with eventual respiratory arrest.

a.  Amyotrophic lateral sclerosis
b.  Bell's palsy
c.  Cerebral palsy
d.  Encephalitis
e.  Epilepsy
f.  Herpes zoster
g.  Hemiplegia
h.  Hydrocephalus
i.  Meningitis
j.  Migraine headache
k.  Multiple sclerosis
l.  Neuralgia
m. Paraplegia
n.  Parkinson's disease
o.  Reye's syndrome
p.  Sciatica
q.  Spina bifida
r.  Transient ischemic attack
s.  Trigeminal neuralgia

17. Refer to the ABHES Course Content Requirements in Appendix C of the textbook. Within the area of *Anatomy and Physiology,* which content requirements are discussed in this unit? _____

_____

18. Crossword Puzzle

ACROSS

4. Posterior lobe of cerebrum
8. Nerve that causes action or movement
9. Contains sensory nerve cell bodies
10. Nerve of vision
11. Acronym for multiple sclerosis
12. Cavity within the brain

DOWN

1. Portion of CNS in cranium
2. Membrane covering CNS
3. Small brain part at top of brain stem
5. The skull
6. Part of peripheral nervous system
7. Portion of cerebrum behind forehead

**CRITICAL THINKING SCENARIOS:  What would your response be in the following situations?**

1. Mr. Burns recently suffered a CVA that caused damage to the right side of his brain. He has difficulty with his left leg and has numbness in his left arm and hand. He cannot understand why his left side is affected.

_____
_____
_____

2. Yesterday your nephew was severely injured in a motorcycle accident. Your brother is very concerned because his son has no apparent sensations or control of his body from the waist down. Can you give him any encouragement? _____

_____
_____

3. A patient phones the office complaining of painful blisters on the right side of his chest. He wants the doctor to call the pharmacy to order something to put on them. _____

_____
_____
_____

4. A female patient calls late Saturday morning complaining of severe throbbing headache with nausea and sensitivity to light. It has been going for for the past 12 hours, and she's afraid she is having a stroke. She is very frightened. _____

_____
_____
_____

5. A male patient tells you that on two separate occasions he has had "spells" of double vision, dizziness, and a tendency to lose his balance and fall. He says it only lasts about a half day so it's probably just old age and he's not going to bother the doctor about it. _____

_____

After your instructor has returned your work to you, make all necessary corrections and place in a three-ring notebook for future reference.

**ASSIGNMENT SHEET**

## Chapter 11:  ANATOMY AND PHYSIOLOGY OF THE HUMAN BODY

## Unit 3:  THE SENSES

### A.  Mixed Quiz

1. List the five senses of the human body and identify the organ(s) responsible for the perception.

   a. _See — eyes_
   b. _hear — ear_
   c. _taste — tounge_
   d. _smell — noise_
   e. _touch — skin_

2. Labeling:  Add labels to each part of the eye. Refer to Figure 11-43 in the textbook.

   | | |
   |---|---|
   | Anterior chamber | Optic nerve |
   | Choroid | Path of light |
   | Ciliary body | Posterior chamber |
   | Conjunctiva | Pupil |
   | Cornea | Retina |
   | Fovea centralis | Sclera |
   | Iris | Vitreous body |
   | Lens | |

Conjuctiva
CORNEA
IRiS
Pupil
Path of Light
Lens
Anterior chamber
Posterior chamber
Suspensory ligament
ciliary body and Muscle

Retina
Retina arteries and veins
Optic nerve
choroid coat
Sclera

Name _____

3. Name the structures of the eye through which light passes in the process of sight.
   a. _Light Rays through the cornea_
   b. _on through the Aqueous humor_
   c. _the pupil_
   d. _the lens_
   e. _onto the vitreous humor_
   f. _Focusing out the breaks & eyeball on the retina_
4. Explain the function of the lens and the process of accommodation. _lens is automatically_
_altered by salavary muscles of the body, to the_
_focus objects into the retina when sum body contracts,_
_the lens becomes rounder in a process_
5. How does the cornea affect vision? _curvature of the cornea corrects_
_some of the unclear image that the edge of lens_
_projects being that cornea light passes through_
6. Name the two humors and describe their purpose. _won't interfere a/vision._
   a. _Aqueous humor_
   1. _salty, clear fluid, maintains curvicture_
   2. _Asoits on the refraction process_
   b. _vitreous tumor_
   1. _Aids in refraction_
   2. _Maintains shape of the eyeball_
7. Matching: Match the disease or disorder of the eye in column II with the major symptoms in column I.

COLUMN I

| | |
|---|---|
| G | 1. Scratch from foreign body or injury to the cornea |
| D | 2. Red-rimmed, crusted eyelids with scales, itching, and burning |
| J | 3. Aching, loss of peripheral vision, visual halos around lights |
| P | 4. Visual deviation of the eyeball, blurred or double vision |
| N | 5. Drooping of the upper eyelid |
| B | 6. Inward turning of one eye with blurred vision |
| F | 7. Redness, pain, occasional discharge caused by an infectious microbe |
| E | 8. Painless, gradual visual blurring and loss of vision |
| H | 9. Pain, especially on blinking; excessive tearing; exudate; irregular cornea; blurred vision |
| K | 10. Red, painful swelling of gland of the eyelid |
| M | 11. Inability to accommodate for near vision |
| O | 12. Visual floating spots, light flashes, and gradual vision loss |
| I | 13. Glare, blurred vision, reduced visual acuity, eventual blindness |
| C | 14. A thin grayish-white circle at edge of cornea |
| A | 15. Gradual loss of central vision |
| L | 16. Vision is blurred except close objects due to misshapen eyeball |

COLUMN II

a. Age-related macular degeneration
b. Amblyopia
c. Arcus senilis
d. Blepharitis
e. Cataract
f. Conjunctivitis
g. Corneal abrasion
h. Corneal ulcers
i. iabetic retinopathy
j. Glaucoma
k. Hordeolum
l. Myopia
m. Presbyopia
n. Ptosis
o. Detached retina
p. Strabismus

8. Labeling: Label the illustration of the outer, middle, and inner ear using the following terms. Refer to Figures 11-50 and 11-51 in the textbook.

| Outer and Middle Ear | Inner Ear |
|---|---|
| Auricle | Cochlea |
| Cochlea | Cochlear nerve |
| Eustachian tube | Lateral semicircular canal |
| External auditory canal | Oval window |
| Incus | Posterior semicircular canal |
| Malleus | Superior semicircular canal |
| Semicircular canals | Vestibular nerve |
| Stapes | Vestibule |
| Tympanic membrane | |
| Vestibulocochlear nerve | |

9. Explain how sounds are heard. _the ear Receives vibrations in the air translates it to sounds. vibrations are picked up by the pinna to the external auditory canal to the tympanic menbrane. Sand waves vibrate the menbrane the malleus to the incus true moves_

10. How is equilibrium maintained? _eustachian tube is responsibl for eaualizing air pressure_

_____

11. Matching: Match the major symptoms in column II with the diseases and disorders of the ear in column I.

COLUMN I

_D_ 1. Auditory canal obstruction

_E_ 2. Ménière's disease

_A_ 3. Motion sickness

_F_ 4. Otitis externa

_B_ 5. Otitis media

_C_ 6. Otosclerosis

_G_ 7. Presbycusis

COLUMN II

a. Loss of equilibrium, headache, nausea and vomiting due to movement

b. Severe, deep, throbbing pain, fever, hearing loss, nausea and vomiting, dizziness, bulging eardrum

c. Slow, progressive conduction hearing loss

d. A degree of hearing loss, possible discomfort; may be a foreign body

e. Severe vertigo, tinnitus, nerve hearing loss, nausea and vomiting

f. Infection in auditory canal, pain, fever, conduction hearing loss

g. Loss of ability to hear high-frequency sounds, tinnitus, possible depression

12. Describe the structure of the olfactory organ and explain how an odor can be detected. _the sense of smell is caused by the factory organ. Nerve fibe respond to stimuli from ions or molecules dissolu in the moisture from the mucous._

13. Define the following terms:
    a. Epistaxis _nose bled_
    b. Allergic rhinitis _Rhinitis to the airbone allergens_
    c. Nasal polyp _benign growths, usually multiple in both sides of nose_

Incus

Malleus

Semicircular canals

Auricle

Branches of vestibulocochlear Nerve

cochlea

External auditory CANAL

Auditory

tymphanic membrane

Stapes and foot plate

Superior Semicicular CANAL

Posterior Semicircular canal

vestibular nerve

cochlear NERVE

Lateral Semicircular CANAL

cochlea

vestibule

oval window

171

14. Labeling: Label the taste receptors of the tongue in the following illustration. Refer to Figure 11-53 in the textbook.

Bitter
Sour
Salt
Sweet

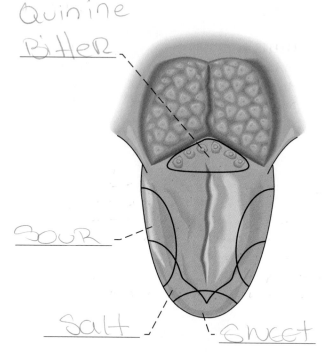

Quinine
Bitter
Sour
Salt
Sweet

15. Identify the touch sensations that are perceivable by the skin.

   a. pressure
   b. hot
   c. pain
   d. touch
   e. cold
   f. traction
   g. tickle

16. Refer to the Role Delineation Chart in Appendix A of the textbook. Within the area of *Administrative Procedures,* which role relates to the content of this unit's *Words to Know?* _____

17. Word Search: Find the following words hidden in the puzzle.

| | | |
|---|---|---|
| BUD | HUMOR | SEE |
| CATARACT | IRIS | SENSATION |
| CHOROID | LENS | SENSES |
| COCHLEA | MOTOR | SENSORY |
| CONJUNCTIVA | NOSE | SIGHT |
| CORNEA | OPTIC | SMELL |
| EAR | OTITIS | STAPES |
| EYE | PUPIL | TASTE |
| GLAUCOMA | RETINA | TOUCH |
| HEAR | SCLERA | VISION |

```
H O P T I C O C H L E A V X G
B U D C U S M E L L B M N E L
I P M H Q H E A R I O V M R A
S E E O Y S E N S A T I O N U
T I B R R C T A S T E S T U C
A O R O E O O R L E Q I O E O
P U P I L R U S E N S O R Y M
E W U D S N C I N T U N E E A
S I G H T E H E S O I L O V N
C A T A R A C T I E I N E S R
C O N J U N C T I V A U A C E
Y T O T I T I S C L E R A M C
```

18. Unscramble

a. _ _ _ _ _ _ _        UAOUEQS

b. _ _ _ _ _ _ _ _        NUSITNTI

c. _ _ _ _ _ _        ASTESP

d. _ _ _ _ _ _ _        ODHOCIR

e. _ _ _ _ _ _ _        HCEOLCA

f. _ _ _ _ _ _ _ _        ALPEIALP

g _ _ _ _ _ _ _ _        ATCRAATC

h. _ _ _ _ _ _ _ _        AMLCIRAL

i. _ _ _ _ _ _ _ _        UESTVOIR

**CRITICAL THINKING SCENARIOS: What would your response be in the following situations?**

1. A little girl in preschool with your child has one eye that turns inward. The mother feels it is just temporary and her daughter will grow out of it—besides, it is only bad when she is tired. _____

_____

_____

2. Your grandmother calls and in the process of your conversation complains that she is getting too old to drive at night. She says the oncoming lights make it very difficult for her to see. _____

_____

_____

_____

3. A patient calls to ask for an appointment to bring in one of her children who has a red, painful eye. It was, swollen a little this morning when he got up. _____

_____

_____

_____

4. A neighbor's 22-year-old son seems to be losing his hearing. His mother blames it on loud rock music. She said the same thing happened to his father when he was about 35 from noisy machinery at work. _____

_____

_____

5. A male patient proudly announced he has quit smoking. You notice he has a small bulge under his lower lip. You suspect it might be some form of smokeless tobacco. _____

_____

_____

After your instructor has returned your work to you, make all necessary corrections and place in a three-ring notebook for future reference.

**ASSIGNMENT SHEET**

**Chapter 11: ANATOMY AND PHYSIOLOGY OF THE HUMAN BODY**

**Unit 4: THE INTEGUMENTARY SYSTEM**

**A. Mixed Quiz**

1. List the five functions of the skin.
   a. _protection_
   b. _perception_
   c. _temperature control._
   d. _absorption._
   e. _excretion._
2. How does the skin regulate body temperature? _____
   _____
3. How does the body cool its surface? _____
   _____
4. List the three layers of skin tissue; identify the characteristic structure of each layer.
   a. _epidermis=(top) full of ridges that fit snugly_
      _over the papillae._
   b. _dermis=(middle) Blood vessels, nerves, hair_
      _follicles, sweat, oil glands,_
   c. _subcutaneous=(Bottom) filled w/ fat globules, Blood vessels,_
5. What causes wrinkles? _nerves._____
   _____
6. Why does exposure to the sun cause the skin to turn darker? _____
   _____
   _____
7. Why does the skin become red when a person blushes? _____
   _____
8. What causes birthmarks? _____
9. What is a mole? _____
10. Define *albinism* and describe the main characteristics of the condition. _____
    _____
    _____

11. Matching: Match the lesion in column I with its correct description in column II.

    COLUMN I          COLUMN II
    _____ Macule      1. A small, circumscribed lesion filled with exudate and lymph.
    _____ Papule      2. A round lesion with a white center and a red periphery that usually itches.
    _____ Pustule     3. A various colored spot that is neither elevated nor depressed.
    _____ Vesicle     4. A solid, elevated circular red mass about a pinhead to a pea in size.
    _____ Wheal       5. A blisterlike, elevated mass containing serous fluid.

12. Identify the ABCD rules of melanoma.
    a. _____
    b. _____
    c. _____
    _____
    d. _____

13. Spelling: Each line contains four different spellings of a word. Underline the correctly spelled word.

| | | | |
|---|---|---|---|
| dermatitus | dermatitis | dermitius | dermotitis |
| epidermis | epedermis | epdermus | epidermus |
| erathema | erithema | erythema | erethema |
| intagumentary | integumentary | integumintary | integumentary |
| psoriasis | psariasis | psoriase | spsorisis |
| sabeceous | sebacous | sebaceous | sebaceus |
| subcutanous | subcutaneous | subcuteneous | subcutaenus |
| urticaria | urtacaria | urtecaria | urticarea |
| varrucai | varrucea | verrucae | varrucae |
| alopecia | alopechia | alepecia | alapechia |
| eggsama | egsema | egzema | eczema |
| mellonoma | melanoma | mellenoma | malemoma |
| leson | leshion | lesion | leishon |

14. Word Puzzle: Use the clues listed to spell out these terms.

```
— — — I — —              Eruption
— — — — N — —            A pigment
— — — T — — — —          A lesion with exudate
— — — — — E — — —        Provides lubrication
— — G — — — —            Color
— — — — U — — — — — — —   A skin layer
— — — M — —              The real thing
— E — — — — —            A blisterlike lesion
— — — — N —              Pale
— — — T — —              Organs working together
— — — A — —              With allergy
— — — R — — — — —        A chronic condition
— — Y — — — — —          Sun effect
```

15. Refer to the CAAHEP Standards in Appendix B of the textbook. Within the area of *Anatomy and Physiology*, which curriculum standards are discussed in this unit? _____

_____

16. Matching: Match the main disease characteristics in column I with the disease or disorder in column II.

COLUMN I                                                                          COLUMN II

_____ 1. Dry skin, redness, itching, edema, scaling.                             a. Scabies

_____ 2. A small red macule becomes a vesicle and then                           b. Psoriasis
         changes into a pustule with yellow crust and outer rim.                 c. Urticaria

_____ 3. A thickened scar.                                                       d. Dermatitis

_____ 4. Itching red papules covered with silvery scales.                        e. Verrucae

_____ 5. Flat lesion that can be dry and scaly or moist and                      f. Ringworm
         crusty. Has characteristic outer ring with clear center.                g. Impetigo

_____ 6. Threadlike red nodules at the inner wrists, elbows,                      h. Keloid
         between fingers, and in axilla.                                         i. Lyme disease

_____ 7. Distinct raised wheals surrounded by reddened areas;                    j. Herpes simplex
         they usually itch.                                                      k. Pediculosis capitus

_____ 8. Rough, elevated, rounded surface, especially on the hands               l. Hirsutism
         and fingers. Some forms appear on soles of feet and on genitalia.       m. Melanoma

_____ 9. A loss of hair, usually on the scalp.                                   n. Eczema

_____ 10. A lesion exhibiting some of the ABCD characteristics.                  o. Alopecia

_____ 11. Red, dry, itching, and scaly skin; occurs in both acute                p. Carbuncule
          and chronic forms, often producing watery discharge.

_____ 12. Cold sores or blisters on the mouth or face.

_____ 13. A deep abscess involving several follicles with multiple
          drainage points.

_____ 14. A bulls-eye rash and a bite site.

_____ 15. Oval, grayish, dandruff-appearing flecks, itching scalp,
          matted hair.

_____ 16. Excessive body hair on females and children, in an adult
          male growth pattern.

17. Matching: Match the definition in column II with the correct term in column I.

COLUMN I                          COLUMN II

_____ 1. Dermis                   a. Reddened, flat area with definite edge

_____ 2. Epidermis                b. Bottom layer of skin

_____ 3. Keloid                   c. Hives

_____ 4. Macule                   d. The middle layer of skin

_____ 5. Melanin                  e. Raised areas surrounded by reddened area

_____ 6. Pustule                  f. Raised lesion containing serous fluid

_____ 7. Subcutaneous             g. Lesion with purulent material

_____ 8. Urticaria                h. The top layer of skin

_____ 9. Vesicle                  i. Pigment in the skin

_____ 10. Wheals                  j. An overgrowth of scar tissue

_____ 11. Whorl                   k. The lack of skin pigment

                                  l. An oil gland

                                  m. Fingerprints

**CRITICAL THINKING SCENARIOS: What would your response be in the following situations?**

1. You are following a co-worker up the stairs when you notice a suspicious-looking mole on the back of her right calf. _____
   _____
   _____

2. Your family spent a recent Fall weekend camping in a beautiful wooded area. Your son had a large round reddened area with a circle-shaped center on his leg, but now it is gone. _____
   _____
   _____

3. Your child comes home from school with a note saying one of her classmates has head lice. _____
   _____
   _____
   _____

After your instructor has returned your work to you, make all necessary corrections and place in a three-ring notebook for future reference.

4. A co-worker has just returned from sick leave due to tuberculosis. She appears well and looks much better than when she was diagnosed. She has been on medication for the past six weeks. You overhear other co-workers say they are not going to get too close to her and make remarks about her being back to work that are very unkind. _____

_____

_____

After your instructor has returned your work to you, make all necessary corrections and place in a three-ring notebook for future reference.

**ASSIGNMENT SHEET**

**Chapter 11:  ANATOMY AND PHYSIOLOGY OF THE HUMAN BODY**

**Unit 8:  THE CIRCULATORY SYSTEM**

**A.  Mixed Quiz**

1.  List the four major parts of the circulatory system.

    a.  _____

    b.  _____

    c.  _____

    d.  _____

2.  Labeling:  Label the following structures of the heart on the illustration below:  apex, right atrium (auricle), left atrium (auricle), right ventricle, left ventricle, aorta, pulmonary semilunar valve, tricuspid valve, inferior vena cava, septum, bicuspid (mitral) valve, aortic semilunar valve, right pulmonary artery, left pulmonary artery, superior vena cava. Refer to Figure 11-115 in the textbook.

(from upper part of body)

Endocardium

Myocardium

(from lower part of body)

3. What is the difference between pulmonary and systemic circulation? _____

_____

_____

4. Describe the heart sounds and what heart action causes the sound. Identify where the sounds may be auscultated.

| Sound | Caused by | Where auscultated |
|-------|-----------|-------------------|
|       |           |                   |
|       |           |                   |

5. Describe the location and action of the pacemaker. _____

_____

_____

6. Explain how the action of the pacemaker is related to the symptoms of heart block and fibrillation. _____

_____

_____

_____

7. What causes arrhythmia? _____

_____

8. Describe the characteristics of bigeminal and trigeminal rhythm. _____

_____

9. What purpose does an artificial pacemaker serve and how does it function? _____

_____

10. Explain how the rate of the heartbeat is controlled. _____

_____

_____

11. List the five types of blood vessels, explaining the structure and function of each type.

| TYPE | STRUCTURE | FUNCTION |
|------|-----------|----------|
| a. _____ | _____ | _____ |
| b. _____ | _____ | _____ |
| c. _____ | _____ | _____ |
| d. _____ | _____ | _____ |
| e. _____ | _____ | _____ |

12. How does a capillary bed function? _____

_____

_____

13. Trace the pathway of blood through the pulmonary and systemic circulation beginning at the vena cava, going to a capillary of the body, and returning to the atrium of the heart. Name the structures of the heart and lungs, and the major vessels. _____

_____

_____

_____

14. From where does the blood in the portal circulation come? Where does it go, and why? _____

_____

15. Fill in the Blank

The lymphatic system consists of lymph vessels, which are located throughout the body. Lymph capillaries _____ and other substances and return them to the circulatory system. The system is a _____ system; there are no vessels bringing _____ to the _____ The capillaries join to become _____ which in turn become larger vessels called _____ The lymphatics eventually form two main _____ a _____ duct and a _____ duct. _____ are located along lymph vessels at various places in the body. During an infection, the nodes become _____ and _____ because of the collection of lymphocytes.

16. List four actions of the spleen.

a. _____

b. _____

c. _____

d. _____

17. Name five things that blood transports through the body.

a. _____

b. _____

c. _____

d. _____

e. _____

18. What is plasma? List 17 things that can be found circulating in plasma. _____

_____

a. _____     g. _____     m. _____

b. _____     h. _____     n. _____

c. _____     i. _____     o. _____

d. _____     j. _____     p. _____

e. _____     k. _____     q. _____

f. _____     l. _____

19. List the three types of blood cells, describing the basic function of each.

a. _____

b. _____

c. _____

20. Why is blood typed and crossmatched before being given to a patient? _____

_____

_____

21. Why is the Rh factor especially important with a pregnancy or a transfusion? _____

_____

_____

_____

_____

22. Spelling: Each line contains four different spellings of a word. Underline the correctly spelled word.

| a. | excelerator | axcelerater | accelerator | accelerater |
|----|-------------|-------------|-------------|-------------|
| b. | aneurysm | aneruism | anurysm | anurism |
| c. | bradicardia | bradycardea | bradecardia | bradycardia |
| d. | endecardium | endocardium | endocardeum | endecardeum |
| e. | erythrocyte | erithrocyte | erythrocite | erithrocite |
| f. | hemaglobin | hemoglobin | hemogloben | hemagloben |
| g. | eschemea | eschemia | ischemea | ischemia |
| h. | murmer | murrmur | murmur | murmmur |
| i. | myocardium | myocardeum | myacardium | myacardeum |
| j. | phelebitis | phlebities | phlebitus | phlebitis |
| k. | tachycardea | tachycardia | tachicardia | tachicardea |
| l. | varecose | varicose | veracose | vericose |
| m. | arrhythmea | arrhythmia | arrhthmia | arrhthmya |
| n. | ischemic | eshcemic | ishemic | ishcemic |

23. Matching: Match the cardiovascular tests in column I with the appropriate purpose for conducting it in column II).

COLUMN I

_____ 1. Arteriograph
_____ 2. Cardiac catheterization
_____ 3. Doppler ultrasonography
_____ 4. Echocardiograph
_____ 5. Electrocardiograph
_____ 6. Holter monitor
_____ 7. Venogram
_____ 8. Muga scan

COLUMN II

a. To evaluate cardiac function and structure, and to detect defects by means of sound waves

b. To detect irregularly occurring symptoms or evaluate status of a recovering cardiac patient

c. Detects condition of deep veins of the legs, especially deep vein thrombosis

d. To inject dye to indicate the status of blood flow, malformed vessels, aneurysm, or hemorrhage

e. To evaluate major blood vessels to determine deep vein thrombosis, peripheral aneurysms, and occluded carotid arteries

f. To identify heart rhythm, electrolyte imbalance, and conduction abnormalities

g. To visualize by fluoroscope the internal heart structure and activity and to visualize the coronary arteries

h. Determine condition of myocardium

24. Refer to the Role Delineation Chart in Appendix A of the textbook. Within the area of *Instruction,* which roles would be benefited by the content of this unit when trying to help patients conform to the physician's orders?

_____

_____

25. Matching: Match the major symptom or description in column II with the disease or disorder in column I.

COLUMN I

_____ 1. Anemia
_____ 2. Aneurysm
_____ 3. Angina
_____ 4. Arrest
_____ 5. Arrhythmia
_____ 6. Arteriosclerosis
_____ 7. Atherosclerosis
_____ 8. Athletic heart syndrome
_____ 9. CVA
_____ 10. CHF
_____ 11. Coronary artery disease
_____ 12. Embolus
_____ 13. Endocarditis
_____ 14. Hypertension
_____ 15. Hypotension
_____ 16. Leukemia
_____ 17. Murmur
_____ 18. MI
_____ 19. Myocarditis
_____ 20. Pericarditis
_____ 21. Phlebitis
_____ 22. Sickle cell anemia
_____ 23. Stasis ulcer
_____ 24. Thrombophlebitis
_____ 25. Varicosities

COLUMN II

a. Sharp, sudden pain at sternum radiating to back of shoulders and arms; decreases when erect or leaning forward

b. A circulating foreign substance in a blood vessel

c. Irregular heart rhythm

d. Fatty deposits on the lining of blood vessels

e. Severe chest pain from a coronary artery spasm

f. Pounding heartbeats after exercise, enlarged heart, slow pulse

g. Blood pressure consistently above normal

h. Congestion of blood in the circulatory system, edema of extremities and lungs

i. Tightness of chest, substernal chest pain radiating down left arm, nausea and vomiting, perspiration, fainting

j. Lack of red blood cells and/or hemoglobin

k. Rigid arterial walls; causes hypertension

l. Confusion, weakness of one side, visual changes, paralysis, personality change

m. A bulging arterial wall that may produce palpitations or tear

n. Complete sudden cessation of heart action

o. Mild chest soreness, fever, dyspnea, palpitations, feeling of pressure

p. Vegetative growths or inflammation of inner heart structures

q. Abnormally shaped red blood cells, enlarged liver, pallor, painful crisis periods

r. Skin breakdown from inadequate circulation

s. Excessive WBCs, bruising, fatigue, painful lymph nodes

t. Inflamed vein lining with thrombus formation, severe pain, fever, chills, and discoloration of involved extremity

u. Dilated, twisted veins, inefficient valves, leg cramps

v. A gurgling or swishing sound heard upon auscultation of the heart

w. Localized inflammation of a vein

x. Severe, crushing pain radiating through chest to neck and jaw and down left arm; nausea, dyspnea

y. Consistently low blood pressure

26. Word Search: Find the following words hidden in the puzzle.

| | | |
|---|---|---|
| ADENITIS | CARDIAC | MURMUR |
| AMBULATE | CORONARY | NODES |
| ANEMIA | DIASTOLE | PLASMA |
| ANGINA | EXUDATE | SPLEEN |
| AORTA | HEART | SYSTOLE |
| ARTERIOLES | HEMOGLOBIN | TACHYCARDIA |
| ARTERY | INFARCT | VAGUS |
| ATRIAL | ISCHEMIA | VALVE |
| ATRIUM | LEUKEMIA | VENTRICLE |
| BICUSPID | LYMPH | VENULE |
| CAPILLARY | MITRAL | |

```
A L E U K E M I A V E N U L E
V N H E M O G L O B I N I W V
A D E N I T I S C H E M I A E
G N A M B U L A T E C T G C N
U E R I I A T I N F A R C T T
S X T T C A T C N G D N E S R
S U O R A R O A T R I U M Y I
C D O A R T E R Y D A N X S C
O A T L E E R D T L S R A T L
R T P Q B R V I C A T X R O E
O E S I E I D A A H O P M L P
N L U P L O C C L L A U E A
A O D Y L L R U P V E Y R Y R
R E D A X E A R S C E P M E P
Y L U E D S E R T P O A U P A
P P L A S M A N Y H I R R Y H
R E L T A C H Y C A R D I A P
```

**CRITICAL THINKING SCENARIOS: What would your response be in the following situations?**

1. A female patient calls and is very concerned because she has just noticed a couple lumps in her left axilla. They are not tender and seem to be shaped like large beans. _____

_____

_____

2. A male patient who has angina calls to report that he has been experiencing severe chest pains off and on for the past two days. He is perspiring profusely and has had constant pain for the past 20 minutes. He has used four nitroglycerin tablets, but they are not working. _____

_____

_____

_____

_____

3. A female patient has been under treatment for two years for hypertension. She has lost 50 pounds and is getting regular exercise and watching her diet. Last time she was in the office, over three months ago, her blood pressure had been normal for about six months and she thought she was cured. Today, it is elevated again.

_____

_____

_____

_____

4. You have gone to your spouse's company picnic. About one-half hour after eating several people began playing ball. A man made a hit and ran to first base, but then he grabbed his chest and fell to the ground. He complained of a crushing chest pain that went up to his jaw and down his left arm. He was also nauseated, perspiring, and short of breath. _____

_____

_____

_____

_____

After your instructor has returned your work to you, make all necessary corrections and place in a three-ring notebook for future reference.

**ASSIGNMENT SHEET**

## Chapter 11: ANATOMY AND PHYSIOLOGY OF THE HUMAN BODY

## Unit 9: THE IMMUNE SYSTEM

*Note:* This material is challenging. Concentrate on what you read and write and it will be easier. Keeping your immune system strong is vital to your health and well-being. The more you understand, the better your chances of avoiding severe illness.

### A. Mixed Quiz

1. What are antigens? _____

2. List five types of antigens. _____

3. Name five kinds of foreign materials. _____

4. What are the body's three *main* lines of defense against antigens? _____

   _____

5. What are the six components of the immune system? _____

   _____

6. Fill in the Blank

   All blood cells originate in the _____ and initially develop from _____ Erythrocytes develop from _____ and mature in the bone marrow. Granulated white blood cells develop from _____ stem cells. One type of agranulocyte, the _____ develops from a _____ stem cell into two major classes, _____ which mature in the _____ and _____ which mature in the _____ Mononuclear phagocyte stem cells become the _____ which circulate in the blood and then enter the tissues to become _____ Phagocytes are cells that _____ and _____ Neutrophils carry _____ with _____ to destroy microorganisms. Neutrophils _____ and _____ invading _____ _____ and other _____ Eosinophils are produced in large _____ in response to _____ infections.

7. Name the organs of the immune system.

   a. _____    f. _____

   b. _____    g. _____

   c. _____    h. _____

   d. _____    i. _____

   e. _____    j. _____

8. How is the stage of cancer determined? _____

   _____

9. Name the four types of T-lymphocyte cells. _____

10. How does a B-lymphocyte destroy an antigen? _____

11. Fill in the Blank

    The process of antibody-mediated response and other chemicals also cause an _____ Basophils and mast cells release _____ which _____ and makes them more _____ This _____ blood flow and allows _____ to seep into the surrounding tissues. This results in _____ _____ and _____

Name _____

12. Natural killer cells (NK) destroy _____ and _____ They contain _____
filled with _____ They are called natural because they do not need to recognize a specific
antigen like other T cells to kill the invading antigen. NK cells _____ to their targets and deliver a
_____ of _____ to produce _____ in a cell's membrane, which _____
the cell.

13. There are two branches of immune response, _____ which results from B cell activity,
and _____ which results from _____ activity. Response can also be _____
which means the _____ encounter, or _____ ( _____ encounters). A primary
response requires _____ to _____ days to develop. Antibody-mediated responses act against
_____ and _____ and _____ It cannot react to
microorganisms already within a cell's _____ Only those in _____ or _____
to a cell's _____ Secondary response requires _____ or _____ days because of the
_____ with memory. _____ responses attack _____
_____ _____ and _____

14. Why do killer cells cause rejection of an organ transplant? _____

_____

15. What stops an immune response? _____

16. a. How do immunizations and vaccines provide protection against antigens? _____

_____

b. Active immunity means _____

c. Passive immunity means _____

17. Name the body fluids in which the AIDS virus survives the best.
a. _____
b. _____
c. _____

18. Identify four early symptoms of HIV infection. _____

19. Name seven additional symptoms of HIV infection that occur later. _____

_____

20. List the three infections that are signs of AIDS. _____

_____

21. Name the diagnostic tests that verify the presence of HIV antibodies or antigens.
a. _____
b. _____
c. _____

22. What actions would prevent acquiring the HIV virus? _____

_____

23. What can trigger allergic symptoms?
a. _____   f. _____
b. _____   g. _____
c. _____   h. _____
d. _____   i. _____
e. _____   j. _____

24. What occurs when a person experiences anaphylactic shock? _____

_____

25. What is cancer? _____

_____

26. Name the four classifications of cancer. _____

27. What do the terms *differentiated* and *undifferentiated* mean? _____
_____

28. Name the 3 types of procedures used to diagnose cancer. _____

29. Identify and explain the goals of cancer therapy.
_____
_____
_____
_____

30. What are the major methods of treatment for cancer? _____
_____

31. What are some promoted alternative "cures." _____

32. List nine complementary therapies. _____
_____
_____

33. What is a clinical trial? _____

34. Name the three forms of lupus. _____
_____

35. Describe rheumatoid arthritis. _____
_____

36. What is lymphedema? _____

37. Word Puzzle: Use the clues listed to spell out these terms.

| Puzzle | Clue |
|---|---|
| _ _ _ I _ _ _ _ | Belongs to immunoglobulin family |
| _ _ _ _ _ _ M _ _ _ | Starts a chain reaction |
| _ _ M _ _ _ _ | Type of immunity |
| _ _ _ U _ | Organism |
| _ N _ _ _ _ _ | Foreign matter |
| _ E _ _ _ _ | Harmless |
| _ _ _ _ _ - _ _ _ _ _ _ _ | T-cell activated |
| _ _ _ _ S _ _ | Small sample |
| _ _ Y _ _ _ | An organ |
| _ _ _ _ _ _ S _ _ _ | Cancer cell |
| _ _ T _ _ _ _ _ _ | Secondary growth |
| _ E _ _ _ _ _ _ | Controlled |
| _ _ _ M _ _ _ _ _ _ _ | A drug treatment |

38. Refer to the Role Delineation Chart in Appendix A of the textbook. Within the area of Patient Care, which role would apply to the content of this unit if it were necessary to refer a patient? _____
_____

## CRITICAL THINKING SCENARIOS: What would your response be in the following situations?

1. You notice one of your co-workers looks and acts very tired. Recently she has lost about 15 pounds and has had a cold. She has a little congestion in her chest, which is making her short of breath and causing her to cough. When you talk to her about it, she breaks down and cries, telling you she is HIV-positive and is having a hard time dealing with it. She doesn't want you to tell anyone, especially the doctor, because she has to work to take care of herself and her child. She's afraid she will lose her job. _____
_____
_____
_____
_____

2. A neighbor has just been diagnosed as having lung cancer. He says he is not going to go through chemotherapy or radiation because he will just end up dying anyhow. He believes these treatments just make you feel worse while you are waiting for the inevitable. Instead, he is going to take the advice of a friend and send away for a cancer cure that's available in Mexico. _____

_____

_____

_____

_____

_____

3. A patient in her late 20s has just been told she has systemic lupus erythematosus. She has heard the disease is life-threatening and she is frightened. _____

_____

_____

_____

After your instructor has returned your work to you, make all necessary corrections and place in a three-ring notebook for future reference.

**ASSIGNMENT SHEET**

**Chapter 11: ANATOMY AND PHYSIOLOGY OF THE HUMAN BODY**

**Unit 10: THE DIGESTIVE SYSTEM**

**A. Mixed Quiz**

1. Define *digestion.* _____

   _____

   a. _____   e. _____
   b. _____   f. _____
   c. _____   g. _____
   d. _____

3. List, in order, the organs of the alimentary tract through which food passes.

   a. _____   d. _____
   b. _____   e. _____
   c. _____   f. _____

4. Labeling: Label the organs of digestion on the illustration using the following terms. Refer to Figure 11-155 in the textbook.

Ascending colon

Cecum

Descending colon

Esophagus

Gallbladder

Liver

Pancreas

Pharynx

Rectum

Sigmoid colon

Small intestine

Stomach

Teeth

Tongue

Transverse colon

Vermiform appendix

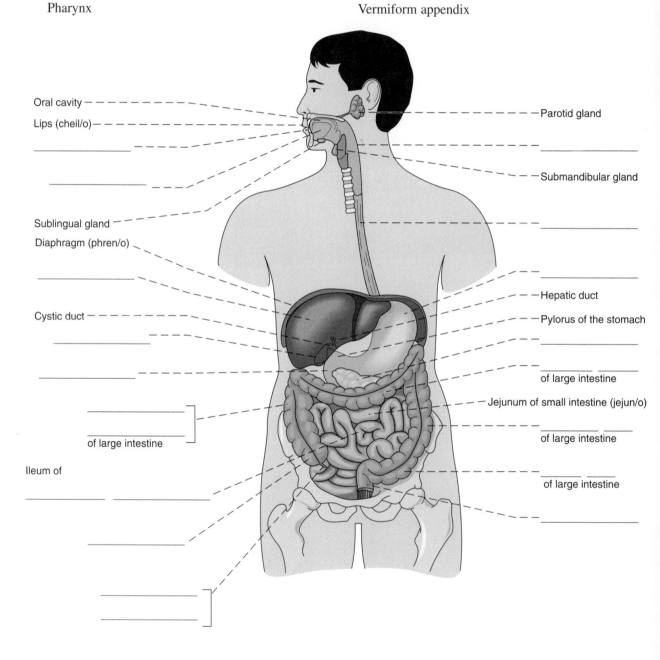

Oral cavity — — — — — — — — — — — — — — — — — — — — — — — — Parotid gland

Lips (cheil/o)— — — — — — — — — — — — — — — — — — — — — — — — —

_____ — — — — — — — — — — — — — — — — — — — _____

_____ — — — — — — — — — — — — — — — — — — — Submandibular gland

Sublingual gland — — — — — — — — — — — — — — — — — — — — — — _____

Diaphragm (phren/o) — — — — — — — — — — — — — — — — — — — — —

_____ — — — — — — — — — — — — — — — — — — — Hepatic duct

Cystic duct — — — — — — — — — — — — — — — — — — — — — — Pylorus of the stomach

_____ — — — — — — — — — — — — — — — — — — — _____

_____ — — — — — — — — — — — — — — — — — — — _____ _____
of large intestine

_____ ⌐ — — — — — — — — — — — — — Jejunum of small intestine (jejun/o)

_____ ⌐

of large intestine ⌐ — — — — — — — — — — — — — _____ _____
of large intestine

Ileum of

_____ _____ — — — — — — — — — — — — — _____ _____
of large intestine

_____ — — — — — — — — — — — — — _____

_____

_____ ⌐

5. List the accessory digestive organs of the mouth; explain their function in the digestive process.

a. _____

b. _____
_____

c. _____
_____
_____

6. a. What are the initial teeth called? _____

b. When do they appear? _____

c. Initial teeth are lost beginning about age _____ and are replaced by _____

d. Identify the four types of "secondary" teeth and their specific duties.

a) _____

b) _____

c) _____

d) _____

7. How is swallowing accomplished? _____
_____
_____

8. Labeling: Label the illustration of the structures involved in swallowing using the following terms. Refer to Figure 11-158 in the textbook.

Epiglottis
Food
Hard palate
Jawbone
Pharynx
Soft palate
Tongue
Trachea

Air

Sinus

(windpipe)                    (food tube)

9. How is food moved through the esophagus? _____
_____

10. Describe the structure of the stomach and explain its function. _____
_____
_____
_____
_____
_____
_____

11. Describe the structure of the small intestine, naming its sections and explaining its function. _____
_____
_____
_____
_____

12. What functions does the liver perform, including the relationship with the portal circulation?
   a. _____
   b. _____
   c. _____
   d. _____
   e. _____
   f. _____
   g. _____
   h. _____
   i. _____
   _____

13. What role does the gallbladder play, and how is it related to the liver? _____
_____
_____
_____

14. Labeling: Label the illustration using the following terms. Refer to Figure 11-161 in the textbook.

Common bile duct
Cystic duct
Duodenum
Gallbladder
Hepatic duct
Liver
Pancreas

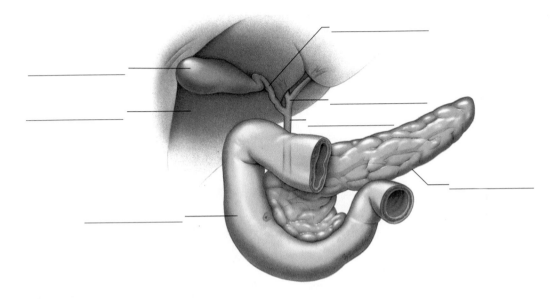

15. Explain why the duodenum is vital to digestion. _____
_____

16. Describe the location and function of the pancreas. _____
_____
_____

17. Where in the body are nutrients absorbed, and how is absorption accomplished? _____
_____
_____
_____

18. Explain the function of the colon and name its five sections.
_____

a. _____     d. _____
b. _____     e. _____
c. _____

19. What function does the rectum perform? _____
_____

20. Describe the structure and function of the anal canal. _____
_____
_____

21. Labeling: Label the illustration below using the following terms. Refer to Figure 11-164 in the textbook.

Anal canal                              Ileum
Anus                                    Internal anal sphincter muscle
Ascending colon                         Rectum
Cecum                                   Sigmoid colon
Descending colon                        Splenic flexure
External anal sphincter muscle          Transverse colon
Hepatic flexor                          Vermiform appendix
Ileocecal valve

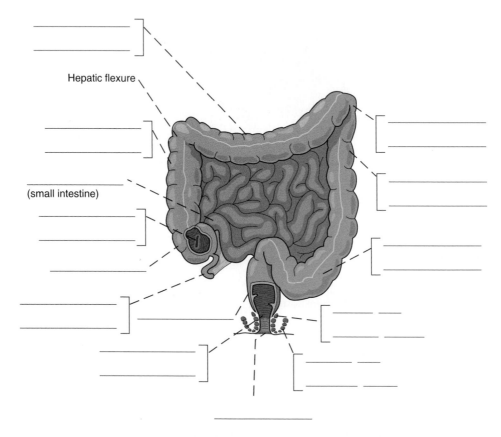

Hepatic flexure

(small intestine)

22. Multiple Choice: Circle the number for each question that best describes results of the test.

a. Cholecystography
   1. properly functioning gallbladder      4. bile duct obstruction
   2. non-functioning gallbladder           5. 2, 3, and 4
   3. cholelithiasis                        6. all of these

b. Barium swallow
   1. condition and function of esophagus   4. esophageal stricture
   2. esophageal varices                    5. duodenal ulcer
   3. diverticulitis                        6. 1, 2, and 4

c. Upper GI series
   1. gastric ulcer                         5. polyp of the colon
   2. tumor of stomach                      6. ulcerative colitis
   3. diverticulitis                        7. all but 5 and 6
   4. duodenal ulcer                        8. all of these

d. Lower GI series
   1. tumors of colon
   2. polyps
   3. ulcerative areas
   4. diverticula
   5. duodenal ulcer

6. gastric ulcer
7. hemorrhoids
8. 1, 2, 3, and 6
9. 1, 2, 3 and 4
10. 5, 6, and 7

e. Gastroscopy
   1. view growth for biopsy
   2. remove foreign objects
   3. obtain cells for study
   4. photograph sites

5. chemical damage determination
6. 1, 2, and 5
7. 2, 3, and 4
8. all of these

f. Nuclear and ultrasonography studies
   1. screen for disease processes
   2. locate infarcts
   3. locate cysts, tumors
   4. outline organ shape

5. detect functioning liver
6. 2, 3, and 4
7. all of these

g. Occult blood test
   1. detects mucus in feces
   2. detects blood in feces
   3. determines location of bleeding
   4. determines enzymes in stool

5. 1, 3, and 4
6. 2
7. 2, 3, and 4
8. all of these

h. Proctoscopy
   1. hemorrhoids
   2. colitis
   3. polyps of the sigmoid
   4. fistulas

5. rectal abscess
6. 1, 2, and 4
7. 1, 4, and 5
8. 2, 3, and 5

i. Sigmoidoscopy
   1. inflammation and infection
   2. ulcerations
   3. tumors
   4. polyps
   5. duodenal ulcers

6. condition of ileocecal valve
7. 2, 4, and 5
8. 3, 5, and 6
9. 1, 2, 3, and 4

23. Refer to the CAAHEP Standards in Appendix B of the textbook. Within the area of *Medical Assisting Clinical Procedures,* which curriculum standard is discussed in this unit? _____

24. Matching: Match the disease or conditions in column I with the appropriate symptoms or description in column II.

COLUMN I

_____ 1. Anorectal abscess or fistula
_____ 2. Cirrhosis
_____ 3. Colitis
_____ 4. Colostomy
_____ 5. Diarrhea
_____ 6. Diverticulitis
_____ 7. Esophageal varices
_____ 8. Anal fissure
_____ 9. Gastroenteritis
_____ 10. Hemorrhoids
_____ 11. Hepatitis
_____ 12. Hiatal hernia
_____ 13. Inguinal hernia
_____ 14. Ileostomy
_____ 15. Pancreatitis
_____ 16. Paralytic ileus
_____ 17. Peptic ulcer
_____ 18. Polyps
_____ 19. Pruritus ani
_____ 20. Pyloric stenosis
_____ 21. Spastic colon
_____ 22. Ulcerative colitis

COLUMN II

a. Frequent, liquid stools
b. Enlarged spleen, ascites, bloody emesis and stools, reduced platelets
c. Dilated anal veins, painful defecation, bleeding
d. Protruding mass at inguinal area or loop of intestine in scrotum
e. Tenderness and discomfort of the colon
f. Jaundice, hepatomegaly, loss of appetite, fatigue, clay-colored stools, weight loss
g. Absence of peristalsis, abdominal distention, distress, vomiting
h. Severe epigastric pain, not relieved by vomiting; a rigid abdomen, rales, tachycardia, fever, cold, perspiring extremities
i. Asymptomatic growths protruding from the intestinal lining
j. Painful, throbbing lump near the anus, with or without drainage
k. Fever, nausea and vomiting, abdominal cramps, travelers' diarrhea
l. Forceful vomiting, dilation of stomach, difficulty emptying contents of stomach into duodenum
m. Recurrent bloody diarrhea with mucus and exudate, weight loss, weakness, anorexia, nausea, vomiting, abdominal pain
n. Itching of anal area, especially following bowel movement, reddened skin, weeping and thickened skin, darkening of tissue
o. Lack of appetite, indigestion, nausea, vomiting, nosebleeds, bleeding gums, enlarged, firm liver, jaundice, ascites
p. Alternating periods of constipation and diarrhea, lower abdominal pain, daytime diarrhea, mucus stools
q. A single or double opening on abdomen through which solid fecal material passes
r. Heartburn, epigastric pain relieved by food, weight gain, bubbling hot water sensation
s. Opening of small intestine into the abdomen through which liquid stool is expelled
t. Bulging pouches in the intestine that cause abdominal pain, nausea, flatus, irregular bowel movements, high white blood cell count
u. Burning rectal pain with a few drops of blood with passing of stool, sentinel pile
v. Heartburn, regurgitation, vomiting, fullness, stomach spasms, difficulty swallowing, gastric reflux

25. Unscramble

a. _ _ _ _ _ _ _ _       EDPAXINP

b. _ _ _ _ _ _ _ _ _       HSIORCISR

c. _ _ _ _ _ _ _       ICOTSIL

d. _ _ _ _ _ _ _ _       EHARIDRA

e. _ _ _ _ _ _ _ _ _       EIGISOTND

f. _ _ _ _ _ _ _ _       UNDMEUOD

g. _ _ _ _ _ _ _ _ _       HSUOGSAEP

h. _ _ _ _ _ _ _ _ _ _       DLBALRAGLDE

i. _ _ _ _ _ _ _ _ _       SETIHATIP

j. _ _ _ _ _ _ _ _ _       EILCOELAC

k. _ _ _ _ _ _ _       UISNNIL

l. _ _ _ _ _ _ _ _       UCJADNIE

m. _ _ _ _ _ _       UANSAE

n. _ _ _ _ _ _ _ _       ARNPAESC

o. _ _ _ _ _ _ _       IDSMGIO

p. _ _ _ _ _ _ _ _       ESOSNTSI

q. _ _ _ _ _ _ _       HCTASMO

r. _ _ _ _ _ _       UOEGTN

s. _ _ _ _ _ _ _       SVIERAC

**CRITICAL THINKING SCENARIOS: What would your response be in the following situations?**

1. Joe is a weight lifter. He has been trying to increase his dead lift amount before the national competition. He has developed a tender area in his right groin that seems to protrude at times. _____

_____

2. Nancy has not felt well the past two days. She had a generalized pain in her abdomen that got increasingly more uncomfortable and then moved to the lower right quadrant. She was nauseated and didn't feel like eating. However, overnight the pain went away and she is feeling better. A friend suggested it was probably just PMS. _____

_____

3. A male patient called to schedule an appointment. He is complaining about what he thinks is an ulcer. Almost every time he eats he gets a feeling of fullness and chest pain. He usually has heartburn and sometimes brings food up into his throat, which causes a burning sensation. You cannot schedule him for two weeks because the doctor is out of town. _____

_____

_____

After your instructor has returned your work to you, make all necessary corrections and place in a three-ring notebook for future reference.

**ASSIGNMENT SHEET**

## Chapter 11:  ANATOMY AND PHYSIOLOGY OF THE HUMAN BODY

## Unit 11:  THE URINARY SYSTEM

### A.  Mixed Quiz

1. List the three main functions of the urinary system, explaining the meaning of each.

   a. _____

   b. _____

   c. _____

2. Identify the organs of the urinary system; describe their physical characteristics.

   a. _____

   _____

   b. _____

   _____

   c. _____

   _____

   d. _____

   _____

3. Labeling:  Label the illustration using the following terms. Refer to Figure 11-172 in the textbook.

   Aorta

   Inferior vena cava

   Hilum

   Left kidney

   Left ureter

   Right kidney

   Urethra

   Urinary bladder

Left renal artery

Left renal vein

Left common
iliac artery

4. How does the urinary system work with the other body systems to accomplish its job? _____

_____

_____

_____

_____

_____

5. How is the interior of the kidney constructed? _____

_____

6. Labeling: Label the illustration with the following terms. Refer to Figure 11-173 in the textbook.

Cortex

Hilum

Medulla

Renal papilla

Renal pelvis

Renal pyramid

Ureter

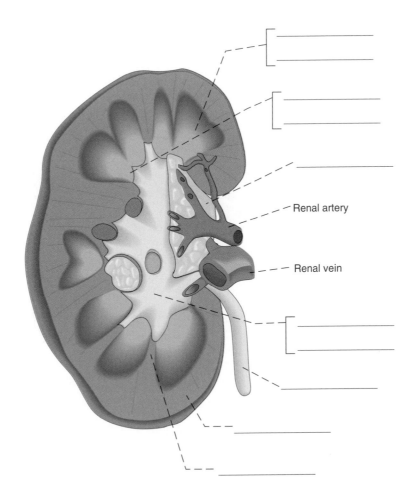

Renal artery

Renal vein

7. List the parts of the nephron and describe the function of each part.

a. _____

b. _____

c. _____

_____

d. _____

8. Labeling: Label the illustration using the following terms. Refer to Figure 11-174 in the textbook.

Afferent arteriole

Ascending limb-loop of Henle

Bowman's capsule

Collecting tubule

Descending limb-loop of Henle

Distal convoluted tubule

Efferent arteriole

Glomerulus

Peritubular capillaries

Proximal convoluted tubule

Interlobular-artery

Interlobular-vein

Juxtaglomerular-apparatus

9. Describe kidney dialysis, and identify two major types or methods. _____

_____

_____

_____

_____

_____

_____

_____

_____

10. What are the two main categories of diagnostic examinations? Give one example of each type.

_____

_____

_____

_____

11. List the symptoms of renal calculi.

a. _____

b. _____

c. _____

d. _____

e. _____

f. _____

g. _____

12. Matching: Match the symptoms in column II with the appropriate disease and disorder in column I.

COLUMN I

_____ 1. Cystitis
_____ 2. Glomerulonephritis
_____ 3. Nephrotic syndrome
_____ 4. Polycystic kidney disease
_____ 5. Pyelonephritis
_____ 6. Renal failure
_____ 7. Stricture
_____ 8. Calculi
_____ 9. Uremia

COLUMN II

a. Urgency, dysuria, nocturia, hematuria, ammoniac or fishy odor to urine, high fever, chills, flank pain, fatigue

b. Small stream of urine, prolonged urination time

c. Oliguria, azotemia, severe electrolyte imbalance, acidosis, uremia, other body system involvement

d. Frequency, dysuria, bladder spasms, sharp stabbing pain upon urination

e. Severe pain beginning in kidney, moving to groin area, nausea, vomiting, chills, and fever

f. Generalized dependent edema, pleural effusion, ascites, lethargy, fatigue, pallor, swollen external sexual organs

g. Urine products in the blood, coma, toxic waste levels in blood, eventual death

h. Moderate edema, proteinuria, hematuria, oliguria, fatigue, urinary casts, hypertension

i. Pointed nose, small chin, floppy low-set ears, inner eyelid folds, eventually widened body, swollen, tender abdomen, life-threatening bleeding, ureteral spasms

Name _____

13. Unscramble

a. _ _ _ _ _ _ _ _    ORATNICU

b. _ _ _ _ _ _ _    DELBRAD

c. _ _ _ _ _ _ _ _    LRAGOIUI

d. _ _ _ _ _ _ _    EYACSLC

e. _ _ _ _ _ _ _ _    YAUPILOR

f. _ _ _ _ _ _ _ _    ISYTICTS

g. _ _ _ _ _ _ _ _    AYISLSDI

h. _ _ _ _ _ _ _    RIYSADU

i. _ _ _ _ _ _ _ _ _    NERTNOITE

j. _ _ _ _ _ _ _ _ _    ENRETSOIC

k. _ _ _ _ _ _ _ _ _    RTEISRTUC

l. _ _ _ _ _ _ _    HUATRER

m. _ _ _ _ _ _ _    ONHEPNR

n. _ _ _ _ _ _ _    UILALCC

o. _ _ _ _ _ _ _ _ _ _    IOYPITLHRST

14. Crossword Puzzle

DOWN
1. To separate waste from the blood
2. Absence of urine
3. Urine left after voiding
4. Artificially clean the blood
5. System in this unit
6. Contains glomerulus
9. A narrowing
11. Painful urination
13. Calyx (pl.)
17. Waste product of the kidneys
19. The organ that removes wastes from the blood

ACROSS
6. Kidney stones
7. The act of passing urine
8. To droop
10. To urinate
12. A narrowing
14. Tube from kidney
15. To produce from the blood
16. Renal capillary
18. Greek word for cup
20. Notched area of kidney
21. Bladder inflammation
22. Urine products in the blood
23. Drains urine from the bladder
24. Pertaining to the kidney
25. Sudden urge to void

15. Word Puzzle:  Use the clues listed to spell out these terms.

       __ __ U __ __ __             Absence of urine

      __ __ __ R __ __ __ __ __      Separate and remove

      __ I __ __ __ __             Retroperitoneal organ

  __ __ __ __ __ N __ __ __ __ __    Expel from body

      __ __ __ A __ __ __ __ __      Presence of blood

  __ __ __ __ __ R __ __ __ __      Cluster of capillaries

      __ Y __ __ __ __             Group of organs

16. Name the three types of incontinence

    a. _____

    b. _____

    c. _____

17. List nine treatments to improve the control of urine.

    a. _____

    b. _____

    c. _____

    d. _____

    e. _____

    f. _____

    g. _____

    h. _____

    i. _____

18. Refer to the CAAHEP Standards in Appendix B of the textbook. Within the area of *Medical Assisting Clinical Procedures,* which three standards relate to the content in diagnostic procedures in this unit? _____

_____

**CRITICAL THINKING SCENARIOS:  What would your response be in the following situations?**

1. A female patient who had a cystoscopic examination last week called saying that for the past couple of days, every time she urinates it is very painful. She is having to pass urine very frequently and it looks like there is a little blood in it now. She wonders if this is normal. _____

_____

_____

_____

2. A male patient is complaining of periods of severe pain in his lower abdomen. He is nauseated and has vomited a couple of times. He also has a fever. He believes he has the flu and is requesting the doctor to phone in a prescription. When questioned he reveals he isn't passing much urine, but he didn't think that was unusual since he is not taking in much fluid. _____

_____

_____

After your instructor has returned your work to you, make all necessary corrections and place in a three-ring notebook for future reference.

Name Angela Mae
Date 1/31/06    Score _____

**ASSIGNMENT SHEET**

**Chapter 11: ANATOMY AND PHYSIOLOGY OF THE HUMAN BODY**

**Unit 12: THE ENDOCRINE SYSTEM**

**A. Mixed Quiz**

1. Explain the difference between an exocrine gland and an endocrine gland, giving an example of each.

   _____
   _____
   _____

2. What types of body functions are affected by hormones?

   a. _____   d. _____
   b. _____   e. _____
   c. _____   f. _____

3. List the nine glands discussed in the unit, identifying the location of each gland.

   a. _____
   b. _____
   c. _____
   d. _____
   e. _____
   f. _____
   g. _____
   h. _____
   i. _____

4. Identify the endocrine glands on the following illustration.

Pineal    Pituitary

Thyroid    Thymus

Parathyroid glands    Posterior view

Cortex
Medulla
Adrenal

(Islets of Langerhans)
Pancreas

testes    ovary

225

5. Complete the following chart.

| GLAND | LOCATION | HORMONES SECRETED |
|---|---|---|
| Pituitary-anterior lobe | | |
| -posterior lobe | | |
| Thyroid | | |
| Parathyroids | | |
| Adrenal-medulla | | |
| -cortex | | |
| Pancreas | | |
| Thymus | | |
| Pineal body | | |
| Ovaries | | |
| Testes | | |

6. Identify the hormones secreted by the gonads and the functions of each. _____
_____ \
_____
_____

7. Explain what hormone secretion abnormality causes the following conditions.
   a. Giantism/Gigantism _____
   b. Dwarfism _____
   c. Acromegaly _____
   d. Goiter _____
   e. Tetany _____
   f. Diabetes _____
   g. Cretinism _____
   h. Cushing's syndrome _____
   i. Myxedema _____
8. How are hormones interrelated? _____
_____
_____
_____

9. What diagnostic examinations are used to confirm the following conditions?

a. Diabetes _____

b. Thyroid dysfunction _____

c. Pregnancy _____

d. Cushing's syndrome _____

10. List the symptoms, characteristics, and usual course of action taken in the following conditions or diseases.

a. _____
_____

b. Cushing's syndrome _____
_____
_____

c. _____
_____

d. _____
_____

11. What role does insulin play in the blood?

a. _____

b. _____

12. Fill in the Blank

Type 2 diabetes usually begins because of _____ The body's cells resist both _____ and _____ Insulin resistance can also result from _____ _____ and some medications, but _____ and the _____ are the main non-genetic factors.

13. Name the three categories of insulin drugs according to their effects. _____
_____

14. Define the following *Words to Know* using the Glossary.

a. Adrenaline _____
_____

b. Diabetes mellitus _____

c. Estrogen _____

d. Gonad _____

e. Hormone _____

f. Hypoglycemia _____

g. Ovary _____
_____

h. Progesterone _____

i. Testes _____

j. Testosterone _____

15. Refer to the Role Delineation Chart in Appendix A of the textbook. Within the area of Instruction, which role would relate to helping patients discussed in this unit to obtain assistance, additional information, or support?

_____

16. Word Search: Find the following words hidden in the puzzle.

ACROMEGALY      ESTROGEN      OVARY
ADRENAL      EXOCRINE      PINEAL
ADRENALINE      GIANTISM      PITUITARY
ALDOSTERONE      GLAND      PUBERTY
CRETINISM      GOITER      TESTES
DWARFISM      GONAD      TETANY
ENDOCRINE      HORMONE      THYMUS

```
R I O G O N A D A W T D C
A C R O M E G A L Y U E P
V D I I W E S D D L T I U
M N R T E S T R O G E N B
C T W E Q Z C E S V T H E
E R E R N I O N T P A O R
N G E S T A L A E I N R T
D L I T T E L L R T Y M Y
O A E A I E C I O U P O T
C N E R N N S N N I I N H
R D O W Q T I E E T N E Y
I D W A R F I S M A E I M
N K L V C O P S M R A E U
E X O C R I N E M Y L W S
```

**CRITICAL THINKING SCENARIOS: What would your response be in the following situations?**

1. A patient who is under care for diabetes calls to get something for the infection in her big toe. She had had an ingrown toenail that she cut out, and it has gotten red and swollen. _____

_____
_____
_____

2. An individual who is new in town calls to make an appointment. His chief complaints: he has no energy and he is always thirsty, which of course makes him drink more and have to urinate more frequently. He says he doesn't think it's anything serious, probably just an enlarged prostate gland, so he can wait a couple of weeks to get in. _____

_____
_____

After your instructor has returned your work to you, make all necessary corrections and place in a three-ring notebook for future reference.

**ASSIGNMENT SHEET**

**Chapter 11: ANATOMY AND PHYSIOLOGY OF THE HUMAN BODY**

**Unit 13: THE REPRODUCTIVE SYSTEM**

**A. Mixed Quiz**

1. What is the difference between asexual and sexual reproduction? _____

   _____

2. Explain the process of differentiation of the reproductive organs; compare the male to female organs.

   _____

   _____

   _____

   _____

   _____

   _____

3. Fill in the Blank

   A male infant develops if the zygote contains a _____ chromosome. At about the seventh or eighth week, the _____ begin to develop within the _____ During the eighth or ninth month, the _____ move from the _____ through the _____ into the

   _____

4. List the nine male sex organs or structures, and describe their function.

   a. _____

   b. _____

   c. _____

   d. _____

   _____

   e. _____

   f. _____

   _____

   g. _____

   _____

   h. _____

   i. _____

5. Labeling: Label the structures on the illustration using the following terms. Refer to Figure 11-204 in the textbook.

Anal opening

Bulbourethral gland or Cowper's gland

Ejaculatory duct

Epididymis

Penis

Prepuce

Prostate gland

Rectum

Scrotum

Seminal vesicle

Spermatic cord

Symphysis pubis

Testis

Vas deferens (two times)

Urethra

Urinary bladder

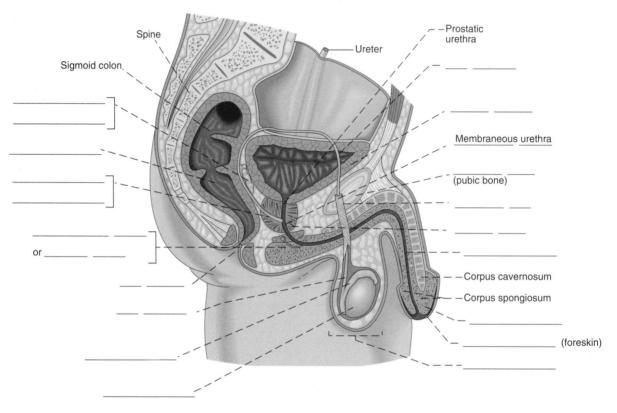

6. How do pituitary hormones affect the function of the testes? _____

_____

_____

7. List the secondary male sex characteristics.

a. _____     e. _____

b. _____     f. _____

c. _____     g. _____

d. _____

8. List, in order, the structures through which sperm pass.

   a. _____

   b. _____

   c. _____

   d. _____

   e. _____

9. What is the composition of semen?

   a. _____

   b. _____

   c. _____

   d. _____

10. List the four diseases and disorders of the male reproductive system; define the condition and identify the main symptoms and/or cause of the condition.

   a. _____
   _____

   b. _____
   _____

   c. _____
   _____
   _____

   d. _____
   _____
   _____

11. List the eight female sexual structures and describe their function.

   a. _____

   b. _____

   c. _____

   d. _____

   e. _____

   f. _____

   g. _____

   h. _____

12. Labeling: Label the internal structure on the illustration using the following terms. Refer to Figure 11-212 in the textbook.

Anus                              Ovary
Cervix                         Symphysis pubis
Corpus of uterus       Ureter
Crus of clitoris         Urinary bladder
Fallopian tube          Vagina
Fundus of uterus

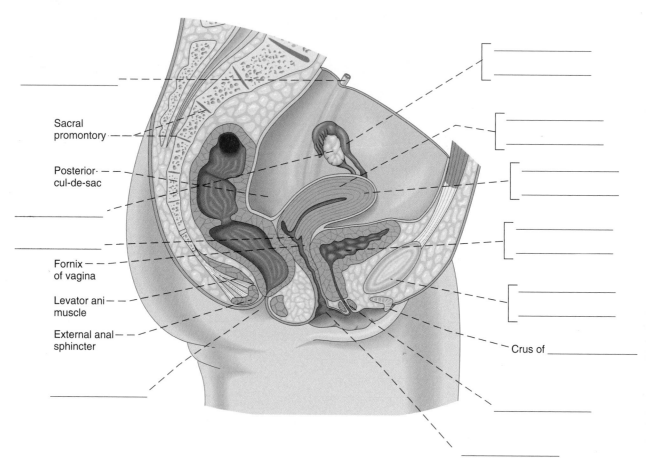

Sacral promontory

Posterior cul-de-sac

Fornix of vagina

Levator ani muscle

External anal sphincter

Crus of _____

13. Labeling: Label the external structure on the illustration using the following terms. Refer to Figure 11-213 in the textbook.

Anus                    Mons pubis
Clitoris                 Perineum
Hymen                   Urethral orifice
Labia majora            Vaginal orifice
Labia minora            Vestibule

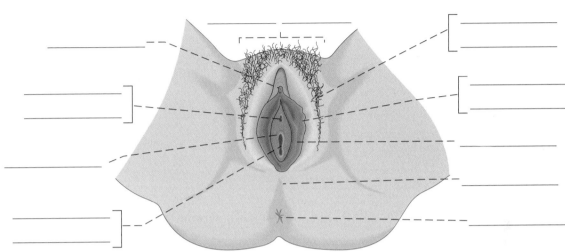

14. How do hormones from the pituitary gland affect the development of the female reproductive organs? _____

_____

_____

15. List the female secondary sex characteristics.

a. _____

b. _____

c. _____

d. _____

e. _____

f. _____

g. _____

h. _____

i. _____

16. Trace the pathway of an egg from expulsion to implantation if fertilized or to the exterior if not.

a. _____

_____

b. _____

_____

17. List the four phases of the menstrual cycle.

a. _____

b. _____

c. _____

d. _____

18. Describe the fertilization of an ovum. _____
_____
_____
_____

19. Identify the period of time during a pregnancy when the following occurs:
    a. Embryonic stage _____
    b. Called a fetus _____
    c. Systems complete, fingernails _____
    d. Sex can be determined _____
    e. Movement felt _____
    f. Heartbeat detectable, halfway _____
    g. Weighs less than 2 pounds _____
    h. Opens eyes _____
    i. Hears sounds _____
    j. Assumes head-down position _____
    k. Reaches 5 pounds _____
    l. Weighs 7 1/2 lbs. and is 20 in. long _____

20. Using Nagle's rule, calculate the expected delivery date for the following first days of last menstrual periods.
    a. February 6, 1998 _____
    b. January 15, 1998 _____
    c. July 4, 1997 _____
    d. September 29, 1997 _____
    e. December 25, 1997 _____

21. List the usual signs and symptoms of early pregnancy.
    a. _____    d. _____
    b. _____    e. _____
    c. _____    f. _____

22. List symptoms that occur later in pregnancy.
    a. _____    e. _____
    b. _____    f. _____
    c. _____    g. _____
    d. _____    h. _____

23. Describe the characteristics of the three stages of labor.
    First    a. _____
             b. _____
    Second   a. _____
             b. _____
             c. _____
             d. _____
    Third    a. _____
             b. _____

24. List eight reasons to use contraceptives.
    a. _____    e. _____
    b. _____    f. _____
    c. _____    g. _____
    d. _____    h. _____

25. List seven routine screening and diagnostic pregnancy tests. _____

_____

_____

26. Name 14 methods of contraception.

a. _____    h. _____

b. _____    i. _____

c. _____    j. _____

d. _____    k. _____

e. _____    l. _____

f. _____    m. _____

g. _____    n. _____

27. Matching: Match the descriptions in column II with the correct test in column I.

COLUMN I                              COLUMN II

_____ 1. IHSG                         a. Examination with an instrument connected to a monitor to view the

_____ 2. Mammograph                      endometrium

_____ 3. Maturation index            b. Determines hormonal level from cells scraped from vaginal walls

_____ 4. Papanicolaou test           c. High-frequency sound waves that detect and aid in the diagnosis of

_____ 5. Pregnancy test                  breast irregularities

_____ 6. Ultrasonography             d. A urine specimen test to detect the presence of HCG

_____ 7. Colposcopy                  e. Evaluates and restores tubal patency

_____ 8. Hysteroscopy                f. Examination of cervical secretions for cancer cells

                                     g. An X ray of the breast

                                     h. An examination of the cervix following a questionable Pap smear

28. List the warning signals taht may indicate a malignancy of the breast.

a. _____

b. _____

c. _____

d. _____

e. _____

f. _____

29. Identify other sites where females may develop cancer.

a. _____

b. _____

c. _____

d. _____

e. _____

30. Refer to the ABHES Course Content Requirements in Appendix C of the textbook. Within the area of *Medical Law and Ethics,* which content requirements are discussed within this unit that might be related to religious and personal convictions? _____

_____

31. Define the following diseases or disorders of the female reproductive.

    a.  Abortion _____

    b.  Cervical erosion _____

    c.  Cervicitis _____

    d.  Cystic breast disease _____

    e.  Cystocele _____

    f.  Dysmenorrhea _____

    g.  Endometriosis _____

    h.  Fibroids _____

    i.  Hysterectomy _____

    j.  Malignancy of the breast _____

    k.  Ovarian cyst _____

    l.  PMS _____

    m.  Polyp _____

    n.  Rectocele _____

32. Identify the main characteristics of each of the following disease conditions.

    a. Chlamydia _____

    b. Gonorrhea _____

    c. Herpes _____

    d. NGU _____

    e. P.I.D. _____

    f. Syphilis (four stages)  (1) _____

                        (2) _____

                        (3) _____

                        (4) _____

    g. Trichomoniasis _____

33. Spelling: Each line contains four different spellings of a word. Underline the correctly spelled word.

| | | | |
|---|---|---|---|
| a. circumcision | circomcision | circumsision | circumcisun |
| b. dysmenorrhea | dismemorrea | dismenorehea | dysmenorrea |
| c. epididimus | epididimis | epididymis | epididymus |
| d. genetalea | genetalia | genitalea | genitalia |
| e. menapause | menopause | menaplaus | menoplaus |
| f. menorrhagia | menarrhagia | menorrhagea | menarrhagea |
| g. prostratectomy | prostatectemy | prostetectomy | prostatectomy |
| h. syfhillis | syphillis | syphilis | syphelis |

236

34. Word Puzzle:  Use the clues listed to spell out these terms.

| | |
|---|---|
| _ _ _ R _ _ | Pelvic organ |
| _ _ _ _ E _ _ _ _ _ | Wall of uterus |
| _ _ _ P _ _ _ _ _ _ _ _ _ _ | Improper location of testes |
| _ _ _ R _ _ _ | Muscle growth |
| _ _ _ _ _ _ O _ _ _ _ _ | Pertains to menstruation |
| _ _ _ D _ _ _ _ _ _ | Coiled tube |
| _ _ _ _ U _ _ _ _ _ _ _ | Foreskin surgery |
| _ _ _ _ _ _ C _ _ | The beginning |
| _ _ _ T _ _ | Group of organs |
| I _ _ _ _ | Protozal |
| _ _ _ _ _ _ _ _ _ _ _ _ _ | Entrance to uterus |
| _ _ _ V _ _ | Entrance to uterus |
| _ _ _ _ E _ _ _ _ | Removal of mammary gland |

**CRITICAL THINKING SCENARIOS:  What would your response be in the following situations?**

1. A 65-five-year-old male patient wants the doctor to call in a prescription for him to get rid of his kidney infection. He has been having to urinate frequently, even getting up at night, and then he still dribbles sometimes in between. His brother had the same problems. _____

_____

_____

2. You have a good relationship with your teenage daughter. She tells you some of the kids at school have been talking about birth control. One of the girls said she didn't need anything because she always douched right after she had sex. She buys those premixed disposable units at the supermarket. She also thinks that will prevent her from getting AIDS. _____

_____

_____

3. A 35-year-old female called to see if she should see the doctor. She had found a lumpy place on her left breast, but it didn't hurt or anything. Her friend told her that it was probably just cysts at her age and not to worry about it. _____

_____

_____

_____

After your instructor has returned your work to you, make all necessary corrections and place in a three-ring notebook for future reference.

## Section 4: THE CLINICAL MEDICAL ASSISTANT

## Chapter 12: PREPARING FOR CLINICAL DUTIES

Review the objectives and text for each unit before completing the assignment sheet for that unit. When you have completed all sheets for the chapter, remove them from this Workbook and give them to the instructor for evaluation.

## Unit 1: GUIDELINES FOR THE PERSONAL SAFETY AND WELL-BEING OF STAFF AND PATIENTS

### A. Brief Answer

1. How can the medical assistant be considerate of patients when assisting with procedures? _____

_____

2. Besides being apprehensive about procedures, what else might a patient be afraid of? _____

_____

3. List the types of patients who will need the undivided attention of the medical assistant. _____

_____

_____

4. How should you speak to patients, and why? _____

_____

5. What special instructions should you give to a patient who is blind? deaf? _____

_____

_____

### B. Multiple Choice: Place the correct letter or letters on the blank line for each question.

___D___ 1. Assistance dogs (or other assistance animals) should be left alone because the animal
  a. might bite
  b. is working
  c. is protecting its owner
  d. may feel threatened or distracted

___C___ 2. The state of being free of all pathogenic microorganisms is
  a. sanitization
  b. asepsis
  c. disinfection
  d. esthetic

___A___ 3. The ideal temperature setting in a medical office is
  a. 72°F
  b. 74°F
  c. 76°F
  d. 78°F

_____ 4. After a tissue has been used to catch a sneeze, it should be
  a. put in your pocket
  b. placed in a sharps container
  c. placed in a waste receptacle

_____ 5. In the medical facility a foamed alcohol preparation is used to ____ hands.
  a. disinfect
  b. clean
  c. sterilize
  d. soothe

_____ 6. To turn water faucets on and off for handwashing you should use a
  a. tissue
  b. gauze square
  c. paper towel
  d. glove

_____ 7. Disposable gloves are available with or without
  a. cuffs
  b. powder
  c. lotion
  d. disinfectant

8. Areas of the skin that should be covered with a bandage after handwashing and drying and before gloving are
   a. moles and scars
   c. burns
   b. breaks, scratches, cuts
   d. all of these

9. Disposable instruments and _____ should be deposited in the sharps container after use.
   a. lancets
   c. bandages
   b. syringes
   d. needles

10. Electrical wiring and appliances should be checked periodically and tagged for ___ as necessary.
    a. repair
    c. expiration date
    b. cleaning
    d. date of purchase

11. Phone numbers that should be posted near the phone are
    a. personal
    c. patients'
    b. retailers
    d. emergency

12. One who wears loose-fitting clothing and jewelry when working with machines or equipment can contribute to
    a. attractiveness
    c. asepsis
    b. accuracy
    d. accidents

## C. True or False: Place a "T" for true or "F" for false in the space provided. For false statements, explain why they are false.

1. There should be a scheduled time weekly for inspection of the entire medical facility.
2. Medical facilities are prime targets of pathogenic organisms.
3. Periodic remodeling of a medical facility should be done only after furniture and carpets become a safety hazard.
4. A disinfectant spray should be kept in a convenient place to disinfect small areas and to help eliminate unpleasant odors.
5. Small toys are not recommended in the pediatric area of the reception room because babies might swallow them.
6. Soap and water should be used every time you wash your hands.
7. If you wear gloves for assisting with invasive procedures, you will not need to wash your hands as often.
8. Emergency exits should be clearly posted with easy-to-follow paths for evacuation in each room of the medical facility.

## D. Brief Answer

1. List the reasons for wearing latex gloves.
   a. Provide protection as a barrier and prevent contamination of the hands when touching any blood or body
   b. Reduce the possibility of pathogens
   c. Diminish the chance of any pathogens being transmitted from you to patients as you do from one patient to another.

2. What information should be documented in case of an accident at a medical facility? a Accident Report, what happen, how was the injury and at what time it occur

3. What should you do (and what should you tell patients to do) if stricken with a case of the flu/bad cold?

4. Why should hand lotion be available to the medical assistant in a medical facility? Prevents skin from becoming dry and chapped

### E. Fill in the Blank

1. A _liquid soap_ eliminates the possibility of dropping a bar of soap in the sink or on the floor when performing the handwashing procedure.

2. When performing the handwashing procedure, a _____ should be used to dislodge microorganisms around cuticles and under the fingernails.

3. Spills should be cleaned up immediately to prevent _____

4. Lab test results should be recorded _____ on charts and in logs to ensure accuracy.

5. _____ chemicals should be kept away from flames and gas lines.

After your instructor has returned your work to you, make all necessary corrections and place in a three-ring notebook for future reference.

**Chapter 12: PREPARING FOR CLINICAL DUTIES**

**Unit 2: INFECTION CONTROL**

**SUGGESTED RESPONSES TO CRITICAL THINKING CHALLENGE IN TEXTBOOK**

1. What is being jeopardized here? _____

_____

2. What gain is there in rushing through your work? _____

_____

3. Is Ella likely to contract what the patient has? _____

_____

4. Who else is being subjected to becoming sick? _____

_____

5. What should she have done? _____

_____

6. Should Ella be reprimanded? _____

_____

7. How do you think the patient felt? _____

_____

8. Would you like to have Ella be your medical assistant if you get sick? Why or why not? _____

_____

_____

_____

_____

**ANSWERS TO WORKBOOK ASSIGNMENT**

**A. Unscramble**

1. _ _ _ _ _ _ _ _ _ _ _ _     HRDBUZISAOAO
2. _ _ _ _ _ _ _ _     TICAREAB
3. _ _ _ _ _ _ _     SELAMIA
4. _ _ _ _ _ _ _ _ _ _     YORMPGOOHL
5. _ _ _ _ _ _ _ _ _ _     UCTESPBSELI
6. _ _ _ _ _ _     ORPSSE
7. _ _ _ _ _ _ _ _ _ _     TNESISAERC
8. _ _ _ _ _ _ _     PSSASIE
9. _ _ _ _ _ _ _ _     EOPHAGTN
10. _ _ _ _ _ _ _ _ _ _ _     EFNCONINTME
11. _ _ _ _ _ _ _     RLEDTPO

**B. Matching:** Match the definition in column II with the correct term in column I.

COLUMN I

- E 1. Cholera
- 6 2. Autotrophs
- k 3. Obligate parasite
- a 4. Tinea pedis
- j 5. Viruses
- l 6. *Escherichia coli*
- m 7. Dysentery
- B 8. Facultative parasites
- d 9. Ticks and fleas
- C 10. Heterotrophs
- f 11. Pathogens
- H 12. Anaerobes

COLUMN II

a. Fungus condition
b. Can live independently
c. Feed on organic matter
d. External parasites
e. From contaminated food/water
f. Disease-producing microorganisms
g. Feed on inorganic matter
h. Grow best in the absence of oxygen
i. Non-pathogen
j. Smallest of microorganisms
k. Completely dependent on host
l. Common cause of urinary tract infections
m. Protozoa

## C. Brief Answer

1. Name the common pathogens known to man. _____

2. What are the growth requirements for microorganisms? _____

_____

3. Explain the infection cycle.
   a. Resourir host
   b. Means of exit.
   c. Means of transmission.
   d. means of entry.
   e. Susceptible host

4. Name a disinfectant and an antiseptic that are commonly used in the medical office. _____

_____

5. What is most commonly used in preparing a patient's skin for injection or surgery procedures? _____

_____

6. Describe the proper method of cleaning instruments. _____

_____

7. Why should precautions be taken in the storage of instruments? _____

8. Explain the precautions to be taken when you are exposed to all blood and body fluids. (These precautions are known as the "blood and body fluid standard precautions.") Why is it vitally important to follow these precautions carefully? _____

_____

_____

_____

_____

9. How are used needles, scalpels, and other sharp instruments to be handled? Why? _____

_____

_____

_____

10. How should waste be treated before it is disposed of from a medical office or clinic? _____

_____

11. Name the two most feared communicable diseases that health care facilities must strive to prevent
transmitting to the public. _____

**D. Matching: Match the disease in column I with the common name in column II.**

|  | COLUMN I | COLUMN II |
|---|---|---|
| c | 1. Varicella | a. Pinworms |
| ___ | 2. URI | b. Scabies |
| g | 3. Conjunctivitis | c. Chickenpox |
| ___ | 4. Pediculosis | d. Scarlet fever |
| g | 5. Herpes simplex | e. Hepatitis B |
| ___ | 6. *Enterobius vermicularis* | f. Common cold |
| ___ | 7. Scarlatina | g. Fever blister |
|  |  | h. Head lice |
|  |  | i. Pinkeye |

**E. Fill in the Blank**

1. Antibacterial agents, antibiotics, or corticosteroids, depending on the causative agent, is the treatment for

_____

2. Cleansing of areas with antibacterial soap and water and topical and/or oral antibiotics is the treatment for

_____

3. Topical application of drying medications and antibiotics for secondary infections is the treatment for

_____

4. 2–3 weeks, usually 13–17 days, is the incubation period for _____

5. In one week nits (eggs) hatch; in two weeks they mature. This describes the incubation period for

_____

6. Bed rest, antipyretics, and topical antipruritics is the treatment for _____

7. 14–50 days is the incubation period for both _____ and _____

8. Blister-like lesions, which later become crusted and itchy, are symptoms of _____

9. Antibiotics, analgesics, antipyretics, increase in fluid intake, and bed rest is the treatment for _____

10. Strawberry tongue, rash of skin and inside of mouth, high fever, nausea, and vomiting are symptoms of

_____

**F. Brief Answer**

1. How is impetigo transmitted? _____

2. What is the treatment for hepatitis A and hepatitis B? _____

_____

3. How long is the incubation period for aseptic meningitis? for bacterial meningitis? _____

_____

4. Explain the treatment for pediculosis and why it is important to follow it carefully. _____

_____

_____

_____

_____

_____

5. What is the incubation period of pinworms and how are they transmitted?

6. What are the symptoms of *Enterobius vermicularis* and how is it treated?

7. List the symptoms of aseptic meningitis and bacterial meningitis.

8. How is aseptic meningitis transmitted? bacterial meningitis?

_8, 9, 12, 15, 17, 20)_

9. What is the treatment of aseptic meningitis? bacterial meningitis?

10. What are the symptoms of influenza? _Sudden onset fever, chills_ _headache, sore muscle, malaise._

11. What is the means of transmission of the common cold?

12. How is conjunctivitis transmitted? _Direct or indirect contact_ _droplet, airborne, secretion of infected perso_

13. What are the symptoms of hepatitis A? of hepatitis B?

14. How is hepatitis A transmitted? hepatitis B? _Direct contant or by fecal-_ _contaminated food or water (B) contaminate_ _serum in blood transfussion or by use of_ _contamniled neddles_

15. What are symptoms of pediculosis and how is it transmitted?

16. List the symptoms of scabies. _intense itching of small raised_ _areas of skin that contain fluid or tiny burrows_

17. How is scabies transmitted? _Direct contact or indirect contact infected clo_

18. How are strep throat and scarlet fever transmitted, and how long are the incubation periods? _Direct_ _and indirect 1-7 days_

19. List the symptoms of strep throat and scarlet fever and the treatment for each. _Fever, Red and_ _sore throat, Antibiotics, analgescis, antipyretics,_ _Direct_

20. List the symptoms of AIDS.

244

21. What is the incubation period for AIDS? _____

_____

22. What are the symptoms of *Haemophilus influenzae* type B? _____

_____

23. How is *Haemophilus influenzae* type B transmitted? _____

_____

**G. Multiple Choice: Place the correct letter or letters on the blank line for each question.**

____ 1. Red, itching, burning eyes with matted eyelashes are symptoms of
    a. impetigo            c. varicella
    b. scarlatina         d. conjunctivitis

____ 2. Crops of pruritic vesicular eruptions on the skin, slight fever, headache, and malaise are symptoms of
    a. cholera             c. pediculosis
    b. varicella          d. scabies

____ 3. This disease is transmitted by direct contact with an infected person who has painful blisters on her lips (pustular/then crusted scabs) and small ulcerated oral lesions.
    a. bacterial meningitis      c. herpes simplex
    b. tinea pedis         d. cholera

____ 4. Bed rest, increased intake of fluids, and antipyretics is the treatment for
    a. Hepatitis B        c. dysentery
    b. influenza          d. bacterial meningitis

____ 5. The treatment listed in #4, plus a decongestant and mild analgesics. is the treatment for
    a. common cold       c. cholera
    b. measles           d. scarlatina

____ 6. The incubation period for scabies is
    a. 2–6 months       c. 2–3 days
    b. 2–6 weeks        d. none of these

____ 7. The incubation period for the common cold is
    a. 12–72 hours      c. 12–72 weeks
    b. 12–72 days       d. all of these

____ 8. A scabicide, oral antihistamines, and salicylates to reduce itching is the treatment for
    a. pediculosis        c. scabies
    b. measles           d. varicella

____ 9. The good health habits of proper rest, nutrition, hygiene, and exercise are helpful in resisting disease and they
    a. promote circulation      c. increase heart rate
    b. destroy pathogens      d. reduce stress

____ 10. Autoclaving is the most effective and desirable form of sterilization because it
    a. is convenient to use      c. disinfects items
    b. has an automatic timer    d. kills and destroys spores

____ 11. All members of the health care team must remember to do ___ before and after gloving.
    a. check the patient's chart    c. inventory supplies
    b. check the day's schedule    d. proper hand washing

_____ 12. When cleaning instruments, a brush should be used to
- a. loosen and remove particles from crevices/hinges
- b. protect you from injury
- c. kill and destroy spores
- d. avoid contamination

_____ 13. Soaking instruments in _____ will help loosen material from metal.
- a. alcohol
- b. cool water
- c. zephrin chloride
- d. hot water

## H. Crossword Puzzle

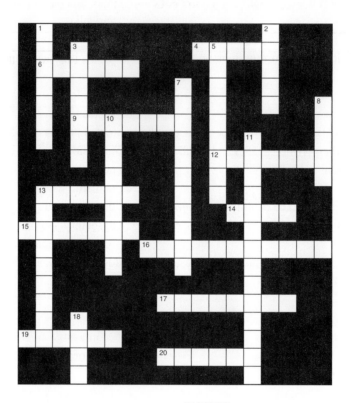

ACROSS
4. Every day
6. Latex barrier for hands
9. Regular habit
12. Free from septic matter
13. Destroyed only by autoclaving
14. Rinse used instruments in _____ water
15. Protection
16. Helps reduce the spread of diseases
17. Do over and over
19. Prior to
20. To do again

DOWN
1. Clean and sanitary
2. Circle
3. Management
5. Destroys microorganisms using steam under pressure
7. Safety measures
8. Used in washing hands/instruments
10. Global
11. Duty
13. Free of all living organisms
18. Infected person/animal

**CRITICAL THINKING SCENARIOS:  What would your response be in the following situations?**

1. One of your co-workers is negligent about handwashing. It bothers you because you realize how easily diseases can be transmitted from person to person. _____

_____

2. You notice that there are several patients in the reception area waiting to be seen by the physician. One of them is sneezing and coughing, and appears to be very ill. _____

3. As you remove a suture pack from the autoclave, you notice that the sterilization indicator tape has not changed color. _____

4. You are checking instruments in preparation for autoclaving. You notice that two of the hemostats have loose hinges and a towel clamp is rusty. _____

_____

## ACHIEVING SKILL COMPETENCY

Reread the performance objective for each procedure and then practice the skills listed below, following the procedure in your textbook.

Procedure 12-1:  Hand Washing

Procedure 12-2:  Wrap Items for Autoclave

When you feel you have mastered the performance of the skill, sign your name on the appropriate evaluation sheet and give it to your instructor to indicate you are prepared to perform the procedure for evaluation.

After your instructor has returned your work to you, make all necessary corrections and place in a three-ring notebook for future reference.

## Chapter 13: BEGINNING THE PATIENT'S RECORD

Review the objectives and text for each unit before completing the assignment sheet for that unit. When you have completed all sheets for the chapter, remove them from this Workbook and give them to the instructor for evaluation.

## Unit 1: MEDICAL HISTORY

### A. Uncramble

1. _ _ _ _ _ _ _           MPYSTMO
2. _ _ _ _ _ _             RVEXET
3. _ _ _ _ _ _             YDRMEE
4. _ _ _ _ _ _             CILETI
5. _ _ _ _ _ _ _           TUSTRAE

### B. Brief Answer

1. Why must assistance be given to patients in completing the medical history form? _____

_____

2. Where should the medical assistant interview patients to obtain medical history information? _____

_____

3. Describe how additional questions on the medical history form regarding AIDS/HIV and hepatitis should be worded. _____

_____

4. What additional questions should be asked of patients regarding AIDS/HIV and hepatitis to determine if further investigation should be made as to the health status of that patient? _____

_____

_____

5. Define the following terms.
   a. CC (chief complaint) _____
   b. PI (present illness) _____

   _____

   c. ROS (review of systems) _____

   _____

   d. PH (past history) _____

   _____

   e. FH (family history) _____

   _____

   f. PSH (personal/sociocultural history) _____

6. Explain why medical history forms vary in detail and length. _____

_____

7. What is a genogram and why is it helpful to physicians? _____

_____

_____

8. Why must the patient's height and weight be recorded at the initial visit? _____

_____

9. Why is it important to keep an accurate record of the patient's weight? _____

_____

10. What is usually requested for adults when taking the chest measurement? _____

_____

## C. Spelling: Each line contains four different spellings of a word. Underline the correctly spelled word and use it in a sentence.

1. measurement     measurement     measuremit     measeurment
2. stadure     statere     stateure     stature
3. infermation     informashion     information     infarmation
4. simptom     symptom     symptome     symptim
5. haight     heite     height     hieght
6. interview     intraview     innerview     inerveiw

1. _____
2. _____
3. _____
4. _____
5. _____
6. _____

## D. Multiple Choice: Place the correct letter or letters on the blank line for each question.

_____ 1. The medical assistant shows respect and compassion by calling them in from the reception area by
    a. title (Mr., Ms., etc)        c. either "dear or honey"
    b. first name only        d. first and last name

_____ 2. If the patient has several chief complaints, the medical assistant should
    a. list all the questions that were asked        c. make a list of the symptoms
    b. tell the patient to tell the doctor        d. record the most serious problem

_____ 3. When a patient tells you of a significant personal change in his or her life (e.g. loss of a loved one, being fired, etc.),
    a. keep it to yourself        c. the physician should be told
    b. note it in the chart        d. just acknowledge what was said

_____ 4. A stress-inducing situation (such as mentioned above)
    a. is irrelevant        c. is the patient's business
    b. can influence treatment        d. none of these

_____ 5. If the patient gains or lose weight, this can
    a. be a hereditary trait        c. change the course of treatment
    b. be an error in the scale        d. be recorded on a genogram

## CRITICAL THINKING SCENARIOS: What would your response be in the following situations?

1. A new co-worker is interviewing a new patient at the reception window, asking medical history questions and completing the form in earshot and in view of everyone in the office. What would you do? _____

_____

2. This same new worker is found erasing several items on the completed medical history form. What advice do you offer and why? _____

_____

## ACHIEVING SKILL COMPETENCY

Reread the performance objectives for these procedures and then practice the skills listed below, following the procedures in your textbook.

Procedure 13-1: Interview Patient to Complete Medical History Form

Procedure 13-2: Measure Height

Procedure 13-3: Weigh Patient on Upright Scale

When you feel you have mastered performance of a skill, sign your name on the appropriate evaluation sheet and give it to your instructor to indicate you are prepared to perform the procedure for evaluation.

After your instructor has returned your work to you, make all necessary corrections and place in a three-ring notebook for future reference.

**Chapter 13:  BEGINNING THE PATIENT'S RECORD**

**Unit 2:  TRIAGE**

### A.  Brief Answer

1. Discuss the origin of triage. _____
2. Where in the medical office should triage be performed? _____
   _____
3. Explain phone triage. _____
   _____
   _____
4. State the purpose of progress notes in the patient chart. _____
   _____
5. What type of questioning should be used during patient interviews to obtain information regarding their medical condition? _____
   _____
6. Discuss what you should cover with patients at each office visit. _____
   _____
7. List the categories for determining the urgency of a patient's condition. _____
   _____
   _____
8. What is the best way to gain patient compliance? _____
   _____

### B.  Fill in the Blank

1. The French word *triage* means to _____
2. In many medical facilities, small _____ provide privacy to patients during triage.
3. In the medical office there should be a _____ of action developed regarding telephone and face-to-face triage.
4. All office personnel must be familiar with standard first aid procedures and _____
5. You should _____ patients to write down their questions to discuss with the doctor so they will not forget.

### C.  Matching:  Match the definition in column II with the correct term in column I.

| COLUMN I | COLUMN II |
|---|---|
| _____ 1. Prioritize | a.  Careful; dedicated and thorough |
| _____ 2. Trivial | b.  Permission to make decision using your own judgment |
| _____ 3. Dispatch | c.  Sort in order of importance |
| _____ 4. Discretion | d.  To combine together in a united whole |
| _____ 5. Conscientious | e.  Of little importance |
| | f.  Send; convey |

After your instructor has returned your work to you, make all necessary corrections and place in a three-ring notebook for future reference.

**Chapter 13: BEGINNING THE PATIENT'S RECORD**

**Unit 3: VITAL SIGNS**

## SUGGESTED RESPONSES TO CRITICAL THINKING CHALLENGE IN TEXTBOOK

1. What areas of the Role Delineation Chart were ignored?

2. How might this incident affect Susan's employment opportunities?

3. What effect could this have on her current and future insurance coverage?

4. How might the medical assistant and the physician be affected?

This unit contains many important concepts and skills to be mastered; therefore, this workbook unit is divided into four parts.

## PART 1—TEMPERATURE CONTROL AND MEASUREMENT

### A. Mixed Quiz

1. Identify the four vital signs, indicating what body function is being measured.
   a. _Blood Precisure_ measures the force of the heart.
   b. _temporature_ measures the body's heat.
   c. _Pulse_ measures the action of the heart.
   d. _Respiration_ measures action of the lungs (breathing).
2. Vital sign findings should be recorded _immediately following measurement to avoid memory error._
3. The body loses heat through _perspiration_ and _breathing / waste_
4. The balance between heat production and heat loss determines the _Body temperature._

5. Temperature is usually the ___Lowest___ in the morning and the ___highest___ in the afternoon and evening.

6. Fill in the Blank
Temperature in the body is controlled by the ___Brain___ in the ___hypothalamus___ of the brain. When receptors sense the presence of excess heat, the ___sweat glands___ produce ___sweat___ which ___evaporates___ from the surface of the skin, causing the body to ___cool___ The surface blood vessels ___dialate___ which allows more blood to be in contact with the surface of the skin. The blood ___loses___ heat, thereby ___cooling___ the blood in the vessels. When receptors sense a lack of heat, the surface blood vessels ___constrict___ to ___heat loss___ heat loss. Small papillary muscles ___contract___ producing ___goose flush___ to help ___warm___ the body. Shivering and chills will cause body heat to ___rise___ ___protective mechanism from cool air___

7. Explain briefly how a fever develops (use five steps).
   a. ___microorganism cause the patient to exp. chills and shivering untill the temp. is warm___
   b. ___white blood cell activity from fighting Bacterial infection___
   c. _____
   d. _____
   e. _____

8. Fill in the Blank
Provide the correct Fahrenheit temperature when referring to classifications of fevers.
   a. Slight = ___99.6___°F
   b. Moderate = ___101.0___°F
   c. Severe = ___102.0___°F
   d. Dangerous = ___104.0___°F
   e. Fatal = over ___106.0___°F

9. The column of mercury shown on the thermometer reads a "normal" 98.6° on the Fahrenheit scale. At each arrow, read the temperature and enter the finding at the corresponding space.

a. ___94.4___ ✓   c. ___97.4___ ✓   e. ___99.2___ ✓   g. ___101.6___ ✓   i. ___103.4___ ✓
b. ___95.6___ ✓   d. ___98.8___ ✓   f. ___100.2___ ✓   h. ___102.2___ ✓   j. ___105.4___ ✓

10. The column of mercury on the thermometer reads a "normal" 37° on the Celsius scale. At each arrow, read the temperature and enter the finding at the corresponding space.

a. ___35.4___   c. ___36.6___   e. ___37.6___   g. _____   i. ___41.1___
b. ___35.8___   d. ___37.2___   f. ___38.4___   h. ___39.4___   j. ___40.9___

11. List the five thermometer types.
   a. _glass mercury_
   b. _plastic disposable_
   c. _Digital_
   d. _electronic probe_
   e. _tympatic infrared_
12. Name situations when oral temperature measurement is contraindicated.
   a. _they have breathing problems_
   b. _when person is ophyso_
   c. _unconsious_
   d. _stroke_
   e. _Breathing_
13. Matching: Match the terms in column I with their meanings in column II.

COLUMN I
_i_  1. Afebrile
_g_  2. Axillary
_F_  3. Febrile
_b_  4. Oral
_j_  5. Sublingual
_k_  6. Fever
_A_  7. Celsius
_L_  8. Rectal
_C_  9. Calibration
_e_  10. Stem
_H_  11. Disinfectant
_d_  12. Contraindicated

COLUMN II
a. A metric measurement
b. By mouth
c. Numbered markings
d. Not appropriate
e. Thermometer section
f. Fever
g. Underarm
h. Germicide → kill germs
i. Without fever
j. Beneath tongue
k. Elevated body heat
l. Anal
m. Fahrenheit
n. Anesthetic
o. Security

14. Convert the following Celsius temperatures to Fahrenheit.
   a. 36.5°C = _____ °F          d. 35.7°C = _____ °F
   b. 39.5°C = _____ °F          e. 36.8°C = _____ °F
   c. 38.8°C = _____ °F          f. 37.4°C = _____ °F

15. Convert the following Fahrenheit temperatures to Celsius.
   a. 96.8°F = _36.9_ °C         d. 99.2°F = _____ °C
   b. 97.4°F = _____ °C          e. 100.2°F = _____ °C
   c. 98.6°F = _____ °C          f. 102.4°F = _____ °C

16. **Word Search:** Find the following words hidden in the puzzle.

ACCURACY · AFEBRILE · ASEPTICALLY · AXILLARY · BULB · BUTTOCKS · CALIBRATION · CENTIGRADE · CHILLS · CHIPPED · COLLAPSE · COOLING · CONTRAINDICATED

DANGEROUS · DEGREES · DISINFECT · ELECTRONIC · ELEVATION · FAHRENHEIT · FATAL · FEBRILE · FEVER · FINDINGS · FRAGILE · GLASS · HEAT

HOLDER · INFECTION · INSERT · INSPECT · LUBRICANT · MERCURY · METRIC · MODERATE · MOUTH · NORMAL · ORAL · RECORD · RECTAL

SECURITY · SEVERE · SHAKE · SLIGHT · STEM · STUBBY · SUBLINGUAL · SUBNORMAL · TEMPERATURE · TENTHS · THERMOMETER

```
A G L A S S I E T V E E O F A T A L M M W Q I S T N D
C H I L L S O T B C L O B T P W I E L E V A T I O N V
O I Y T W C B N Y I C F I H E M K V Z T O P W I M G X
L G F J M I T O G P H C N E C M M I W R W S T U B B Y
L V A C C U R A C Y I U S R C V P S Y I E A S H A K E
A E A J K U R L R Y P T P M P O E E C C R V Y T Z X P
P N F A H F P U I X P B E O Q H C S R B K N L R W V C
S W E R T I C D L P E Y C M R T O W I A J L V C X I N
E N B P R R B V A G D D T E I Y Q L P U T M V X W O F
W I R C E B V X U N J H V T L W A L D I W U L W I O E
M V I M C O W G T E G H I E M C A L O E W P R T Z C V
B C L I T E N I P I U E S R C M V X U Y R W C E N L E
C F E S A I J L L Y T Q R X R S Z Y I N S E R T D E R
K H J R L N B S A W Q Z R O P U T V W L F U C B L S W
B G D O M U R B C I W R N P U F X C V N L I Y I V C S
U K O M L U B R I C A N T G H S W Q I K N A R X C V T
T C C O N T R A I N D I C A T E D E P O T B R C X I E
T D F A S C V B B N I O Y U I O R W R C E I O Y E C M
O S U B N O R M A L M T Q W E E O T C F K L H H T Y U
C E N T I G R A D E I O S D V C C S U B L I N G U A L
K E R E Y U I O O R S D D E L E I O L S D E M N V C S
S E R N K L M O U T H I S E L K L U S D R E C O R D I
U T Y T F G H C R T Y U I E R I B I O H E A T Y U I O
W E R H A S E P T I C A L L Y A K L A W E R T Y O I R
A S D S L S Z X C V B N M S D F T F I N D I N G S I A
D I S I N F E C T A N T E D E G R E E S G J K L Z X L
```

## ACHIEVING SKILL COMPETENCY

Reread the performance objective for each procedure and then practice the skills listed below, following the procedures in your textbook.

Procedure 13-8:  Measure Oral Temperature with Disposable Plastic Thermometer
Procedure 13-9:  Measure Oral Temperature Electronically
Procedure 13-10: Measure Core Body Temperature with Infrared Tympanic Thermometer

When you feel you have mastered performance of a skill, sign your name on the appropriate evaluation sheet and give it to your instructor to indicate you are prepared to perform the procedure for evaluation.

## PART 2—THE PULSE AND ITS MEASUREMENT

### B. Mixed Quiz

1. Define *pulse* and explain how it occurs. the Rhythmic expansion of an artery that may be felt with the finger.

2. Name and locate the five pulse points.
   a. Radial = thumb side of the inner surface of the wrist, over the Radius B
   b. Brachial = on the inner medial surface of the elbow
   c. Carotid =
   d. femoral point =
   e. dorsalis pedis =

3. How is pulse rate determined? What is the normal adult rate? the # of times the heart beats per min is counting the pulse in the radial artery

4. List five factors that influence heart rate.
   a. exercise / Activity
   b. size
   c. Age
   d. sex of the person / more female
   e. physical condition

5. Stimulation of the sympathetic nervous system increases heart rate. The parasympathetic nervous system decreases the heart rate.

6. List eight situations that cause the heart rate to increase.
   a. Fear
   b. Anxiety
   c. Pain
   d. Anger
   e. Thyroid disease
   f. Anemia
   g. shock
   h. Fever

7. List four situations that cause the heart rate to decrease.
   a. certain medication
   b. heart disease
   c. Emotional depressi
   d. drugs

8. Name the two qualities of the heartbeat that must be observed, defining the terms and listing the words used to describe the characteristics.
   a. Volume = the strength of the pulse / normal, full, bounding, weak, thre
   b. Rhythm = Relular spacing of the beats / arRhythmia

9. List eight times when apical pulse measurement would be indicated.
   a. difficulty feeling Radial pulse
   b. Missing beats
   c. Rapid Rate
   d. Slow Rate
   e. thready Quality
   f. 9 Irregular Quality
   g. existing pulse deficit
   h. suspected pulse deficit

10. True or False: Place a "T" for true or an "F" for false in the space provided. For false statements, explain why they are false.
    T — a. A patient should be sitting or lying down when the pulse is measured.
    F — b. The radial pulse can be found at the inner wrist area on the little finger side. – thumb side
    F — c. The radial pulse is best felt by placing your thumb over the artery.
    F — d. The pulse that can be felt in the radial artery is caused by the contraction of the aorta.
    F — e. Apical pulse is located at the right fifth intercostal space.
    F — f. A quick way to estimate the location of the apex is to position the right hand over the patient's chest and listen at the point under the thumb.

11. Fill in the Blanks

Pulse deficit can be determined by measuring ___apical___ pulse and ___radial rate___ pulse at the ___same time___ If a patient has a pulse deficit, the auscultated apical pulse rate is ___higher apical___ than the ___radial___ pulse rate. This occurs because some of the contractions are ___not strong enough.___

12. Matching: Match the terms in column I with the correct meaning in column II.

COLUMN I

___C___ 1. Antecubital
___h___ 2. Apex
___b___ 3. Arrhythmia
___i___ 4. Auscultate
___j___ 5. Brachial
___A___ 6. Bradycardia
___g___ 7. Carotid
___l___ 8. Femoral
___b___ 9. Palpate
___M___ 10. Pulse deficit
___f___ 11. Radial
___e___ 12. Tachycardia

COLUMN II

a. Excessively slow heart rate
b. Feel by touching
c. Inner elbow area
d. A pulse point on the instep of the foot
e. Excessively rapid heart rate
f. A pulse point at the inner wrist
g. A pulse point near the trachea
h. Lower edge of the heart
i. To listen
j. A pulse point at the inner elbow
k. Without a regular pattern of beats
l. A pulse point at the groin
m. The difference between apical and radial pulse
n. Weak heart volume

13. Unscramble

a. _ _ _ _ _     RTEHA
b. _ _ _ _     EBTA
c. _ _ _ _ _ _ _ _     TCNTAROC
d. _ _ _ _ _ _ _ _     LYOISTSC
e. _ _ _ _ _ _     LIACAP
f. _ _ _ _ _     SLUEP
g. _ _ _ _ _ _ _ _ _ _     HRAMTIRHYA
h. _ _ _ _ _ _ _     ATCRDIO
i. _ _ _ _ _ _     ALRIDA
j. _ _ _ _ _ _ _ _     HLRAIBAC
k. _ _ _ _ _ _ _     MROAFLE
l. _ _ _ _ _ _     EYTARR
m. _ _ _ _     TREA
n. _ _ _ _ _ _     YHTRMH
o. _ _ _ _ _ _     LVEMOU

## ACHIEVING SKILL COMPETENCY

Reread the performance objective for these procedures and then practice the skills listed below, following the procedures in your textbook.

Procedure 13-11: Measure Radial Pulse

Procedure 13-12: Measure Apical Pulse

When you feel you have mastered performance of a skill, sign your name on the appropriate evaluation sheet and give it to your instructor to indicate you are prepared to perform the procedure for evaluation.

## PART 3: RESPIRATIONS: OBSERVATION AND MEASUREMENT

### C. Mixed Quiz

1. One respiration is the combination of one total _inspiration_ and one total _experiration_
   Two other terms that are frequently used and have the same meaning are _inhale_ and
   _exhale_

2. When are respirations usually measured? _One part of total vital signs assessment._

3. Why are respirations measured as if the pulse is being measured? _So the patient isn't aware that you're watching their breathing_

4. The quality of respirations must be observed. Normal respirations are _quiet effortless_ and
   _Regular space._

5. Excessively rapid and deep respirations are known as _hyperventilation._

6. Patients with difficult or labored breathing are said to have _dyspnea_

7. Noisy respirations are called rales, and are often present with diseases such as _Pneumonia_
   _Bronchitis_ and _asthma_

8. Quality characteristics that are evaluated when respirations are measured are:
   a. Depth of inhalation which, is described as _normal shallow_ or
      _deep_ .
   b. Rhythm of respiration, which is described as _Regular_ or _Irregular_

9. Absence of breathing is known as _apnea_

10. Describe the breathing pattern known as Cheyne-Stokes. _Occurs with acute Brain, heart, or lung damage or disease with intoxicants._

11. Normal respiration rate for an adult is _12 — 20_ per minute.

12. Respiration rate is affected by:
    a. _Age_
    b. _emotions_
    c. _exercises_
    d. _diseases_
    e. _activities_

13. Fill in the temperature-pulse-respiration ratio below.

| Temperature | Pulse | Respiration |
|---|---|---|
| 99°F | | |
| 100°F | | |
| 102°F | | |
| 104°F | | |

14. Crossword Puzzle

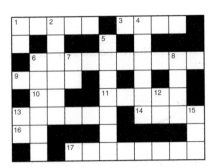

ACROSS

1. Organ which pumps blood
3. Contraction phase
6. Without rhythm
9. Lower heart edge
10. Part of the verb "to be"
11. One of the vital signs
13. Heart
14. A period of time
16. Father
17. A pulse point

DOWN

1. Mercury (abbr)
2. Sudden heart failure
4. Breathe out
5. Difficult breathing
6. Auscultated heart beat
7. Prescription (abbr)
8. A plan or thought
12. Senior (abbr)
13. Anterior-posterior (abbr)
15. Solution (abbr)

15. Speling: Each line contains four different spellings of a word. Underline the correctly spelled term.

| | | | |
|---|---|---|---|
| a. Cheyne-Stokes | Chain-Stokes | Cheyne-Stoakes | Chenye-Stokes |
| b. dispnea | dispena | dyspnea | dyspnae |
| c. eshale | exhale | exhail | exhaile |
| d. expirashun | experation | expieration | expiration |
| e. enhale | enhail | inhale | inhail |
| f. inspiration | enspiration | ensperation | insperation |
| g. resperation | respiration | rexpiration | rexperation |

**ACHIEVING SKILL COMPETENCY**

Reread the performance objective for the procedure and then practice the skill listed below, following the procedure in your textbook.

Procedure 13-13: Measure Respirations

When you feel you have mastered performance of a skill, sign your name on the appropriate evaluation sheet and give it to your instructor to indicate you are prepared to perform the procedure for evaluation.

## PART 4: BLOOD PRESSURE

### D. Mixed Quiz

1. Name the four vital signs.

   a. _____

   b. _____

   c. _____

   d. _____

2. Define *blood pressure.* _____

   _____

3. What does blood pressure measurement evaluate?

   a. _____

   b. _____

   c. _____

   d. _____

4. Where is blood pressure measured? (be specific) _____

5. Name the two organs that maintain blood pressure in the body.

   a. _____

   b. _____

6. Explain briefly how blood pressure is maintained. _____

   _____

   _____

   _____

7. Name the two phases of the blood pressure, describing the corresponding action which occurs and the relative amount of pressure with each phase. _____

   _____

8. Blood pressure is measured in _____

9. Blood pressure is measured by a _____ which has either an _____ dial or a column of _____

10. Normal adult systolic pressure is _____ normal diastolic pressure is _____

11. Blood pressure that is consistently high is called _____

12. Blood pressure that is consistently low is called _____

13. An elevated pressure without apparent cause is said to be _____ or _____ hypertension.

14. List six possible causes of hypertension.

   a. _____    d. _____

   b. _____    e. _____

   c. _____    f. _____

15. Define *pulse pressure.* _____

16. Using the "general rule of thumb," is the pulse pressure of the following examples too low, normal, or too high? (*Note:* A normal pulse pressure does not mean the blood pressure is within a normal range.)

   a. 130/86 _____

   b. 160/90 _____

   c. 110/74 _____

   d. 200/110 _____

   e. 186/98 _____

   f. 120/100 _____

   g. 174/116 _____

260

17. Several equipment factors influence accurate measurement. Explain what each item indicates or would cause to occur.
    a. Leaking mercury or bubbles would cause _____
    b. Too small a cuff would cause _____
    c. Too large a cuff would cause _____
    d. Mercury meniscus below "O" indicates _____
18. True or False: Place a "T" for true or an "F" for false in the space prvoided. For false statements, explain why they are false.
    _____ a. Completely deflate the cuff before applying.
    _____ b. Blood pressure may be measured over a silky sleeve.
    _____ c. The cuff is placed around the arm with the arrow at the brachial artery.
    _____ d. Inflate cuff slowly until you no longer hear beats.
    _____ e. When you miss the systolic reading, immediately reinflate the cuff before all air pressure escapes.
    _____ f. The patient's arm should be extended straight down at the side when in sitting position.
    _____ g. Palpatory readings are done only when the pressure cannot be auscultated.
19. What does it mean to take a baseline reading? _____
_____
20. Define *auscultatory gap.* _____
21. What would cause you to think a patient might have an auscultatory gap: _____
_____

22. Crossword Puzzle

DOWN
1. Bone
2. Article; used in language
3. Silver-colored liquid
4. To take nourishment
5. Lowered
6. 365 days
7. Felt in arteries
10. Contraction phase
13. Pulse point at wrist
14. Noisy respirations
16. The number of times
17. Three dimensional X ray (abbreviation)
20. Pelvic exam (acronym)

ACROSS
2. End of prayer
5. Difficult breathing
8. Second word in music scale
9. Right (abbreviation)
11. Blood _____
12. External organ of hearing
15. Most desirable option
18. Mother
19. Bottom edge of heart
21. Stories
22. Barium enema (acronym)

12. Unscramble

    a. _ _ _ _ _ _ _                          ENIDOAR

    b. _ _ _ _ _ _ _ _ _ _ _ _                TUTENBLAIAC

    c. _ _ _ _ _ _ _ _ _ _                    LSAIDOTCI

    d. _ _ _ _ _ _ _ _                        HRABLICA

    e. _ _ _ _ _ _ _ _ _                      SLATSNEIE

    f. _ _ _ _ _ _ _ _ _ _                    ETUSLTAUAC

    g. _ _ _ _ _ _ _ _ _ _ _ _                OEPTYEHRNSIN

    h. _ _ _ _ _ _ _                          YRUMREC

    i. _ _ _ _ _ _ _ _                        LTYSCOSI

    j. _ _ _ _ _ _ _                          TPEALPA

13. Refer to the ABHES Course Content Requirements in Appendix C of the textbook. Within the area of *Medical Office Clinical Procedures,* which content requirement is discussed in this unit? _____

_____

## ACHIEVING SKILL COMPETENCY

Reread the performance objective for the procedure and then practice the skill listed below, following the procedure in your textbook.

Procedure 13-14:  Measure Blood Pressure

When you feel you have mastered performance of a skill, sign your name on the appropriate evaluation sheet and give it to your instructor to indicate you are prepared to perform the procedure for evaluation.

After your instructor has returned your work to you, make all necessary corrections and place in a three-ring notebook for future reference.

**ASSIGNMENT SHEET**

## Chapter 14:  PREPARING PATIENTS FOR EXAMINATION

Review the objectives and text for each unit before completing the assignment sheet for that unit. When you have completed all sheets for the chapter, remove them from this Workbook and give them to the instructor for evaluation.

## Unit 1:  PROCEDURES OF THE EYE AND EAR

**A. Multiple Choice:  Place the correct letter or letters on the blank line for each question.**

_____  1. Patients should be screened for visual acuity

    a. wearing their corrective lenses         c. early in the morning

    b. only in natural lighting               d. without their corrective lenses

_____  2. Patients should hold the Jaeger near vision card at what distance away from the eyes?

    a. 0.4 to 0.6 inches              c. 14 to 16 feet

    b. 4 to 6 inches                   d. 14 to 16 inches

_____  3. A person with normal hearing should be able to hear all frequencies up to ____ decibels?

    a. 0.15                       c. 15

    b. 1.5                       d. none of these

_____  4. The medical assistant who will be administering the color vision acuity screening must first

    a. be tested to determine if she has normal color vision acuity

    b. take the test wearing corrective lenses

    c. tell patients to cover the right eye and test the left, then reverse, then both

    d. determine if an eye irrigation is necessary

_____  5. It very important to administer the color vision acuity test to patients with

    a. cardiac problems             c. thyroid conditions

    b. diabetes                  d. glaucoma

_____  6. What instrument measures one's hearing ability?

    a. otoscope                  c. autoclave

    b. audiometer              d. tuning fork

## B.  Brief Answer

1. List patient education advice you can offer during procedures of the eye and ear. _____

_____

_____

2. What must the medical assistant remember to do with the ophthalmoscope and otoscope in preparing for eye and ear examinations: _____

_____

3. What types of patients will require being tested for visual acuity with the Snellen chart? _____

_____

4. Why must the patient keep both eyes open during the visual acuity screening even though one eye is covered?

_____

5. What is the Ishihara screening method, and why is it administered to patients? _____

_____

6. Why is it necessary for the medical assistant to wear latex gloves when performing procedures on the eye and ear? _____

_____

7. What is the purpose of an eye irrigation? _____

_____

8. Define instillation of eye or ear drops. _____

_____

9. What is cerumen? _____

10. Why must impacted cerumen be softened and irrigated from the ear? _____

_____

_____

11. Explain why the tip of an eye (medication) dropper or the tip of a tube of eye ointment must never touch the secretions of the eye or the eye itself. _____

_____

_____

12. Describe the Rinne test for hearing. _____

_____

_____

13. Describe the Weber test for hearing. _____

_____

14. List common behaviors that may indicate hearing loss. _____

_____

_____

15. List common complaints that may indicate visual disturbances. _____

_____

16. What is the purpose of the audiometer? _____

_____

## C. Crossword Puzzle

ACROSS

3. Red blindness
9. Green blindness
12. Regarding the ear
13. Please ____ the eye chart
14. Medical term for earwax
16. Another word for lavage
18. To open and close eyes fast
19. Visual acuity charts
21. Instrument used to measure hearing
23. Blue blindness
25. Used to protect hands from body fluids/standard precautions
27. Measuring intraocular pressure
28. One of a pair of the organs of sight
29. Used with otoscope to examine the ear
30. Small amount of sterile cotton (holds medication in ear)

DOWN

1. Carefully
2. Color blindness (both red and green)
4. Abbreviation for left eye
5. Abbreviation for right eye
6. To state further
7. Organ of hearing
8. Means "to wash out"
10. Unit for measuring volume of sound abbreviation for both eyes
11. Abbreviation for both eyes
15. Study of the fundus of the eye
17. To introduce a solution into a cavity
20. Instrument used to examine the ear
21. Clearness/sharpness of perception
24. The external ear
26. Capacity for sight

**A. Matching: Match the definition in column II with the correct term in column I.**

COLUMN I
_____ 1. Pelli-Robson chart
_____ 2. For babies
_____ 3. Numerator of 20/100
_____ 4. Ear instillation
_____ 5. For adults
_____ 6. Observe patient
_____ 7. Snellen chart
_____ 8. Eye instillation
_____ 9. Denominator of 20/100
_____ 10. Wick
_____ 11. Jaeger system

COLUMN II
a. For behaviors indicating visual disturbances
b. Pull up and back to straighten the ear canal
c. A screening for near vision acuity
d. Cotton saturated with medication for ear
e. Required distance one stands from visual acuity chart
f. To treat infection, anesthetize, dilate pupil, relieve irritation
h. Means that one stood 20 feet from chart and read the line that one should be able to read at a distance of 100 feet
g. Measure contrast sensitivity for earlier diagnosis of eye disease
i. Pull down and back to straighten the ear canal
j. Determines color vision acuity
k. To treat infection, relieve pain, soften cerumen
l. A screening for distance visual acuity

**CRITICAL THINKING SCENARIOS: What would your response be in the following situations?**

1. Mr. Harold tells you that his ears often get plugged up and he can't understand it because he uses a cotton-tipped applicator every day after his shower to get all the ear wax out. _____

_____

2. Myra is a teenage patient who comes in frequently to see the doctor for her allergies. She always has her head set and radio on full volume. _____

_____

**ACHIEVING SKILL COMPETENCY**

Reread the performance objective for the procedures and then practice the skills listed below, following the procedure in the textbook.

Procedure 14-1: Irrigate the Eye
Procedure 14-2: Irrigate the Ear
Procedure 14-3: Instill Eardrops
Procedure 14-4: Instill Eyedrops
Procedure 14-5: Screen Visual Acuity with Snellen Chart
Procedure 14-6: Screen Visual Acuity with Jaeger System

When you feel you have mastered performance of a skill, sign your name on the appropriate evaluation sheet and give it to your instructor to indicate you are prepared to perform the procedure for evaluation.

After your instructor has returned your work to you, make all necessary corrections and place in a three-ring notebook for future reference.

## ASSIGNMENT SHEET

## Chapter 14: PREPARING PATIENTS FOR EXAMINATION

## Unit 2: POSITIONING AND DRAPING FOR EXAMINATIONS

### A. Brief Answer

1. Explain the purpose of each of the following examination positions.

   a. Horizontal recumbent or supine. _Position is used for examination and treatment of the anterior surface of the body and for x-rays,_

   b. Dorsal recumbent. _to indicate that the legs are flexed. Position allows for relaxation of the abdominal area. Position may be also used for vaginal or rectal examination._

   c. Prone. _Position is used for examination of the back or spine, with gown open in the back_

   d. Standing erect or anatomical. _____

   e. Sims' or lateral. _____

   f. Knee-chest. _Used for rectal examination and specifically for sigmoidoscopy_

   g. Genupectoral. _used as therapy for postpartum prolapsed uterus._

   h. Fowler's. _Used for patient's with respiratory or cardiovascular problems_

   i. Semi-Fowler's. _____

   j. Lithotomy. _Position used for vaginal or rectal examination this can also be used for examination of the genital area_

   k. Trendelenburg or shock _the position, the patient is supine with feet w/ feet elevated slightly this position may easily be accomplished with a power table_

   l. Jackknife. _(comfortable)_

2. What safety precautions must be observed for protection of both the patient and the medical assistant? _female medical assistant should remain in the room when a female is being examined by a male physician._

3. Why is a drape used when positioning patients? _to show respect for privacy of the patient, and for comfort patient._

4. What support is used for the feet in the lithotomy position? _stirrups_

5. Name the drape used for proctological examinations. _fenestrated drape_

**B. Matching:** Match the position in column II with the correct term in column I.

COLUMN I

_____ 1. Back and posterior
_____ 2. Exercise postpartum
_____ 3. Proctoscopic
_____ 4. Eye, Ear, Nose, Throat
_____ 5. Anterior
_____ 6. Pelvic
_____ 7. Shock
_____ 8. Abdominal exam
_____ 9. Gynecologist
_____ 10. GP/Internal Medicine
_____ 11. Ophthalmologist, thoracic surgeon, ENT specialist
_____ 12. Proctologist
_____ 13. No specialty
_____ 14. GP/Orthopedist/Internist
_____ 15. GP/Internal Medicine/Gynecologist

COLUMN II

a. Genupectoral
b. Sims'/knee-chest
c. Semi-Fowler's/Fowler's
d. Horizontal/recumbent/supine
e. Prone
f. Trendelenburg
g. Dorsal recumbent
h. Lithotomy

**C. Multiple Choice:** Place the correct letter on the blank line for each question.

_____ 1. Patient lying flat on table with buttocks at lower end of the table and feet supported in stirrups
   a. prone        c. lithotomy
   b. Sim's        d. Fowler's

_____ 2. Patient on back with feet elevated
   a. Sim's        c. prone
   b. supine        d. Trendelenburg

_____ 3. Patient sitting with head of table elevated at 45° angle
   a. lithotomy        c. semi-Fowler's
   b. lateral        d. supine

_____ 4. Patient lying flat on back with feet flat on table and knees flexed
   a. knee-chest        c. dorsal recumbent
   b. prone        d. Sim's

_____ 5. Patient flat on stomach with the head to one side
   a. Trendelenburg        c. lateral
   b. prone        d. horizontal recumbent

_____ 6. Patient on knees and chest with knees separated and head to one side
   a. dorsal recumbent        c. knee-chest
   b. Sim's        d. lateral

_____ 7. Patient on left side with left leg flexed slightly and right leg flexed sharply to the chest
   a. lithotomy        c. Sim's
   b. supine        d. supine

_____ 8. Patient lying flat on back with legs together
   a. horizontal recumbent        c. dorsal recumbent
   b. Sim's        d. prone

**D. Identification:** Identify the following examination positions. Refer to pages 611–617 in the textbook.

1. a <u>Horizontal Recumbent</u>

1. b <u>dorsal Recumbent</u>

1. c _____

2. <u>PRONE POSITION</u>

3. <u>Sims position</u>

4. <u>Knee-chest</u>

45°
angle

5. a ___ Semi ___

90°
angle

5. ___ high ___

6. Lithotomy ___

7. Trendelenburg ___

## E. Crossword Puzzle

**ACROSS**

2. Pelvic
5. Chest, proctoscopic exam
8. Back, posterior
9. Same as Sims'
10. Same as supine
11. Eye, ear, nose, throat

**DOWN**

1. Proctoscopic exam
3. Shock
4. Anterior
6. Relax abdomen
7. Eye, ear, nose, throat

## CRITICAL THINKING SCENARIOS: What would your response be in the following situation?

1. A female patient in her 80s seems to be very confused as you explain to her that you want her to undress and wear a gown and drape in preparation for a complete physical examination. _____

_____

## ACHIEVING SKILL COMPETENCY

Reread the performance objective for each procedure and then practice the skills listed below, following the procedures in your textbook.

Procedure 14-8:   Assist Patient to Horizontal Recumbent Position
Procedure 14-9:   Assist Patient to Prone Position
Procedure 14-10:  Assist Patient to Sims' Position
Procedure 14-11:  Assist Patient to Knee-Chest Position
Procedure 14-12:  Assist Patient to Semi-Fowler's Position
Procedure 14-13:  Assist Patient to Lithotomy Position

When you feel you have mastered performance of a skill, sign your name on the appropriate evaluation sheet and give it to your instructor to indicate you are prepared to perform the procedure for evaluation.

After your instructor has returned your work to you, make all necessary corrections and place in a three-ring notebook for future reference.

## ASSIGNMENT SHEET

### Chapter 14: PREPARING PATIENTS FOR EXAMINATIONS

### Unit 3: PREPARING PATIENTS FOR EXAMINATIONS

## SUGGESTED RESPONSES TO CRITICAL THINKING CHALLENGE IN TEXTBOOK

1. What are Martina and Sylvia guilty of doing? _____

2. Should they apologize to Cassie? _____

3. Should the office manager or physician be informed of this behavior? _____

4. Do you think Sylvia and Martina meant any malice? _____

5. Is there any legal action that should be initiated in this situation? _____

6. Should Cassie have responded immediately to what she overheard? _____

7. What would you do in this situation? _____

## ANSWERS TO WORKBOOK ASSIGNMENT

### A. Brief Answer

1. Define *subjective* and *objective symptoms* and give three examples of each.

   Those symptoms that the patient feels but that cannot be seen by another, objective symptoms that can be seen by another and by the patient

2. List each section of a physical examination and describe how the physician conducts the exam.

3. Describe the role of the medical assistant in the patient examination process.

   Explains proceedings, answers any questions and may begin patient education where appropriate.

4. List various patient education tips for various sections of the patient examination.

   Verify what patient feels is the problem, allow patient time to use the restroom, ask to urinate in a specimen cup if needed. Bring one.

5. What are the nine sections of the abdominal cavity? Bring one.

   Right Hypochondriac, Epigastric, left hypochondriac, Right umbilical, Left Lumbar, Right inguinal, Hypogastric, left in

6. List the internal organs located in each of the nine sections of the abdomen. _____

7. Define the Problem Oriented Medical Record (POMR) system.

*Referred to as pos, used for a new patient now to do*

8. Explain how data are recorded with the POMR system.

9. List the warning signs for adults and children.

10. What are the standard physical examination schedules for adults and children?

**B. Matching:** Match the definition in column II with the correct term in column I.

COLUMN I

_____ 1. Sphygmomanometer
_____ 2. Speculum
_____ 3. Tonometer
_____ 4. Tape measure
_____ 5. Stethoscope
_____ 6. Guaiac test paper
_____ 7. Tuning fork
_____ 8. Percussion hammer
_____ 9. Ophthalmoscope
_____ 10. Otoscope
_____ 11. Goose neck lamp
_____ 12. Tongue depressor

COLUMN II

a. Used to elicit an involuntary response
b. Provides light necessary for inspection
c. Used to view tiny capillaries behind retina
d. Used to check sense of smell
e. Instrument used to examine inner ear
f. Used for indirect auscultation
g. Instrument used to inspect a body cavity
h. Permits visual inspections of mouth/throat
i. Measures intraocular pressure to determine glaucoma
j. Physician uses this instrument to assess patient's hearing
k. Test for occult blood in stool
l. For measuring chest and extremities
m. Used to obtain blood pressure readings in both arms

## C. Identification: Identify these instruments used in examinations.

1. PERCUSSION hammer
2. tuning fork
3. flexible tape measure
4. laryngeal miror
5. plastic/disposable
6. otoscope read attached to Base handle

7. MERCURY gravity
8. ANEROID sphygmomanom
9. ophthalmoscope
10. stethoscope
11. tonometer.

1    2    3    4    5    6

7    8    9    10    11

## D. Fill in the Blank

1. Direct percussion is termed __immediate__ and is done by striking the finger against the patient's body.
2. Pitch, quality, duration, and resonance are terms that refer to __PERcussion__
3. Direct __Auscultation__ is done by placing your ear directly over a body area to hear sounds within.
4. __Assesment__ of problems in the SOAP method of recording patient information means documenting measurement of the patient's symptoms.
5. Referrals, medications, surgery, therapy, exercise, or other orders to return a patient to better health are all part of the __plan for treatment__ in the SOAP method.

**E. Matching:** Match the definition in column II with the correct term in column I.

COLUMN I

- i  1. Percussion
- l  2. Progress notes/report
- k  3. Palpation
- g  4. Objective symptoms
- j  5. Manipulation
- a  6. First part of physical exam
- m  7. Romberg test
- n  8. General appearance
- p  9. Set of procedures
- f  10. Auscultation
- o  11. Red ink
- d  12. Inspection
- b  13. Writer
- h  14. Mensuration
- e  15. Subjective findings

COLUMN II

a. Includes measurement, vital signs, and vision screening
b. Takes dictation during patient's exam
c. Plan of treatment
d. Visual exam of body's various parts
e. You can't see; patient feels
f. Listening to body sounds
g. Heel-to-shin test
h. Measurement of chest and extremities
i. The tapping of the fingers over a body area to produce sounds
j. The forceful passive movement of a joint to determine range of motion
k. Applying fingers/hands against the skin to feel underlying tissues/abnormalities
l. Record patient's subsequent visits on these
m. Check balance to detect muscle abnormality
n. Describes patient's overall state of health
o. Alerts of allergy or other vital information
p. Complete physical exam
q. Can be seen by all

**F. Multiple Choice:** Place the correct letter or letters on the blank line for each question.

b  1. The lack of same size, shape, and position of parts or organs on opposite sides is termed
   a. anatomical
   b. asymmetry
   c. acquired
   d. atypical

d  2. A medical term that means to empty, especially the bowels, is
   a. evoke
   b. emesis
   c. exudate
   d. evacuate

a,d  3. Progress notes are also referred to as
   a. chart notes
   b. evaluation forms
   c. exam reports
   d. progress reports

a,c  4. To help patients relax during the pelvic exam, tell them to breathe ____ through the mouth.
   a. slowly
   b. quickly
   c. deeply
   d. shallowly

b  5. The heel-to-shin test is generally performed while the patient is in the ____ position.
   a. Trendelenberg
   b. supine
   c. prone
   d. Fowler's

a,c  6. The Romberg test is performed by the physician to detect
   a. coordination
   b. flexibility
   c. muscle abnormality
   d. infection

b  7. Patients who are scheduled for a Pap test should be reminded that they should not engage in sexual intercourse or _____ for 24 to 48 hours before the appointment.
   a. fast
   b. douche
   c. void
   d. exercise

c  8. To detect disease and abnormalities in children, an exam every _____is recommended.
   a. 3 months
   b. 6 months
   c. year
   d. time child is sick

Name _____

After your instructor has returned your work to you, make all necessary corrections and place in a three-ring notebook for future reference.

**ASSIGNMENT SHEET**

**Chapter 14: PREPARING PATIENTS FOR EXAMINATION**

**Unit 4: ASSISTING WITH SPECIAL EXAMINATIONS**

**SUGGESTED RESPONSES TO CRITICAL THINKING CHALLENGE IN TEXTBOOK**

1. What would you do if someone either clocked in for you or asked you to do it for them? _____
_____

2. What did Suzanne do? Was it anything she shouldn't have done? Why? _____
_____
_____

3. What do you think Jackie was trying to do? _____

4. Why do you suppose that Suzanne is worried about this situation? _____
_____
_____

5. What should Suzanne do about this? _____
_____

6. Why was Suzanne feeling so guilty and worried about? _____
_____
_____

**A. Word Puzzle: Solve this word puzzle using the *Words to Know* in this unit.**

```
_ _ _ _ _ _ S _ _ _
_ _ _ _ _ _ _ P _
_ _ E _ _ _ _ _ _
_ _ C _ _ _
_ _ _ I _ _ _ _ _
_ _ _ A _ _ _ _ _ _ _ _
_ _ _ _ L _ _ _ _
```

**B. Multiple Choice: Place the correct letter or letters on the blank line for each question.**

_____ 1. When charting the patient's LMP, you should record
   a. the last day of her period
   b. the first day of her last period
   c. the date of her period
   d. none of these

_____ 2. Patients are asked to wear disposable gowns and drape sheets
   a. to keep warm
   b. to protect the patient's clothes
   c. to look nice
   d. for privacy

_____ 3. If the physician requests a Pap and Maturation Index for a patient, she or he wants
   a. to check for diabetes
   b. a hormonal evaluation
   c. a pregnancy test
   d. to rule out infection

_____ 4. Because some patients get nauseated and may vomit while they are in the reception area, it is wise to keep a disposable _____ _____ in the receptionist's drawer.
   a. trash bag
   b. box of tissues
   c. emesis basin
   d. paper bag

_____ 5. To reduce the possibility of accidental injury when a baby is to be transported to a scale to weigh her, the _____ should take her and place her on the scale.
   a. the physician
   b. the PA
   c. the medical assistant
   d. the caregiver

_____ 6. A baby's head circumference should be measured until he is
   a. 6 months
   b. 12 months
   c. 24 months
   d. 36 months

_____ 7. Health care professionals are responsible for reporting suspected cases of child _____ to the proper authorities.
   a. abuse
   b. scabies
   c. neglect
   d. growth patterns

_____ 8. Measuring a baby's recumbent length (stature) is taken from
   a. forehead to heel
   b. head to toe
   c. vertex of head to heel

_____ 9. Measurements taken of infants and children should be recorded in the child's
   a. chart
   b. growth graph
   c. caregiver's record book
   d. all of these

_____ 10. The caregiver must sign the _____ before immunizations can be given to a child.
   a. release form
   b. consent form
   c. insurance form
   d. data sheet

**C. True or False: Place a "T" for true or "F" for false in the space provided. For false statements, explain why they are false.**

_____ 1. The sigmoidoscope is used to inspect the abdominal muscles.

_____ 2. Only patients who have used evacuants successfully can be examined with a sigmoidoscope.

_____ 3. During a sigmoidoscopy, air is sometimes introduced to distend the wall of the colon for easier placement of the lumen of the endoscope.

_____ 4. A suction pump may be necessary to remove fecal matter, blood, and mucus during a sigmoidoscopy so that the structures of the colon can be examined.

_____ 5. If a biopsy is taken during the examination of the colon, a patient information sheet should accompany the specimen to the lab.

_____ 6. The metal tip of the suction machine should be washed and dried carefully and put back for the next patient exam.

_____ 7. Patients are placed in either Sims' or knee-chest position for a sigmoidoscopy.

_____ 8. If patients complain of constipation, you should remind them to exercise, drink plenty of water, and add fruits and vegetables, grains, nuts, and cereals to their diet.

_____ 9. All patients age 50 and over should have an occult blood test every five years.

_____ 10. Patients who have a family history of cancer in their family should be alert to the warning signs of cancer and have regular checkups.

**D. Word Puzzle:** Solve this puzzle using the *Words to Know* in this unit.

1.      _ _ S _ _ _ _ _
2.      _ _ _ _ I _ _ _
3.      _ _ _ _ G _ _ _ _ _
4.      _ _ _ M _ _ _ _
5.      _ _ _ O _
6.      _ _ _ _ I _ _ _ _ _
7.      _ _ D _ _ _ _ _ _ _ _
8.      _ O _ _ _ _
9.      _ _ _ _ _ _ _ _ S
10.     _ _ C _ _ _
11.     _ _ _ _ _ O _ _ _ _
12.     _ _ _ _ _ _ P _ _ _ _ _
13.     _ Y _ _ _ _ _ _

**E. Brief Answer**

1. What instructions must be given to patients in preparation for a sigmoidoscopy? _____
_____

2. What might result if patients are not completely informed about preparations for a diagnostic examination such as a sigmoidoscopy? _____
_____

3. What advice can you give to patients in regard to flatulence they may experience following a sigmoidoscopy?
_____

**F. Identification:** Identify these instruments.

1._____

2. _____

## G. Matching: Match the definition in column II with the correct term in column I.

COLUMN I

_____ 1. Triage
_____ 2. Pap test
_____ 3. Women age 35+
_____ 4. Proper preparation
_____ 5. Douching
_____ 6. LMP
_____ 7. Maturation index
_____ 8. Plain enema
_____ 9. Slow deep breaths
_____ 10. Flatulence
_____ 11. Constipation
_____ 12. BSE

COLUMN II

a. Necessary for successful examination
b. Relax abdominal muscles
c. Record first day of last menstrual period
d. Normally relieved with lots of fluids
e. Ascertain reason for patient's visit
f. Part of preparation for sigmoidoscopy
g. Cytological test to detect cervical cancer
h. Advise female patients to do routinely following period
i. Used to obtain a smear of interior cervix
j. Should schedule routine mammographies
k. Washes away natural vaginal secretions
l. Hormonal evaluation
m. For relief, lie in prone position with pillow across mid abdomen

## H. List all necessary supplies/equipment for:

1. Pap test/pelvic examination

_____

_____

_____

_____

_____

2. Sigmoidoscopy

_____

_____

_____

_____

## CRITICAL THINKING SCENARIOS:  What would your response be in the following situation?

1. A female patient in her mid-30s is scheduled for a complete physical examination, including a Pap test. As you are getting the gown and drape sheet out, she tells you that she is so glad she had time this morning to douche before taking her shower because she wanted to be fresh and clean for the exam. _____

_____

_____

_____

## ACHIEVING SKILL COMPETENCY
Reread the performance objective for each procedure and then practice the skills listed below, following the procedure in your textbook.

Procedure 14-14: Assist with a Gynecological Examination and Pap Test

Procedure 14-20: Assist with Sigmoidoscopy

When you feel you have mastered performance of a skill, sign your name on the appropriate evaluation sheet and give it to your instructor to indicate you are prepared to perform the procedure for evaluation.

After your instructor has returned your work to you, make all necessary corrections and place in a three-ring notebook for future reference.

# ASSIGNMENT SHEET

## Chapter 15: SPECIMEN COLLECTION AND LABORATORY PROCEDURES

Review the objectives and text for each unit before completing the assignment sheet for that unit. When you have completed all sheets for the chapter, remove them from this Workbook and give them to the instructor for evaluation.

### Unit 1: THE MICROSCOPE

#### A. Unscramble

1. _ _ _ _ _ _                TENUMI
2. _ _ _ _ _ _ _ _ _          NRBILOUCA
3. _ _ _ _ _ _ _ _ _ _        HECNTIACIN
4. _ _ _ _ _ _ _ _ _          NEIMPSCE
5. _ _ _ _ _ _ _              YMGNFAI
6. _ _ _ _ _ _ _ _ _ _        CPIETOIRFN

#### B. Fill in the Blank

1. The _____ is used to examine objects that cannot be seen with the naked eye.
2. Eyeglasses are not necessary when performing microscopic work because the microscope may be focused to _____ for all visual defects except _____
3. A monocular microscope has _____ eyepiece and a binocular microscope has

   _____
4. The microscope should be transported carefully by holding it by the _____ and supporting it with your other hand under the _____
5. The shortest objective lens of the microscope magnifies objects _____ larger than can be seen with the naked eye.
6. The _____ power lens of the microscope magnifies objects 40 times larger than can be seen with the naked eye.
7. The _____ regulates the amount of light directed on the magnified specimen.
8. The _____ may be raised or lowered in focusing the specimen.
9. The ocular lenses of the microscope should be cleaned with _____
10. The _____ dial helps focus the specimen in detail.

## C. Identification: Label the parts of the microscope. Refer to Figure 15-2 in the textbook.

1. _____
2. _____
3. _____
4. _____
5. _____
6. _____
7. _____
8. _____
9. _____
10. _____

## D. Fill in the Blank

1. Gloving is always a must when handling _____ blood or body fluid specimens.

2. When splashing of any blood/body fluids could be possible while you are working, you should wear _____  _____  _____ (or _____ ), and _____.

3. Basic proper handwashing _____ and _____ all procedures must become a habit for all health workers for self-protection from disease _____

4. Any break in the skin should be covered with a bandage after handwashing and before _____ for self-protection against possible _____

5. It is important to recap or close bottles, jars, tubes, and the like, immediately after use to avoid _____  _____ and _____

6. Immediate recording of lab results helps to ensure _____

7. For better _____ you should work in a well-lighted, properly ventilated, uncluttered, quiet area.

8. _____ should never be broken off or handled after use, but placed intact in a puncture-proof biohazardous container.

9. All _____ waste should be discarded in proper containers.

10. The health care worker should make _____ of all electrical appliances and equipment for frayed wires or faulty operation and _____ for repair if needed.

11. Accidents should be reported to your _____ immediately.

12. Emergency telephone numbers should be posted near the _____ in the lab.

13. Before using any electrical appliance or equipment, you should make sure that your hands are

    _____

14. First aid items should be available in the lab for _____ use.

15. Loose-fitting or bulk clothing and jewelry should not be worn when working in the lab because it could contribute to _____

16. Every lab should have an emergency _____ which is functional in preventing further damage to the eyes from chemical splashes.

17. Broken glass or any sharp, unusable item should be placed in a sturdy cardboard box or puncture-proof container marked _____ and placed in the proper waste receptacle.

18. The health care worker must _____ lean into the work area when working with flame or chemicals to avoid self-injury or accidents.

19. Chemicals should be poured at _____ to avoid injury and accidents.

20. _____ eat, drink, chew gum, smoke, or place hands or fingers to mouth or place any item in your mouth while working.

21. It is a good practice to designate a _____ and a _____ area in your lab and enforce this policy to avoid confusion about items.

## E. Brief Answer

1. List the basic recommended standard precautions for health care providers.

    a. _____

    b. _____

    c. _____

    d. _____

    e. _____

    f. _____

2. How can health care providers set a good example for patients regarding health habits? _____

    _____

    _____

3. When and how and why should you clean up spills in the lab or facility? _____

    _____

    _____

4. How do you clean up spilled blood (or other body fluids)? _____

    _____

    _____

    _____

5. Why should patients be given both verbal and written instructions for procedures/tests? _____

    _____

    _____

    _____

    _____

## ACHIEVING SKILL COMPETENCY

Reread the performance objective for this procedure and then practice the skill listed below, following the procedure in your textbook.

Procedure 15-1:  Use a Microscope

When you feel you have mastered performance of a skill, sign your name on the appropriate evaluation sheet and give it to your instructor to indicate you are prepared to perform the procedure for evaluation.

After your instructor has returned your work to you, make all necessary corrections and place in a three-ring notebook for future reference.

**Chapter 15: SPECIMEN COLLECTION AND LABORATORY PROCEDURES**

**Unit 2: CAPILLARY BLOOD TESTS**

**A. Word Puzzle:** Use the *Words to Know* for this unit to spell out these terms.

1.  — — — — — — — — E — — — — — — — — — — —
2.  — — — — — — — — R — —
3.  — — — — Y — — — — — — — — — — —
4.  — — T — —
5.  — H — — — — — — — — — — — —
6.  — — R — — — — — — —
7.  — — — — O — — — — — — —
8.  P — — — — —
9.  — — — O — — — — — —
10. — I — — — — — — — — — —
11. — — E — — — —
12. — — — — S —
13. — I — — — — —
14. — — — — — — S

**B. Fill in the Blank**

1. Laboratory instructions must be followed exactly in _____ _____ and sending all specimens for analysis.
2. The medical assistant should alert the physician of abnormal laboratory findings by circling or underlining them in _____
3. Skin puncture is performed to obtain a _____ blood specimen.
4. Capillary blood tests are performed when _____ of blood is required.
5. _____ is a congenital disease due to a defect in the _____ of the amino acid, phenylalanine.
6. PKU tests are required by law in _____ and in _____
7. H and H is an abbreviation for _____ and _____
8. A skin puncture site should be approximately _____ deep to allow sufficient blood flow for capillary tests.
9. The microhematocrit tube fills quickly by _____
10. The three layers that blood is separated into after centrifugation in a microhematocrit tube are _____ _____ and _____
11. The hematocrit is expressed as the _____ of the total blood volume in cubic centimeters of erythrocytes packed by _____
12. When performing skin puncture procedures, the first drop of blood is blotted away because it may contain _____ or _____
13. The normal hematocrit range for adult males is _____ and for adult females _____
14. The function of the red blood cell is to transport _____ to and carry _____ from the cells.

15. Patients who complain of lack of energy or fatigue may possibly be suffering from _____

16. _____ should be worn when working with blood or any body fluids.

17. The purpose of a GGT (standard glucose tolerance test) is to determine a patient's ability to metabolize

_____

18. Many physicians order a _____ GTT.

19. Patients scheduled for a GTT must _____ 8 to 12 hours before the test.

20. Patients may feel weakness and may faint during a _____

21. During a GTT, the blood glucose level falls as _____ is secreted into the blood in reaction to the glucose that has been ingested.

22. The normal blood glucose range is _____

23. The _____ is made preferably with fresh whole blood.

24. Name the five types of white blood cells in a differential count.

a. _____

b. _____

c. _____

d. _____

e. _____

25. Draw, color, and label each of the blood cells of the differential WBC count.

26. Draw, color, and label RBCs and platelets (refer to Fig. 15-21).

## C. Labeling: Label this centrifuged microhematocrit tube. Refer to Figure 15-10 in the textbook.

## D. True or False: Place a "T" for true or "F" for false in the space provided. For false statements, explain why they are false.

_____ 1. A blood smear should have an even distribution of cells and end in a feathered tip.

_____ 2. A blood smear can be made with either venous or capillary blood.

_____ 3. The best blood smears are those that are made with old blood from the refrigerator.

_____ 4. Both fasting blood and urine samples are taken in a GTT.

_____ 5. Patients may come and go during a GTT as long as they are on time every hour to have the test performed.

**E. Matching: Match the definition in column II with the correct term in column I.**

COLUMN I

_____ 1. Capillaries
_____ 2. 12 to 16 grams/100 ml blood
_____ 3. Hematology
_____ 4. PKU test
_____ 5. Skin puncture sites
_____ 6. Hematocrit
_____ 7. Centrifugal action
_____ 8. Fasting
_____ 9. 14 to 18 grams/100 ml of blood
_____ 10. Phenylalanine
_____ 11. Fasting blood glucose range
_____ 12. Hemoglobin
_____ 13. 5,000 to 10,000
_____ 14. Anemia
_____ 15. Differential

COLUMN II

a. Limited to neonates
b. Packed red blood cells
c. Separates blood components
d. Arteries
e. Convey blood from arteries to other venules
f. An amino acid
g. Normal hemoglobin range for females
h. Study of blood and its components
i. Ring/great finger, ear lobe, infant's heel or great toe
j. Erythrocytes
k. Decrease in the number of RBCs
l. Normal hemoglobin range for males
m. Nothing to eat or drink for specified time
n. 80 to 120 mg/100 ml of blood
o. Normal WBC count range
p. Carbon dioxide
q. Iron-carrying protein components in blood
r. Test to determine the number of each type of WBC

**F. Identification: Identify these blood cells. Refer to Figure 15-21 in the textbook.**

1. _____

2. _____

3. _____

4. _____

5. _____

6. _____

7. _____

## G. Crossword Puzzle

ACROSS

1. Test to determine the number and percentage of WBCs
5. Must never open while spinning
6. Physicians' office laboratory
9. The body's system that removes worn-out RBCs
12. Leukocyte
13. Immediately!
14. Sugar
15. Used for skin puncture
16. Volume of packed RBCs
17. Secreted by the Islets of Langerhans
20. Sum of all physical and chemical changes in the body

DOWN

2. Formation of RBCs
3. Relinquish; exemption
4. Newborn infant
7. Occupational Safety and Health Administration
8. Process of WBCs eating foreign cells
10. Clinical Laboratory Improvement Amendment
11. Place where diagnostic tests are performed
13. Needles used for skin puncture should be this
18. Glucose tolerance test
19. Erythrocyte

## H. Brief Answer

1. What is the purpose of wearing latex gloves in performing laboratory procedures? _____

_____

2. List the regulatory bodies that govern the POL, and explain why this is necessary. _____

_____

_____

3. List lab practices that yield quality assurance in the POL. _____

_____

4. What are waivered tests? _____

_____

5. List three laboratory tests from each of the sections in Table 15-1 of your textbook. Use reference books to explain the purpose of each test and patient preparation as indicated for each. _____

_____

6. What are the practices health care providers should follow to ensure reliable and accurate data and quality health care to patients? _____

   a. _____

   b. _____

   c. _____

   d. _____

   e. _____

7. For tests performed in the POL, what should the log book include?

   a. _____

   b. _____

   c. _____

   d. _____

   e. _____

8. Explain briefly what POCT (point of care testing) is. _____

_____

9. Explain why QA (quality assurance) and QC (quality control) are essential in laboratory procedures.

_____

_____

_____

10. Why is a GTT (glucose tolerance test) routinely performed on women in the sixth month of pregnancy?

_____

## ACHIEVING SKILL COMPETENCY

Reread the performance objectives for these procedures and then practice the skills listed below, following the procedure in your textbook.

   Procedure 15-2: Puncture Skin with Sterile Lancet

   Procedure 15-3: Obtain Blood for PKU Test

   Procedure 15-4: Determine Hematocrit (Hct) Using Microhematocrit Centrifuge

   Procedure 15-5: Hemoglobin (Hb) Determination Using the Hemoglobinometer

   Procedure 15-6: Screen Blood Sugar (Glucose) Level

   Procedure 15-7: Making a Blood Smear

When you feel you have mastered performance of a skill, sign your name on the appropriate evaluation sheet and give it to your instructor to indicate you are prepared to perform the procedure for evaluation.

After your instructor has returned your work to you, make all necessary corrections and place in a three-ring notebook for future reference.

ASSIGNMENT SHEET

## Chapter 15:  SPECIMEN COLLECTION AND LABORATORY PROCEDURES

## Unit 3:  VENOUS BLOOD TESTS

**A.  Spelling:  Each line contains four different spellings of a word. Underline the correctly spelled word.**

| | | | |
|---|---|---|---|
| 1. Coageulate | Coagulate | Coagulade | Cogulate |
| 2. Consiousness | Conseousness | Consciousness | Consciouseness |
| 3. Elasticity | Elasticiety | Elastisity | Elosticity |
| 4. Angorge | Engarge | Ingorge | Engorge |
| 5. Hemolysis | Himolysis | Hemolisis | Hemolyesis |
| 6. Hemotoma | Hematoma | Himotoma | Hemitoma |
| 7. Legable | Ledgible | Legoble | Legible |
| 8. Prothrombin | Prothromben | Prothrombon | Prothrambin |
| 9. Tournequet | Tourniquiet | Tourniquet | Tournaquat |
| 10. Venipuncture | Veniapuncture | Venapuncture | Venipunkture |

**B.  Brief Answer**

1.  A means of promoting better palpation and sometimes visual position of the vein is a _____

2.  Applying _____ immediately following venipuncture will reduce the possibility of a hematoma.

3.  The two methods for obtaining venous blood specimens are

    a. _____

    b. _____

4.  Blood drawn in blue-stoppered tubes should be tested within _____ hours.

5.  Tubes used to collect whole blood for various tests contain a(n) _____

6.  _____ is a clear, light yellow liquid obtained from whole blood that has been allowed to clot and then is

    _____

7.  Information necessary to perform various blood tests for patients should contain

    a. _____

    b. _____

    c. _____

    d. _____

    e. _____

    f. _____

    g. _____

    h. _____

    i. _____

8.  Cell deterioration may be prevented by _____ the blood specimen if it must be kept for over

    _____ hours.

9.  The SED rate is useful in the diagnosis and evaluation of diseases of the _____ and in

    _____ _____ and collagen patients.

10.  List the four most commonly used colors to code blood specimen tubes and tell what they stand for.

    a. _____

    b. _____

    c. _____

    d. _____

## C. Matching: Match the commonly performed lab test in column I with normal values in column II.

COLUMN I

_____ 1. Hemoglobin
_____ 2. BUN
_____ 3. LDL cholesterol
_____ 4. Sed rate
_____ 5. CO
_____ 6. Triglyceride
_____ 7. RBC count
_____ 8. Creatinine
_____ 9. Potassium
_____ 10. Total cholesterol
_____ 11. Hematocrit
_____ 12. Uric acid
_____ 13. WBC count
_____ 14. Glucose
_____ 15. Pro time
_____ 16. HDL cholesterol
_____ 17. ESR Wintrobe method
_____ 18. Sodium
_____ 19. Platelet count
_____ 20. Chloride

COLUMN II

a. 4 to 5 mEq/L
b. 5,000 to 10,000/cu mm
c. 130 to 200 mg/dl
d. 35.5 to 49%
e. 11 to 13 sec
f. 80 to 120 mg/dl
g. 132 to 142 mEq/L
h. 3.5 to 7.5 mg/dl
i. 0 to 10 mm/hr
j. 90 to 130 mg/dl
k. 8 to 20 mg/dl
l. 12 to 16 g/dl
m. 98 to 106 mEq/L
n. 0 to 15 mm/hr
o. 40 to 150 mg/dl
p. 3.5 to 5.5 × 10/cu mm
q. 150,000 to 350,000/cu mm
r. 0.7 to 1.4 mg/dl
s. 25 to 32 mEq/L
t. 0 to 20 mm/hr
u. 45 to 65 mg/dl

## D. Brief Answer

1. In compliance with quality control and quality assurance regulations, what information must be kept in the POL log book?

   a. _____
   b. _____
   c. _____
   d. _____
   e. _____
   f. _____

2. Explain how to package blood specimens for shipment to out-of-town/state laboratories. _____
   _____
   _____
   _____

3. What is the purpose of a Saf-T-Clik® shielded blood needle adapter? _____
   _____

4. How does the Saf-T-Clik® shielded blood needle adapter work? _____
   _____

**E. Multiple Choice: Place the correct letter on the blank line for each question.**

_____ 1. The surgical puncture of a vein is called
   a. intravenous
   b. intradermal
   c. venipuncture
   d. venolysis

_____ 2. The medical term for a collection of blood just under the skin is
   a. hemolysis
   b. hematoma
   c. angioma
   d. antigen

_____ 3. The breakdown of blood cells is called
   a. hemodialysis
   b. angioblast
   c. hemolysis
   d. angiosis

_____ 4. If a lab result is needed immediately, write _____ on the request form.
   a. immediately
   b. as soon as possible
   c. same day
   d. stat

_____ 5. The rate at which red blood cells fall in a particular calibrated tube within an hour is called a(n)
   a. analysis
   b. sed rate
   c. hemoglobin
   d. prothrombin

_____ 6. When an ESR is performed, you should do it within two hours with
   a. whole blood
   b. crenated blood
   c. blood plasma
   d. platelets

_____ 7. During the venipuncture procedure, the tourniquet should never be left on the patient's arm for more than
   a. 30 seconds
   b. 60 seconds
   c. 2 minutes
   d. 5 minutes

**E. True or False: Place a "T" for true or "F" for false in the space provided. For false statements, explain why they are false.**

_____ 1. Veins carry blood to the heart.

_____ 2. Some patients feel anxious about blood tests and may experience nausea.

_____ 3. A patient should have the arm supported for the venipuncture procedure.

_____ 4. Laws regarding venipuncture are the same everywhere.

_____ 5. Veins have some elasticity and will give somewhat when depressed.

_____ 6. Gentle mixing of blood with an anticoagulant in a figure-eight motion helps prevent hemolysis.

_____ 7. The needle guard should be kept over the needle to protect it from contamination and to prevent injuries.

_____ 8. The bevel of the needle should be down when inserting it for the venipuncture procedure.

_____ 9. Following the syringe method of venipuncture, the entire syringe and needle must be placed (intact) in a puncture-proof receptacle.

_____ 10. The same pair of gloves may be worn all day as long, as one performs proper handwashing technique before and after each procedure.

_____ 11. All breaks in the skin must be covered with a bandage to protect the health care worker from transmitting or contracting disease.

_____ 12. Health care workers should make it a habit to practice standard precaution recommendations.

## ACHIEVING SKILL COMPETENCY

Reread the performance objective for this procedure and then practice the skills listed below, following the procedure in your textbook.

Procedure 15-8:   Obtain Venous Blood with Butterfly Needle Method

Procedure 15-9:   Obtain Venous Blood with Sterile Needle and Syringe

Procedure 15-10: Obtain Venous Blood with Vacuum Tube

When you feel you have mastered performance of a skill, sign your name on the appropriate evaluation sheet and give it to your instructor to indicate you are prepared to perform the procedure for evaluation.

After your instructor has returned your work to you, make all necessary corrections and place in a three-ring notebook for future reference.

# ASSIGNMENT SHEET

## Chapter 15: SPECIMEN COLLECTION AND LABORATORY PROCEDURES

## Unit 4: BODY FLUID SPECIMENS

### A. Matching: Match the terms in column I with their meanings in column II.

COLUMN I

_____ 1. Amber
_____ 2. Caustic
_____ 3. Occult
_____ 4. Crenated
_____ 5. Feces
_____ 6. Micturition
_____ 7. Dextrose
_____ 8. Random
_____ 9. Supernatant
_____ 10. Turbidity
_____ 11. Urinalysis
_____ 12. UTI
_____ 13. LMP
_____ 14. QNS

COLUMN II

a. Quantity not sufficient
b. Urination
c. Clear urine after centrifugation
d. Cloudiness
e. Examination of urine
f. Last menstrual period
g. Rusty color of urine
h. Diagnostic
i. Shrunken (RBC)
j. Hidden
k. Glucose/sugar
l. Can burn
m. Stool
n. Unplanned
o. Calibrated
p. Urinary tract infection

### B. Brief Answer

1. Explain
   a. Clean-catch midstream urine specimen. _____
   _____
   b. Catheterization. _____
   _____
   c. Infant urine collection. _____
   _____

2. The three parts of a complete urinalysis are:
   a. _____
   b. _____
   c. _____

3. Distilled water has a specific gravity of _____

4. _____ is a chemically treated paper that reacts with urine to determine the presence of waste substances in the body.

5. Urine specimens should be kept _____ until analysis can be performed to avoid the growth of _____ or _____.

6. Each specimen sent for laboratory analysis must have a _____ completed and attached to it for proper processing.

7. When performing urinary catheterization, the health care worker must always wear _____

8. Standard precautions state that all health care workers should wear gloves when working with any _____ and _____.

## C. Multiple Choice: Place the correct letter on the blank line for each question.

_____ 1. To avoid bacteria growth and decomposition of cells, urinalysis should be performed within
    a. 1 hour                          c. 2 hours
    b. 45 minutes                d. 4 hours

_____ 2. Catheterization is performed
    a. to obtain a sterile urine specimen for analysis     c. to instill medication into the bladder
    b. for relief of urinary retention               d. all of these

_____ 3. The normal range of specific gravity of urine is
    a. 1.000–1.500               c. 1.020–1.025
    b. 1.010–1.025               d. 1.030–1.035

_____ 4. Urine with a strong ammonia-like odor may be alkaline from a high concentration of
    a. bacteria                   c. sugar
    b. fungus                    d. blood

_____ 5. The pH range for normal urine is
    a. 1 to 3                     c. 5 to 7
    b. 3 to 5                   d. 7 to 9

_____ 6. Ketone (acetone) bodies present in urine are the result of metabolized
    a. fat                      c. starches
    b. sugar                   d. bulk

_____ 7. Before performing any urine test the specimen should first be
    a. centrifuged               c. stirred
    b. heated                  d. refrigerated

_____ 8. Cancer is detected from sputum specimens by the
    a. Gram stain               c. Wright stain
    b. gentian violet stain        d. Papanicolaou stain

_____ 9. Examination of fecal material (stool specimens) may determine the presence of
    a. microbial organisms       c. occult blood
    b. ova                     d. all of these

## D. Brief Answer

1. What patient education would you give to patients regarding:
    a. the respiratory system  _____

    _____

    b. the digestive system  _____

    _____

2. How do you collect a specimen for drug/alcohol analysis?  _____

_____

3. What should you make patients aware of in completing the form for substance analysis?  _____

_____

4. List all who should receive a copy of the substance analysis form.
    a. _____     d. _____
    b. _____     e. _____
    c. _____

5. What information should be included regarding samples for substance analysis?

    a. _____

    b. _____

    c. _____

    d. _____

    e. _____

6. What does the substance analysis screen for? _____

_____

7. Refer to the ABHES Course Content Requirements in Appendix C of the textbook. Within the area of *Medical Office Clinical Procedures,* which two content requirements are discussed in this unit? _____

_____

**CRITICAL THINKING SCENARIOS:  What would your response be in the following situations?**

1. A 10-year-old patient needs to have his hemoglobin checked. He wants you to use his little finger to obtain the blood sample. _____

_____

2. A patient calls to ask if she can run errands in between the times that you take blood and urine samples for her GTT scheduled for tomorrow morning. _____

_____

3. A patient calls to inform you that the scheduled first morning urine sample will have to be dropped off after work tomorrow. _____

_____

**ACHIEVING SKILL COMPETENCY**

Reread the performance objectives for these procedures and then practice the skills listed below, following the procedure in your textbook.

Procedure 15-11:  Catheterize Urinary Bladder

Procedure 15-12:  Test Urine with Multistix® 10 SG

Procedure 15-13:  Determine Glucose Content of Urine with Clinitest Tablet

Procedure 15-14:  Obtain Urine Sediment for Microscopic Examination

Procedure 15-15:  Instruct Patient to Collect Sputum Specimen

Procedure 15-16:  Instruct Patient to Collect Stool Specimen

    When you feel you have mastered performance of a skill, sign your name on the appropriate evaluation sheet and give it to your instructor to indicate you are prepared to perform the procedure for evaluation.

    After your instructor has returned your work to you, make all necessary corrections and place in a three-ring notebook for future reference.

## Chapter 15: SPECIMEN COLLECTION AND LABORATORY PROCEDURES

## Unit 5: BACTERIAL SMEARS AND CULTURES

### SUGGESTED RESPONSES TO CRITICAL THINKING CHALLENGE IN TEXTBOOK

1. What was Judy's thinking when she realized there were no gloves in the room? _____
   _____

2. What should she have done? _____

3. Why was she in such a hurry? _____

4. How do you think she felt when she realized that she could have been at risk? _____
   _____

5. Should the doctor be notified? _____

6. What would you have done in this situation? _____
   _____

### A. Fill in the Blank

1. _____ is a gelatinlike substance, mixed with sheep's blood that encourages the growth of microorganisms in a petri dish.

2. Gram-positive bacteria take a _____ color from the gram-stain procedure.

3. _____ bacteria take a red or pink color from the counterstain in the gram-stain procedure.

4. The purpose of gram-staining is to make heat-fixed bacteria visible for _____ examination.

### B. Brief Answer

1. Explain how to obtain a bacteriological smear. _____
   _____

2. Explain how to heat-fix a bacteriological smear for staining. _____
   _____

3. Why is heat-fixing necessary? _____
   _____

4. What is the purpose of culturing? _____
   _____

5. Why are culture plates placed upside down in the incubator? _____
   _____

6. Name the diseases caused by gram-positive bacteria. _____
   _____

7. Name the diseases caused by Gram-negative bacteria. _____
   _____
   _____

8. Why is it necessary to stain bacteria? _____

_____

9. How are bacteria identified? _____

_____

10. Why must all solutions be recapped immediately after each use? _____

_____

11. Why must gloves be worn when working with bacterial smears and cultures? _____

_____

_____

_____

12. What patient education could you offer a patient while preparing or obtaining a throat culture? _____

_____

_____

_____

_____

**C. Matching: Match the term in column II with the correct definition in column I.**

COLUMN I

_____ 1. Breaks infection cycle
_____ 2. Staphylococci
_____ 3. Nasopharyngeal culture
_____ 4. Diplococci
_____ 5. Streptococci
_____ 6. Incubation period for cultures
_____ 7. Blue flame
_____ 8. Alcohol/acetone
_____ 9. Destroys specimen
_____ 10. Spore-forming bacteria

COLUMN II

a. Bacteria that form pairs
b. 23–48 hours
c. Hottest
d. Proper handwashing and sterile technique
e. Excessive heating
f. Form grapelike clusters
g. NPC
h. Bacteria appearing in chains
i. Crystal violet
j. Helpful in removing dye
k. Immersion oil
l. Have capsule-like coverings

## D. Crossword Puzzle

Across

5. Means passed through a flame
7. Nutrient for microorganisms
8. Gram-positive bacteria stain
10. Gram-negative bacteria stain
12. Cultures streaked with a fine wire _____
14. Means of isolating disease-causing organisms
15. Must be sterile to obtain sample
16. Clear plastic dish with lid
20. Wear latex gloves to obtain a bacteriological _____
21. Have certain characteristic formations and shapes
23. Blue part is the hottest
24. Acronym for identification
25. Fill with dye for gram stain

Down

1. What a bacteriological smear is made on
2. Bacteria are classified by
3. Purpose of the bacteriological smear is to identify _____
4. Take care in handling
6. Crystal violet
9. Gelatin-like substance
11. Provides proper growth temperature for cultures
13. Roll specimen onto slide to _____ microorganisms
17. Use in gram-stain procedure
18. Bacteria in clusters
19. Purpose of procedure is for identification of bacteria
22. Allow specimens to _____ dry

**E. Identification:** Identify these bacterial shapes. Refer to Figure 15-52 in the textbook.

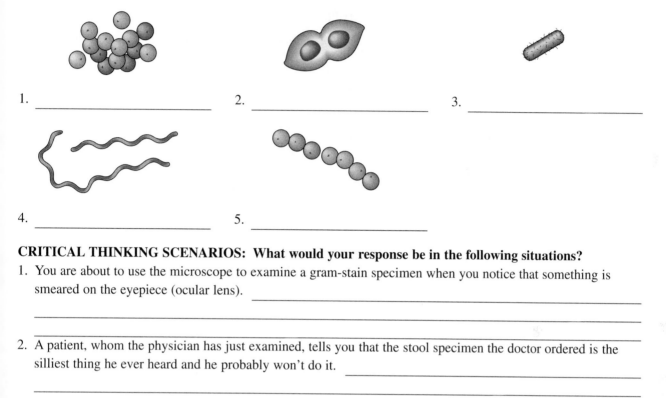

1. _____    2. _____    3. _____

4. _____    5. _____

**CRITICAL THINKING SCENARIOS:** What would your response be in the following situations?

1. You are about to use the microscope to examine a gram-stain specimen when you notice that something is smeared on the eyepiece (ocular lens). _____
   _____
   _____

2. A patient, whom the physician has just examined, tells you that the stool specimen the doctor ordered is the silliest thing he ever heard and he probably won't do it. _____
   _____
   _____
   _____

**ACHIEVING SKILL COMPETENCY**

Reread the performance objectives for these procedures and then practice the skills listed below, following the procedure in your textbook.

Procedure 15-18: Prepare Bacteriological Smear

Procedure 15-19: Obtain a Throat Culture

Procedure 15-20: PrepareGram Stain

When you feel you have mastered performance of a skill, sign your name on the appropriate evaluation sheet and give it to your instructor to indicate you are prepared to perform the procedure for evaluation.

After your instructor has returned your work to you, make all necessary corrections and place in a three-ring notebook for future reference.

## ASSIGNMENT SHEET

### Chapter 16: DIAGNOSTIC TESTS, X RAYS, AND PROCEDURES

Review the objectives and text for each unit before completing the assignment sheet for that unit. When you have completed all sheets for the chapter, remove them from this Workbook and give them to the instructor for evaluation.

### Unit 1: DIAGNOSTIC TESTS

**A. Word Search: Find the words hidden in the puzzle.**

ALLERGY
INJECTION
DILUTE
INTERPRET
ANTIBODY
HYPERSENSITIVE
EXTRACT
CONTACT DERMATITIS
NOTE
EOSINOPHIL
KIT

HISTAMINE
SERUM
ADRENALINE
ITCH
SYMPTOM
WHEAL
SYSTEMATIC
VENOM
GAUGE
TIME
SHOCK

```
G E D C A R T J P F J K T G K L B T
A O I N J E C T I O N M U N G J L H
L R L K R A O A J L S V D H L K B W
L K U C J S N B I N T E R P R E T C
E X T R A C T E J P Z N P F L O B P
R Z E C R H A N T I B O D Y D S R W
G L V A M B C R D O A M K A B I F D
Y B Q D P T T N S E R U M W G N C C
N S T R B C D A J T J T W H C O U K
H Y P E R S E N S I T I V E K P I Z
I N S N A P R S Y Z L T I A D H U O
S R E A G K M K M K Y C O L P I H K
T I M L L R A B P M E H T K F L N T
A L O I O H T C T O G A G O W O R I
M S Y N T D I F O E A B C S E S U M
I B K E Z N T N M Z U H I H O H H E
N O T E D E I G R E G K Z O A O E K
E V E S B O S Y S T E M A T I C E C
K I Q T Z L P C R E O D U P N K I T
```

**B. True or False:** **Place a "T" for true or "F" for false in the space provided. For false statements, explain why they are false.**

_____ 1. A positive allergic reaction to a skin test is shown by a raised area on the skin called a wheal.

_____ 2. Wheals are measured in inches.

_____ 3. Reactions to scratch tests usually occur within the first 20 minutes.

_____ 4. Intradermal tests are sometimes used by physicians to determine medicine sensitivity or immunization needs.

_____ 5. The patch test is read after a 12-hour and a 20-hour time period.

_____ 6. Cockroaches, their egg casings, and fecal matter are major sources of allergens in large cities.

_____ 7. Patients may have allergies only from irritants such as tobacco smoke, perfumes, cleaning supplies, and paint fumes.

_____ 8. Patients who have food allergies should read the content label of all foods and over-the-counter medications before ingesting.

_____ 9. If a patient is to report a skin test reaction by phone after the usual time it should react, explain that the size of the wheal/welt should be compared to a well-known item.

**C. Fill in the Blank**

1. _____ are utilized to determine allergic reactions in patients.

2. Desirable sites for the _____ test are the arms and back.

3. The _____ test is done to determine the cause of contact dermatitis.

4. In performing the intradermal test, the antigen is introduced into the dermal layer of skin in dosages of _____ to _____ by sterile technique.

5. For accurate test results, the expiration date of the _____ should be checked each time before use.

6. It may be necessary to _____ small children to perform skin tests successfully.

7. A life-threatening allergic reaction must be counteracted with an injection of _____ to prevent anaphylactic shock.

8. Symptoms of _____ initially include intense anxiety, weakness, sweating, and shortness of breath.

9. Patients refer to desensitizing injections of allergy serum as _____

10. It is a good practice to alternate arms of patients who have frequent allergy serum injections to prevent _____

11. The medical assistant's role in diagnostic tests and procedures is to _____ and _____ patients.

**D. Matching:** **Match the definition in column II with the correct term in column I.**

COLUMN I

_____ 1. Antibody

_____ 2. Immune

_____ 3. Venom

_____ 4. Histamine

_____ 5. Systemic

_____ 6. Antigen

_____ 7. Extract

COLUMN II

a. Released in allergic/inflammatory reactions

b. Of or pertaining to the whole body

c. Immunizing agent that produces antibodies

d. Protected or exempt from a disease

e. A protein substance carried by cells to counteract effects of an antigen

f. Pertaining to tissue

g. A poisonous secretion

h. A substance distilled or drawn out of another substance

## E. Brief Answer

1. Describe patient education regarding allergy injections.

   _____

   _____

   _____

2. Explain how you would advise a new allergy patient about scheduling desensitizing injections and other instructions.

   _____

   _____

   _____

   _____

## ACHIEVING SKILL COMPETENCY

Reread the performance objectives for these procedures and then practice the skills listed below, following the procedure in your textbook.

Procedure 16-1: Perform a Scratch Test

Procedure 16-2: Apply a Patch Test

When you feel you have mastered the performance of the skill, sign your name on the appropriate evaluation sheet and give it to your instructor to indicate you are prepared to perform the procedure for evaluation.

After your instructor has returned your work to you, make all necessary corrections and place in a three-ring notebook for future reference.

**ASSIGNMENT SHEET**

**Chapter 16: DIAGNOSTIC TESTS, X RAYS, AND PROCEDURES**

**Unit 2: CARDIOLOGY PROCEDURES**

**A. Matching: Match the definition in column II with the correct term in column I.**

COLUMN I

_____ 1. Artifacts
_____ 2. Somatic
_____ 3. Segment
_____ 4. Repolarization
_____ 5. Purkinje
_____ 6. Augmented
_____ 7. Sedentary
_____ 8. Galvanometer
_____ 9. Precordial
_____ 10. Voltage
_____ 11. Interval
_____ 12. Electrode
_____ 13. Standardization
_____ 14. Impulse
_____ 15. Stylus

COLUMN II

a. Enlarged
b. Electrocardiogram
c. Little activity
d. Additional electrical activity
e. Changes impulses into mechanical motion
f. Chest leads
g. Difference in electrical potential
h. Fibers that cause muscles of the ventricle to contract
i. Momentary surge of current
j. Provides a reliable reading
k. Muscle voltage artifacts
l. Provides printed representations of ECG paper
m. Period when heart momentarily relaxes
n. Bectrolyte
o. Metal sensors that pick up electrical impulses
p. Portion of EKG between two waves
q. Length of a wave

**B. Multiple Choice: Place the correct letter on the blank line for each question.**

_____ 1. The ECG is interpreted by the _____ .
    a. lab technician               c. physician
    b. medical assistant         d. nurse practitioner

_____ 2. The routine ECG consists of _____ leads.
    a. 6                     c. 8
    b. 10                  d. 12

_____ 3. The patient must be _____ for a good tracing to be obtained.
    a. sleeping              c. relaxed
    b. standing            d. unconscious

_____ 4. Metal electrodes should be cleaned with _____ .
    a. mild detergent/scouring powder    c. baking soda/water
    b. alcohol/ether            d. mild detergent/silver polish

_____ 5. A proper amount of _____ must be used with each metal electrode to provide maximum electrical conduction.
    a. alcohol              c. oil
    b. electrolyte          d. powder

_____ 6. The _____ of the ECG is necessary to enable a physician to judge deviations from the standard.
    a. length               c. standardization
    b. quality             d. augmentation

_____ 7. The usual standardization mark is _____ in size.
    a. 1 mm wide and 10 mm high          c. 1 mm wide and 5 mm high
    b. 2 mm wide and 5 mm high           d. 2 mm wide and 10 mm high

_____ 8. If the tracing is too large, the _____ button should be turned down to one half.
    a. sensitivity                       c. selector
    b. stylus                           d. on/off

_____ 9. The tracing paper is normally run at a speed of _____ mm/second.
    a. 15                              c. 50
    b. 25                              d. 75

## C. Labeling: Label these diagrams of the ECG cycle.

1. Place the correct letter for each wave of the ECG tracing on the line next to the number in the following. Refer to Figure 16-17 in the textbook.

2. Label the numbered lines below with the correct name of each area of the electrical conduction through the heart. Refer to Figure 16-16 in the textbook.

## D. Fill in the Blank

1. All muscle movement produces _____
2. The current enters the electrocardiograph through the wires to reach the _____
3. The amplifier _____ the electrical impulses.
4. Electrical impulses are transformed into mechanical motion by the _____
5. A _____ produces printed representations on ECG paper.
6. An electrical impulse originates in the modified myocardial tissue in the _____
7. The first impulse recorded on the ECG paper from the atrial contraction is known as the _____
8. When the muscles of the ventricles contract, the _____ of waves is produced on the ECG paper.
9. During the recovery of the ventricles, the _____ is produced.
10. A routine ECG consists of _____ leads.

11. _____ means to make larger.

12. Chest leads are also called _____ leads.

13. AC or _____ current interference is caused by additional electrical activity.

14. The standardization mark is included in an EKG to provide a _____ reading.

## E. Crossword Puzzle

**ACROSS**

1. Time of recovery before heart contracts again
3. Pick up electrical current from patient
5. Produces a printed representation on ECG paper
8. Precordial is another name for _____ leads
10. Irregular heartbeat
12. Ambulatory ECG
13. Inactivity
14. Slight/distant

**DOWN**

2. Instrument used to record electrical impulses of the heart
3. Permanent record of heart's electrical activity
4. An ECG tech does lots of these
5. These provide a basis for physicians to judge deviations from the standard
6. Immediately!
7. Acronym for electrocardiogram
9. Used to provide maximum electrical conduction
11. Study of the heart

**F. True or False:** **Place a "T" for true or "F" for false in the space provided. For false statements, explain why they are false.**

_____ 1. In the electrical conduction system, the first area of the heart to receive the electrical impulse is the Purkinje fibers.

_____ 2. Shivering from being nervous or cold can cause somatic tremor.

_____ 3. A rhythm strip indicates to the physician the size of a patient's heart.

_____ 4. For better electrode contact, the skin sites should be rubbed vigorously to increase circulation.

_____ 5. For single- and multi-channel computerized electrocardiographs, you simply press "auto" to run a 12-lead ECG.

_____ 6. It is necessary to shave dense chest hair for placement of electrodes.

_____ 7. Stress test ECGs are performed routinely on all patients.

_____ 8. A fetal monitor is a walking or 24-hour ECG.

_____ 9. Patients should keep a diary of their activities and symptoms during a 24-hour electrocardiogram.

_____ 10. It is important to check the batteries and proper working order of the Holter monitor before applying the device to a patient.

**G. Labeling:** **Fill in the missing information from this diagrammatic representation of cardiac impulses on EKG tracing:** (A) course of electrical impulses, (B) cardiac muscle reaction to impulses, (C) ECG tracing of impulse waves, (D) phases of cardiac cycle. Refer to Figure 16-17 in the textbook.

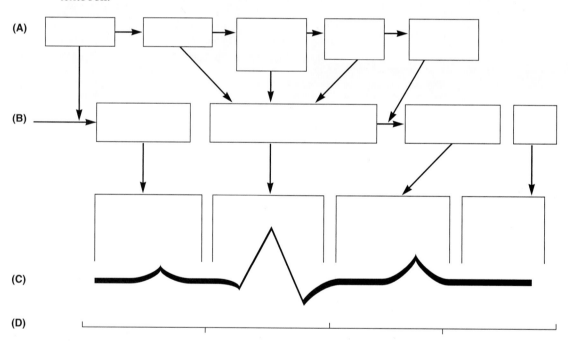

**H. Labeling: Label the ECG Tracings.** Are they abnormalities or interference artifacts?

1. _____

2. _____

3. _____

4. _____

Name _____

5. _____

6. _____

7. _____

8. _____

310

**CRITICAL THINKING SCENARIOS:  What would your response be in the following situation?**

1. A patient is being prepped for an ECG and appears to be very apprehensive. She is apparently intimidated by the machine and the wires and expresses a great fear of electric shock.

_____

_____

**ACHIEVING SKILL COMPETENCY**

Reread the performance objective for this procedure and then practice the skill listed below, following the procedure in your textbook.

Procedure 16-3:  Obtain a Standard 12-Lead Electrocardiogram

When you feel you have mastered the performance of the skill, sign your name to the evaluation sheet and give it to your instructor to indicate you are prepared to perform the procedure for evaluation.

After your instructor has returned your work to you, make all necessary corrections and place in a three-ring notebook for future reference.

**ASSIGNMENT SHEET**

**Chapter 16: DIAGNOSTIC TESTS, X RAYS, AND PROCEDURES**

**Unit 3: DIAGNOSTIC PROCEDURES**

**A. Fill in the Blank**

1. Vital capacity should equal _____ capacity plus _____ reserve.

2. _____ mouthpieces are used with vital capacity tests to prevent disease transmission.

3. Advising patients to list their concerns and bring them to their next appointment will _____
   the number of phone consultations.

4. In the performance of procedures, the medical assistant must be aware of explaining what is _____
   of the patient, for cooperation is essential in successful completion of the procedure.

5. As a _____ patients should be made aware of the expected amount of time a procedure will take
   so that their transportation can be planned accordingly.

**B. Matching:** **Match the definition in column II with the correct term in column I.**

COLUMN I

_____ 1. Dyspnea
_____ 2. Maturity
_____ 3. Ultrasound
_____ 4. Intermittent
_____ 5. Spirometry
_____ 6. Resonance
_____ 7. Expirations
_____ 8. Patient education
_____ 9. Claustrophobia

COLUMN II

a. Coming and going
b. To sound again
c. Breathing out; exhaling air
d. Fear of being enclosed
e. Yields more accurate test results
f. Full development
g. Difficulty breathing
h. Measures hearing
i. Measurement of air capacity of lungs
j. Vibrations of sound waves

**C. Word Search:** Find the words hidden in the puzzle. After you complete the puzzle, use the words numbered 5, 7, 8, 9, 11 in a sentence.

1. TEST
2. CONTRAST
3. EARLY
4. POLYPS
5. INVASIVE
6. PATIENT
7. ECHOES

8. CLAUSTROPHOBIA
9. SPIROMETER
10. IMPLANTS
11. MAGNETIC
12. IMAGE
13. SONOGRAM

```
C M H M M M R E S A D A S D O S A C P F
J S S A R B R M S P I R O M E T E R B S
I M A G E H R B G L A L D J T N D H L K
L J A N I T K A L C P T I N V A S I V E
Y A C E X N L M P D H J T F R L F C L R
C P A T I E N T O Q A H C F B P Y C M B
M H M I F G S B M S N Y C P L M E G M C
R E C C L A U S T R O P H O B I A P D W
T K L A B E T V A U G C Q Z N P F E R K
S O N O G R A M H U R B C A T T A W B C
W M K B P C T A A G A S D U S R R A J T
P L B T L S G I R S P M H D L C B A P E
Z T F L O K A S H O H M I Y Q T C F S S
R S E O H C E Z S P Y L O P K L H B K T
```

5. Invasive _____
7. Echoes _____
8. Claustrophobia _____
9. Spirometer _____
11. Magnetic _____

**D. True or False:** Place a "T" for true or "F" for false in the space provided. For false statements, explain why they are false.

_____ 1. In the spirometry procedure a clip is placed on some patients' noses to encourage them to breathe in deeply through the mouth.

_____ 2. One of your important duties in performing spirometry is to coach patients to expel completely all the air from their lungs quickly.

_____ 3. An oscilloscope is an instrument that shows a picture of converted electrical impulses from the patient during echocardiography.

_____ 4. High-frequency sound waves are conducted through the use of a transducer in ultrasonic scanning.

_____ 5. Thermography is a measurement of heat patterns given off by the skin.

_____ 6. Diaphanography is performed by transillumination.

**CRITICAL THINKING SCENARIOS:  What would your response be in the following situation?**

1. The patient that you just scheduled for an MRI lets you know in no uncertain terms that she is extremely claustrophobic and just might not go if she's having a bad day.

   _____
   _____
   _____
   _____

After your instructor has returned your work to you, make all necessary corrections and place in a three-ring notebook for future reference.

**ASSIGNMENT SHEET**

**Chapter 16: DIAGNOSTIC TESTS, X RAYS, AND PROCEDURES**

**Unit 4: DIAGNOSTIC RADIOLOGICAL PROCEDURES**

**SUGGESTED RESPONSES TO CRITICAL THINKING CHALLENGE IN TEXTBOOK**

1. What was Johnetta's first mistake? _____

_____

_____

2. When should she have made the appointment? _____

_____

3. Did she even look at the chart before filing it? _____

_____

4. Why didn't she tell the physician? _____

_____

5. How serious is this situation? _____

6. What should Johnetta do? _____

_____

_____

_____

7. Is the clinical supervisor at fault for anything? _____

_____

8. What would you have done in this situation? _____

**ANSWERS TO WORKBOOK ASSIGNMENT**

**A. Word Puzzle: Use the *Words to Know* to spell out these terms.**

1. \_ \_ \_ \_ \_ \_ \_ M \_ \_ \_ \_ \_ \_ \_
2. \_ \_ \_ \_ A \_ \_ \_ \_
3. \_ \_ M \_ \_ \_ \_ \_ \_ \_ \_
4. \_ \_ \_ M \_ \_ \_ \_ \_
5. \_ \_ \_ O \_ \_ \_ \_ \_ \_ \_
6. \_ \_ \_ \_ G \_ \_ \_
7. \_ \_ R \_ \_ \_
8. \_ \_ \_ \_ \_ A \_ \_ \_ \_ \_
9. \_ \_ \_ \_ \_ \_ P \_ \_ \_ \_
10. \_ \_ H \_ \_ \_ \_ \_
11. \_ \_ \_ Y

## B. Brief Answer

1. What are roentgen rays?

   _____

   _____

2. What are therapeutic X rays used for?

   _____

3. What type of symptoms do patients experience if the gallbladder malfunctions?

   _____

4. What food should patients avoid if they have gallbladder trouble?

   _____

5. Why must the digestive tract be free of foods during an upper GI series?

   _____

   _____

6. Why is air contrast sometimes ordered with a barium enema examination?

   _____

   _____

7. What is an IVP?

   _____

   _____

8. What is another term for KUB?

   _____

9. How are patients X-rayed for mammography?

   _____

   _____

10. Describe the method of radiology called a CAT (computerized axial tomography) scan.

    _____

    _____

11. Describe echocardiography.

    _____

    _____

12. List the steps to prepare patients for a barium enema.

    _____

    _____

    _____

13. Describe a barium swallow or upper Gl Series.

    _____

    _____

    _____

14. Explain why pregnant women should not have X rays.

    _____

15. List X-ray procedures that do not require patient preparation.

    _____

16. Refer to the ABHES Course Content Requirements in Appendix C of the textbook. Within the area of *Medical Office Clinical Procedures*, which two content requirements are discussed in this unit? _____

    _____

**C. Matching:** Match the definition in column II with the correct term in column I.

COLUMN I                               COLUMN II

_____   1. Therapeutic X rays       a. Defines structures of the urinary system

_____   2. Mammography           b. Do not require patient preparation

_____   3. Evacuants               c. Barium and water mixture

_____   4. UGI series                d. Flat plate of abdomen

_____   5. CAT scan                e. Breast self-examination

_____   6. Bone studies           f. Performed with sterile catheter in conjunction with cystoscopy

_____   7. IVP                    g. Laxatives and enemas

_____   8. KUB                   h. X ray of different angles of breast tissue

_____   9. Contrast media         i. Used to treat cancer

_____  10. Retrograde pyelogram     j. Generates images of tissue in slices about one centimeter thick

                                            k. Barium swallow

**D. Multiple Choice:** Place the correct letter on the blank line for each question.

_____   1. A diagnostic aid frequently requested by physicians that needs no patient preparation is the:

         a. IVP                             c. UGI

         b. chest X ray                 d. cholecystogram

_____   2. Diagnostic X rays are _____ in pregnant female patients, especially during the first trimester.

         a. contraindicated             c. important

         b. indicated                   d. common

_____   3. Carbonated and alcoholic beverages should be avoided prior to X rays of the visceral organs because they produce

         a. rashes                       c. delays

         b. stones                     d. flatus

_____   4. A voiding cystogram may be ordered along with a(n)

         a. UGI                         c. IVP

         b. KUB                      d. BaE

_____   5. Nuclear medicine is the branch of medicine that uses _____ in the diagnosis and treatment of patients.

         a. xeroradiography           c. radioactive materials

         b. radionuclides            d. both b and c

_____   6. Which X ray is helpful in determining the position of an IUD?

         a. IVP                        c. MRI

         b. UGI                      d.KUB

_____   7. Breast self-examination is recommended for women of all ages

         a. daily                       c. monthly

         b. weekly                  d. yearly

_____   8. All women should have a baseline mammography between the ages of

         a. 25 and 39                c. 45 and 49

         b. 35 and 39                d. 55 and 59

_____ 9. To reduce the possible effects of swelling and soreness often caused by compression of the breasts during mammography you should instruct patient to omit _____ from their diets 7 to 10 days prior to the examination.

    a. salt                            c. fats

    b. caffeine                    d. cholesterol

_____ 10. Compression of the breasts during mammography allows a much clearer picture of breast tissue and also requires less

    a. analgesics                   c. radiation

    b. time                         d. flatus

**CRITICAL THINKING SCENARIOS: What would your response be in the following situation?**

1. A male patient in his late 50s phones to tell you of his discomfort following his barium enema this morning. He says he feels bloated and constipated.

_____

_____

_____

After your instructor has returned your work to you, make all necessary corrections and place in a three-ring notebook for future reference.

**ASSIGNMENT SHEET**

## Chapter 17: MINOR SURGICAL PROCEDURES

**SUGGESTED RESPONSES TO CRITICAL THINKING CHALLENGE IN TEXTBOOK**

1. Who was at fault here? _____

2. What was Barry's first mistake? _____
_____

3. Was Renita responsible for any problems? _____
_____

4. What should Barry have done? _____
_____
_____

5. Do you think Barry handled the reprimand from the doctor well? _____
_____

6. Since Barry didn't know that there were no sterile packs in the drawer, should the doctor blame him?
_____
_____

7. Did Renita really do Barry a favor? _____
_____

**ANSWERS TO WORKBOOK ASSIGNMENT**

**A. Word Puzzle: Use the list of *Words to Know* from this unit to spell out these terms.**

1. _ _ _ _ _ _ _ I _ _ _ _ _ _ _
        N
2.       _ C _ _ _ _ _ _
        I
3.     _ _ _ _ S _ _ _ _ _
        I
4.     _ _ _ _ O _ _ _ _
        N
5. _ _ _ _ _ _ _ _ A _ _ _ _
        N
        D
        D
6.       R
7.       A _ _ _ _ _ _ _ _ _
   _ _ _ _ _ _ _ I _ _ _
8.       N
   _ _ _ _ _ _ _ A _ _ _ _
9.       G
     _ _ E _ _ _ _ _ _ _

## B. Brief Answer

1. List what you must tell a patient in preparation for minor office surgery.

   a. _____

   b. _____

   c. _____

   d. _____

2. What two things should the medical assistant do the day before the scheduled surgery?

   a. _____

   b. _____

3. What is the purpose of the skin preparation before a surgical procedure?

   a. _____

   b. _____

4. Why must the medical assistant be extremely careful to avoid nicking the patient's skin when performing a skin preparation? _____

   _____

5. What must the medical assistant do if asked to assist directly with a surgical procedure?

   _____

6. Other than directly assisting with a surgery procedure, when else should the medical assistant wear surgical gloves, and why? _____

   _____

7. List the items included in the basic setup for most minor surgical procedures. _____

   _____

   _____

   _____

8. What types of surgical procedures may the medical assistant be asked to assist with in the medical office/clinic? _____

   _____

   _____

9. What is the usual recommended post-op diet? _____

10. Why are follow-up visits necessary in patient care? _____

11. Other than the scheduled post-op visit, what can the medical assistant do to follow up with patients?

    _____

12. What, in general, can the medical assistant advise patients to do following minor surgery?

    _____

13. How should the medical assistant instruct patients to care for the site of surgery? _____

    _____

14. What is the purpose of an electrocautery device in minor office surgical procedures? _____

    _____

15. Give pre-op instructions to a patient scheduled for a minor surgical procedure. _____

_____

   a. _____

   b. _____

   c. _____

   d. _____

   e. _____

When the patient arrives for the appointment:

   a. _____

   b. _____

   c. _____

   d. _____

16. Give post-op instructions to a patient following a minor office surgery.

   a. _____

   b. _____

   c. _____

   d. _____

   e. _____

   f. _____

   g. _____

17. List standard precaution barriers that must be worn by health care providers for invasive procedures.

_____

18. Explain how to care for surgical instruments before and following use. _____

19. List the important information that must be recorded on the patient's chart regarding a surgical procedure.

_____

20. List the items needed for a skin prep tray. _____

_____

21. Explain how to remove sutures properly and why. _____

_____

_____

_____

22. Describe how to remove skin staples. _____

_____

23. Describe skin closures and how they are applied. _____

24. Refer to ABHES Course Content Requirements in Appendix C of the textbook. Within the area of *Medical Office Clinical Procedures,* which content requirements are discussed in this chapter?

_____

_____

**C. Matching:** **Match the definition in column II with the correct term in column I.**

COLUMN I

_____ 1. Local anesthetic
_____ 2. Medical history
_____ 3. I & D
_____ 4. Before surgery
_____ 5. Formalin solution
_____ 6. Necessary
_____ 7. 30° angle
_____ 8. Application of antiseptic
_____ 9. Sterile transfer forceps
_____ 10. After surgery
_____ 11. 6 minutes
_____ 12. IUD
_____ 13. Antiseptic
_____ 14. D & C
_____ 15. Contaminated

COLUMN II

a. Preoperative
b. Used to place specimen in formalin solution
c. Surgical consent form
d. Dilation and curettage
e. Postoperative
f. Incision and drainage
g. Skin preparation
h. Administered by physician
i. May help in determining possible allergic reactions
j. Reduces microbial growth
k. Used to preserve tissue specimen
l. Expiration date
m. Angle of shaving surgery site
n. Intrauterine device
o. Circular motions
p. Unsterile
q. Thorough surgical scrub

**D. Identification:** Identify the following surgical instruments. Refer to Table 17-1 in the textbook.

1. _____

2. _____

3. _____

4. _____

5. _____

6. _____

7. _____

8. _____

9. _____

10. _____

11. _____

12. _____

323

**E. Multiple Choice: Place the correct letter on the blank line for each question.**

_____ 1. This process uses subfreezing temperature to destroy/remove tissue.
    a. electrocautery                  c. diathermy
    b. cryosurgery                  d. chemotherapy

_____ 2. Electrocoagulation is performed with a(n)
    a. cryo unit                     c. hyfrecator
    b. autoclave                   d. scalpel

_____ 3. A fenestrated sheet is one that has a(n)
    a. fold                        c. stain
    b. pleat                      d. opening

_____ 4. Autoclaved items remain sterile if they have been properly processed and protected from moisture for
    a. 3 days                    c. 3 weeks
    b. 30 days                  d. 3 months

_____ 5. Reducing the possibility of infection for a surgical procedure skin preparation includes
    a. cleaning the site with a soapy solution    c. applying antiseptic solution
    b. shaving the skin               d. all of these

_____ 6. A serious hereditary blood clotting disease that occurs mostly in males is called
    a. hemophilia               c. hematuria
    b. hemophobia            d. hemiplegia

_____ 7. A thorough initial surgical scrub must be performed for _____ minutes.
    a. two                      c. six
    b. four                    d. eight

_____ 8. Assisting with surgical procedures not only requires knowledge and skill, but
    a. self-discipline            c. empathy
    b. personal integrity        d. all of these

_____ 9. Tell patients who are to have skin staples removed that it is normal to feel a _____ sensation during the procedure.
    a. burning                c. nauseating
    b. tugging              d. stinging

_____ 10. Patients are normally requested to fast before surgical procedures because it lessens the possibility of the patient
    a. bleeding a lot          c. being late
    b. talking too much      d. becoming nauseated

_____ 11. Included in the list of symptoms following a surgical procedure that should be reported to the physician are
    a. unusual pain, burning, or uncomfortable sensation   c. fever, nausea, and vomiting
    b. bleeding or discharge       d. all of these

_____ 12. The use of sterile needles to stimulate the energy force (chi) of the body is
    a. debridement           c. electrocautery
    b. cryosurgery           d. acupuncture

_____ 13. The process of using sterile technique with sterile instruments to remove necrotic tissue from a wound or a burn is called
    a. cauterization
    b. dermabrasion
    c. debridement
    d. diathermy

_____ 14. The medical term for the healing of a wound commonly known as a scab is
    a. erythroderma
    b. eschar
    c. esthesia
    d. extima

_____ 15. Medical/surgical scissors are labeled as _____ to describe the points of the blades.
    a. sharp-sharp
    b. sharp-blunt
    c. blunt-blunt
    d. all of these

_____ 16. You should always check the patient's emergency room report for the following information regarding suture removal:
    a. the date and the number of sutures put in
    b. date of patient's tetanus booster
    c. the length of time the sutures were to be left in
    d. all of the above

_____ 17. An ace wrap is a supportive bandage that
    a. gives an attractive appearance to the injury
    b. increases circulation of the injured area
    c. gives support to the injured limb
    d. b and c

**F. Word Search:** **Find the following words hidden in the puzzle.**

PATIENT
GLOVES
BIOPSY
AUTHORIZE
PRE-OP
CAUTERIZE
HEMOPHILIA
POLYP
ANESTHESIA

ELECTROCAUTERY
SUTURE
HISTOLOGY
WART
FENESTRATED
ANTISEPTIC
CRYOSURGERY
TAUT
POST-OP

```
G L E X A T R E P A T I E N T R E A
L Q M L Q K B I O P S Y N L R E A S
O Z A B S M Z T L B S R A T K M F D
V K Z N U P A R Y T Z E D G F R B H
E R P K T H O T P M A G M K E B J I
S E W O U I B T G I E R P W N L A S
L Z F Q R H S S S F G U L B E R T T
K I H C E T G E T O L S B F S K C O
P R E O P W H M P X P O D P T S E L
Z O T S A T A U T T K Y N L R F C O
P H W B S G L R O Z I R Z S A X B G
Q T X E E L E C T R O C A U T E R Y
S U N O P Y A I L I H P O M E H E P
C A U T E R I Z E T X C M J D O F D
```

**G. Fill in the Blank:** Fill in what's missing in this list of sterile items used in a basic setup for most minor surgical procedures.

1. scalpel handle and _____
2. hemostats
3. _____
4. needles and _____
5. suture scissors
6. _____
7. probe
8. gauze squares
9. vial of _____ medication
10. _____
11. _____
12. towels
13. _____
14. tray

**CRITICAL THINKING SCENARIOS:** What would your response be in the following situations?

1. As you are performing a skin prep on a patient for removing a sebaceous cyst from his scalp, he tells you that he is rather nervous about this procedure because he is a hemophiliac. _____

_____

2. A young lady returns to have sutures removed. As you take the bandage off you notice that the sutured laceration site is infected. _____

_____

3. You have not been able to clean and sterilize the instruments on the counter because you have been so busy with patient care. A co-worker picked up these instruments and says the doctor needs them for a surgical procedure stat! _____

_____

4. You have set up the suture tray for the physician to suture a 7-year-old's laceration of the right forearm. This child is curious about everything he sees and asks many questions. The child's mother is with him. You must leave the room to answer a phone call. When you return, the child's mother is in the rest room and the child is touching some of the instruments on the suture tray. _____

_____

_____

_____

## ACHIEVING SKILL COMPETENCY

Reread the performance objectives for these procedures and then practice the skills listed below, following the procedure in your textbook.

Procedure 17-1:  Prepare Skin for Minor Surgery
Procedure 17-2:  Put on Sterile Gloves
Procedure 17-3:  Assist with Minor Surgery
Procedure 17-4:  Assisting with Suturing a Laceration
Procedure 17-5:  Remove Sutures

When you feel you have mastered the performance of the skill, sign your name on the appropriate evaluation sheet and give it to your instructor to indicate you are prepared to perform the procedure for evaluation.

After your instructor has returned your work to you, make all necessary corrections and place in a three-ring notebook for future reference.

**ASSIGNMENT SHEET**

## ASSISTING WITH MEDICATIONS

... ...e objectives and text for each unit before completing the assignment sheet for that unit. When you have comp...eted all sheets for the chapter, remove them from this Workbook and give them to the instructor for evaluation.

## Unit 1: PRESCRIPTION AND NONPRESCRIPTION MEDICATIONS

**A. Word Puzzle: Use the clues below to spell out these terms.**

| | | |
|---|---|---|
| 1. | _ D _ | Medication reference |
| 2. | _ _ _ _ R _ _ _ _ | Mastery |
| 3. | _ _ _ _ _ U _ _ | To plan |
| 4. | _ _ G _ _ _ _ _ _ _ | Rule |
| 5. | _ _ _ _ E _ _ _ | Distribute |
| 6. | _ _ _ _ N _ | Quantity |
| 7. | _ _ _ _ _ _ _ F _ _ _ _ _ _ _ | Categorize |
| 8. | _ _ _ _ _ O _ _ _ _ | Monitored |
| 9. | _ _ _ _ R _ _ _ | Correct |
| 10. | _ _ _ _ _ _ C _ _ _ _ _ | Study of medicines/drugs |
| 11. | _ _ _ _ E _ _ _ _ _ _ _ _ | To shorten |
| 12. | _ _ _ _ M _ _ _ _ _ | One show fills prescriptions |
| 13. | _ _ E _ _ _ _ _ _ _ _ _ _ | Written order for medicine |
| 14. | _ _ _ _ N _ _ | A permit |
| 15. | _ _ T _ | Numerical calculations |
| 16. | _ _ _ _ _ A _ _ _ _ | Medicines |
| 17. | _ _ D _ _ _ | Command |
| 18. | _ _ _ _ M _ _ _ _ _ _ _ _ _ | Big word for drugs/medicines |
| 19. | _ _ _ _ _ _ I _ _ | Highly controlled substances |
| 20. | _ _ _ _ _ _ _ N _ _ | Consultation |
| 21. | _ _ _ I _ _ _ _ | Enrollment |
| 22. | _ _ _ S _ _ _ _ _ | To write an order for medicine |
| 23. | _ _ _ _ T _ _ _ _ _ | Chemical |
| 24. | _ _ _ _ _ R _ _ | Means |
| 25. | _ _ _ A _ _ | Amount of medicine to take |
| 26. | _ T _ | Needs no prescription |
| 27. | _ _ _ _ _ I _ _ _ _ | To give |
| 28. | _ _ O _ _ | Call |
| 29. | _ _ _ N _ _ _ | Caution |

**H. Math Review: Solve the following word problems.**

1. Jessica, a medical assistant, earns $7.50 per hour for the first 40 hours per week. When she exceeds 40 hours in any work week, she is paid time and a half. One week during the winter flu season she worked 53 hours. When she received her paycheck, the gross amount was $397.53

   a. When Jessica works overtime, what is the hourly rate of pay?
   
   _____

   b. Based on the 53 hours, 13 of which were overtime, what should the gross amount be on her paycheck?

   _____

   c. Is the gross amount on the paycheck she received correct?

   _____

2. The Medical Supply Company is offering a 15% discount on sterile gloves purchased during their anniversary month. The regular cost of the sterile gloves is $37.50 per 100 gloves.

   a. What is the cost of 300 gloves without the discount?

   _____

   b. What is the cost of 300 gloves with the discount?

   _____

   _____

   c. How much is saved with the discount?

   _____

3. A medical assistant can type 250 words in 3 minutes. At the same rate, how long would it take this medical assistant to type 5000 words?

   _____

   _____

   _____

4. Two of Mrs. Smith's children have been diagnosed with conjunctivitis. The physician wrote a prescription for an antibiotic ophthalmic solution. It reads: 2 gtts TID in each affected eye for 5 days.

   a. If each child needs drops instilled in each eye, how many drops would be needed?

   _____

   _____

   _____

   b. How many household teaspoons would this be?   _____

5. A medical assistant was asked by her physician-employer to check over a small order from the medical supply house that had arrived while the staff was out to lunch. To expedite the task, the physician handed the medical assistant a copy of the original order (see illustration following):

THE ORIGINAL ORDER

| ITEMS | PER UNIT | TOTAL |
|---|---|---|
| 2 boxes disposable gloves; 100 ct. | $3.75 | $7.50 |
| 3 boxes syringes; 50 ct. | 25.00 | 75.00 |
| 10 thermometers | 1.50 | 10.50 |
| 12 boxes tissues | 0.25 | 3.00 |
| 5 cartons tongue dep.; 100 ct. | 1.38 | 6.90 |
| 6 bottles hand soap | 1.77 | 17.70 |
| | | $130.60 |

THE FINAL BILL

| ITEMS | PER UNIT | TOTAL |
|---|---|---|
| 2 ctns., surg. gloves | $5.75 | $11.50 |
| 3 ctns., disp. syr. | 25.00 | 75.00 |
| 100 thermometers | 1.50 | 150.00 |
| 12 boxes tissues | 0.25 | 3.00 |
| 5 cartons tongue dep. | 1.38 | 6.90 |
| 19 bottles, hand soap | 1.77 | 17.70 |
| | | $264.15 |

The first obvious problem is that the totals do not match on the order and on the bill. An item count further reveals some discrepancies between the quantities shown on the bill and the items actually received. Specifically, only 10 boxes of tissues and 4 cartons of tongue depressors were delivered.

a. Double check each item on the original order; if any mathematical errors are found, correct them.

THE ORIGINAL ORDER

| ITEMS | PER UNIT | TOTAL |
|---|---|---|

b. Double check the final bill as shown: if any mathematical errors are found, correct them.

_____

c. Still working with the bill as shown, are there any further discrepancies beyond mathematical errors?

1. _____

_____

2. _____

3. _____

4. _____

d. Now reconcile the count discrepancies with the corrected amounts shown on the bill.

_____
_____
_____
_____
_____
_____
_____

e. What procedure should be followed in paying the supplier for items actually ordered and received? What should be done with overages? with shortages? with incorrect items?

_____
_____
_____

6. Mrs. Brown, a patient of Dr. Johnston, has been diagnosed as suffering from refractory rickets. Dr. Johnston has prescribed the following treatment:

Ergocalciferol USP, Vitamin $D_2$ Tab, 100,000 USP units q6h for 14 days.

Ergocalciferol USP, Vitamin $D_2$ is available in either 50,000 USP units tablets or 8,000 USP units/ml drops. Dr. Johnston has decided to start Mrs. Brown on tablets. After 14 days of treatment, Dr. Johnston will test to determine if Mrs. Brown's serum calcium levels have returned to within normal limits. If so, therapy may be continued at a lower dosage.

a. How many tablets should be given q6h?

_____

b. How many tablets should be given Qid? _____

c. How many tablets should be ordered for the 14-day treatment? _____

7. After the 14-day treatment that Mrs. Brown took in problem 6, Dr. Johnston finds that her serum calcium levels are returning to normal limits. He decides to continue her on a treatment of Ergocalciferol USP, Vitamin $D_2$ at a reduced level for a period of one month. However, instead of tablets, the medication will be administered in liquid form. His new prescription is as follows:

Ergocalciferol USP, Vitamin $D_2$ gtt, 48,000 USP units, Bid for 30 days.

As stated in problem 6, Ergocalciferol USP, Vitamin $D_2$, is available in 8,000 USP units/ml drops; 60 ml bottle with dropper.

a. How many drops will be required for each dosage?

_____

b. How many drops are required for Mrs. Brown's daily dosage? _____

c. How many bottles of Ergocalciferol USP, Vitamin $D_2$ , will be needed to fill the entire prescription?

_____

_____

8. Bill Jones, a young boy weighing 73 $\frac{1}{4}$ pounds, has a mild ulcerative colitis condition which has been bothering him for several weeks. The physician recommended a treatment of Azulfidine and wrote the following prescription:

Azulfidine 30mg/kg, q6h for 7 days.

Azulfidine is available in 500 mg 100s tablets.

a. How many ml of Azulfidine will Bill receive per day?

1. _____

2. _____

b. How many tablets will be needed per dosage? For the whole prescription?

1. _____

2. _____

_____

9. Brad has a history of chronic asthma. As a treatment of first choice, Brad's doctor has prescribed theophylline anhydrous. Since this is a rather strong medication, the dosage is individualized for Brad based on his body weight and age. Brad is 15 years old and weighs 121 pounds. The recommended dosage for ages 12–16 years is 18mg/kg/day. The prescription is as follows:

18mg/kg/day p.o., not to exceed 900 mg/day.

Theophylline is available in 125 mg capsule form.

a. How many mg of theophylline would Brad receive based on 18mg/kg/day p.o.?

_____

_____

_____

b. Would this amount be the proper dosage?

_____

c. If not, what would be the amount of theophylline in mg Brad would receive per day based on the prescription?

_____

10. Bobby, a 10-year-old boy, was diagnosed as having strep throat. The physician ordered penicillin G potassium U 5,000,000 IM, stat. The recommended pediatric dosage is U 3,000,000–1,200,000 per day. Penicillin G potassium is available in U 5,000,000/ml. How many ml has the doctor prescribed for Bobby?

_____

**ASSIGNMENT SHEET**

## Chapter 19: EMERGENCIES, ACUTE ILLNESS, ACCIDENTS, AND RECOVERY

Review the objectives and text for each unit before completing the assignment sheet for that unit. When you have completed all sheets for the chapter, remove them from this Workbook and give them to the instructor for evaluation.

## Unit 1: MANAGING EMERGENCIES IN THE MEDICAL OFFICE

### Mixed Quiz

1. What is a universal emergency medical identification symbol and what does it do?

_____

_____

2. Identify five medical conditions for which a patient should wear an identification symbol.

a. _____

b. _____

c. _____

d. _____

e. _____

3. When is a situation considered to be an emergency? _____

_____

4. List the 16 items identified in the text that should be included in an emergency kit or cart.

a. _____

b. _____

c. _____

d. _____

e. _____

f. _____

g. _____

h. _____

i. _____

j. _____

k. _____

l. _____

m. _____

n. _____

o. _____

p. _____

5. What is an AED unit, and what three functions can it perform?

_____

_____

6. Refer to the CAAHEP Standards in Appendix B of the textbook. Within the area of *Medical Assisting Clinical Procedures,* which curriculum standard is discussed in this unit? _____

7. True or False: Answer the following statements with "T" for True or "F" for False, where true indicates the data is necessary to document in an emergency situation and false indicates the data is *not* necessary to document in an emergency situation.

a. _____ Name of injured patient or employee
b. _____ Date of incident
c. _____ Social Security number of person injured
d. _____ Time of injury or emergency
e. _____ Name and phone number of next-of-kin
f. _____ Location of accident or injury
g. _____ Description of condition surrounding accident or injury
h. _____ Description of past like incidences
i. _____ Employer's name, address, and phone number
j. _____ Identification of accident or incident witnesses
k. _____ Signature of examining physician
l. _____ Description of action taken, including disposition of the patient
m. _____ Signature of person filing report

8. Enter below the phone number for emergency medical services in your location. (Don't assume the universal 911 number is in effect in your area. Be certain!

_____

9. Determine the procedure to follow in your area when an individual dies without benefit of recent medical attention either within a physician's office or at another site.

_____

10. What follow-up record-keeping action is necessary following death of a patient?

_____
_____

11. Word Puzzle: Using the *Words to Know*, spell out the following terms.

| | |
|---|---|
| _ _ E _ _ _ | An emetic |
| _ _ _ _ M _ | Injury |
| _ E _ _ _ _ _ _ _ _ _ _ _ _ | Revive |
| _ _ R _ _ _ _ | A physician |
| _ _ _ _ _ G _ | A dressing |
| _ _ E _ _ _ | Cause vomiting |
| _ _ _ _ _ _ N _ | A happening |
| _ _ C _ _ _ _ _ | Unexpected injury |
| _ Y _ _ _ _ | An emblem |

12. Unscramble

_____ EULNRISVA
_____ IANRCOTITFECI
_____ OCRERON
_____ TIDNICNE
_____ OLYSBM
_____ CTICEAND

After your instructor has returned your work to you, make all necessary corrections and place in a three-ring notebook for future reference.

**ASSIGNMENT SHEET**

**Chapter 19: EMERGENCIES, ACUTE ILLNESS, ACCIDENTS, AND RECOVERY**

**Unit 2: ACUTE ILLNESS**

**Mixed Quiz**

1. Matching: Match the common term used to describe the severity of illness in column I with the correct meaning in column II.

| COLUMN I | COLUMN II |
|---|---|
| _____ Chronic | a. Occurring quickly and without warning |
| _____ Insidious | b. Extensive, advanced |
| _____ Urgent | c. May cause death |
| _____ Sudden | d. Long, drawn out, not acute |
| _____ Acute | e. Hidden, not apparent |
| _____ Severe | f. Requires intervention as soon as possible |
| _____ Life-threatening | g. Rapid onset, severe symptoms, and short course |

2. List the nine steps or stages that might occur with a major seizure.

    a. _____
    b. _____
    c. _____
    d. _____
    e. _____
    f. _____
    g. _____
    h. _____
    i. _____

3. Fill in the Blank: Listed below are symptoms of diabetic coma and insulin shock. Enter "C" for coma or "S" for shock before the symptom to indicate which condition may be present.

    _____ a. Drooling
    _____ b. Perspiration
    _____ c. Dry mouth
    _____ d. Not hungry
    _____ e. Full, bounding pulse
    _____ f. Dry, flushed skin
    _____ g. Fruity odor to breath
    _____ h. Weak, rapid pulse
    _____ i. Intense thirst
    _____ j. Double vision

4. Fill in the Blank

    A temporarily diminished supply of _____ to the _____ may cause _____
    The medical term for this condition is _____ A patient should be positioned with
    _____ to improve circulation to the _____ Symptoms of approaching syncope
    are _____ and complaints of _____ or _____
    When using aromatic spirits of ammonia capsules, it is important to _____
    _____

5. List the prime symptoms of heart attack.

a. _____

b. _____

c. _____

d. _____

e. _____

f. _____

g. _____

h. _____

i. _____

6. Fill in the Blank: Indicate whether the following symptoms are possible heat stroke (S) or heat exhaustion (E). Place an "S" or "E" in front of the symptoms.

_____ Pale, cool skin

_____ Profuse perspiration

_____ Rapid pulse, possible Cheyne-Stokes respirations

_____ Dry, red face

_____ Body temperature above average

_____ Dilated pupils

_____ Hypertension

_____ Headache

_____ Mental confusion, giddiness

_____ Thirst, nausea, vomiting

7. List the six successive symptoms of frostbite and identify the most often damaged body parts.

a. _____

b. _____

c. _____

d. _____

e. _____

f. _____

8. Name the three types of visible bleeding and the characteristics of each type.

a. _____

b. _____

c. _____

9. Labeling: Label the pressure points where severe arterial bleeding can be controlled. Refer to Figure 19-5 in the textbook.

10. What are the symptoms of internal bleeding, and how is it initially and eventually treated?

a. _____
b. _____
c. _____
d. _____
e. _____
f. _____
g. _____
h. _____
i. _____

11. Identify six routes by which poison can enter the body.

a. _____
b. _____
c. _____
d. _____
e. _____
f. _____

12. Determine the phone number for your local poison control center. Write it on the line below and add it to the emergency medical service number on your personal reference card.

_____

13. List the seven most common causes of obstructed airway.

a. _____
b. _____
c. _____
d. _____
e. _____
f. _____
g. _____

14. What are the three names for the method used to relieve an obstructed airway?

a. _____
b. _____
c. _____

15. List six conditions that may cause respiratory distress.

a. _____
b. _____
c. _____
d. _____
e. _____
f. _____

16. Name the components of the AED unit. _____

17. What three things need to be examined in a scheduled equipment check? _____

_____

18. List the sequence of events required for survival of cardiac arrest.

a. _____
b. _____
c. _____
d. _____
e. _____
f. _____

19. What is the critical concern in cases of cervical spinal injury?

_____

20. Identify the six symptoms of shock.

a. _____
b. _____
c. _____
d. _____
e. _____
f. _____

21. What are the usual causes of shock?

_____

_____

22. What is anaphylactic shock?

_____

23. Name substances that can cause anaphylactic shock.

    a. _____

    b. _____

    c. _____

    d. _____

    e. _____

    f. _____

    g. _____

    h. _____

    i. _____

    j. _____

24. What are the symptoms of stroke?

    a. _____

    b. _____

    c. _____

    d. _____

    e. _____

    f. _____

    g. _____

    h. _____

    i. _____

23. Spelling: Each line contains three different spellings of a word. Underline the correctly spelled word.

| | | |
|---|---|---|
| asperation | aspirashun | aspiration |
| diaphoresis | diephoresis | diaforesis |
| incidious | insidious | insideous |
| profalatic | profalytic | prophylatic |
| exhaustion | eghaustion | egaustion |
| ammonea | ammonia | amoania |
| seezure | seazure | seizure |

24. Refer to the Role Delineation Chart in Appendix A of the textbook. Within the area of *Patient Care,* which role relates to the content of this unit? _____

## ACHIEVING SKILL COMPETENCY

Reread the performance objectives for the procedures and then practice the skills listed below, following the procedure in your textbook.

    Procedure 19-1:  Give Mouth-to-Mouth Resuscitation

    Procedure 19-2:  Give Cardiopulmonary Resuscitation (CPR) to Adults

    Procedure 19-3:  Give Cardiopulmonary Resuscitation (CPR) to Infants and Children

When you feel you have mastered the performance of a skill, sign your name on the appropriate evaluation sheet and give it to your instructor to indicate you are prepared to perform the procedure for evaluation.

    After your instructor has returned your work to you, make all necessary corrections and place in a three-ring notebook for future reference.

**ASSIGNMENT SHEET**

**Chapter 19: EMERGENCIES, ACUTE ILLNESS, ACCIDENTS, AND RECOVERY**

**Unit 3: FIRST AID IN ACCIDENTS AND INJURIES**

**Mixed Quiz**

1. How is a bee stinger removed?

   _____

2. When is anti-rabies serum required following an animal bite?

   _____

3. Name the three types of burns, and give examples of each.

   a. _____

      _____

   b. _____

   c. _____

4. What is the first priority in the treatment of burns?

   _____

5. Compare the first aid treatment for the three degrees of burns

   _____

   _____

   _____

   _____

6. Describe the symptoms of a dislocation.

   _____

7. What is the benefit of adding moisture to a heat treatment?

   _____

8. What action does the application of cold treatments have on the body?

   _____

9. What action does the application of heat treatments have on the body?

   _____

   _____

10. Name four types of wounds.

    a. _____

    b. _____

    c. _____

    d. _____

11. Refer to the CAAHEP Standards in Appendix B of the textbook. Within the area of *Medical Assisting Clinical Procedures*, which three curriculum standards are discussed in this unit? _____

    _____

12. Word Puzzle: Use the *Words to Know* to spell out these terms.

| | |
|---|---|
| _ _ _ A _ _ _ _ | A scrape or scratch |
| _ _ _ _ _ C _ _ | Acid or alkaline substance |
| _ _ _ C _ _ _ _ _ _ | Having a current |
| _ _ _ _ _ I _ _ _ _ | Prevent from moving |
| _ _ _ _ D | An injury |
| _ _ _ E _ _ _ _ _ _ | A tear |
| _ _ N _ _ _ _ _ | A hole |
| _ _ _ _ T _ _ _ | Rub briskly |
| _ _ _ _ S _ _ _ | Smooth cut |

12. Word Search: Find the following words hidden in the puzzle.

ANAPHYLACTIC
BANDAGE
BITE
BURN
CHEMICAL
ELECTRICAL
FRICTION
IMMOBILIZE
INCISION
INJURIES
LACERATION

MOLTEN
PUNCTURE
SHOCK
SPLINTER
SPRAIN
STINGS
STRAIN
SUPERFICIAL
THERMAL
WOUND

```
S U P E R F I C I A L E
R I P D J V S H O C K L
L I W N I S P R A I N E
A N A P H Y L A C T I C
C C C H E M I C A L M T
E I P S T I N G S C M R
R S F R I C T I O N O I
A I M O L T E N Q O B C
T O M T H E R M A L I A
I N J U R I E S V X L L
O Q W O U N D B P B I H
N I W S T R A I N U Z P
W R G P U N C T U R E Y
X B A N D A G E P N I U
```

After your instructor has returned your work to you, make all necessary corrections and place in a three-ring notebook for future reference.

**ASSIGNMENT SHEET**

**Chapter 19: EMERGENCIES, ACUTE ILLNESS, ACCIDENTS, AND RECOVERY**

**Unit 4: RECOVERING FUNCTION AND MOBILITY**

**SUGGESTED RESPONSES TO CRITICAL THINKING CHALLENGE IN TEXTBOOK**

1. What factors might be involved in Mary's problem with using a cane? _____

_____

2. What options does Shelly have to help Mary with her mobility? _____

_____

_____

3. Does Shelly have an obligation to question the physician's order? _____

_____

4. What risk factors may be involved in this situation? _____

_____

5. Are there any options at home to be considered? _____

_____

_____

_____

_____

_____

**Mixed Quiz**

1. Identify seven situations when the use of some form of device may be indicated to assist patients with mobility.

   a. _____

   b. _____

   c. _____

   d. _____

   e. _____

   f. _____

   g. _____

2. Identify six basic benefits from regular exercise.

   a. _____

   b. _____

   c. _____

   d. _____

   e. _____

   f. _____

3. What is a range-of-motion exercise? _____

_____

4. What is a flexibility exercise? _____

_____

5. What two precautions must be observed when applying a sling? _____

_____

6. Identify two guidelines concerning fitting a cane. _____

_____

7. Explain the proper height for crutches. _____

_____

8. List four factors that will increase safety for the patient at home. _____

_____

_____

9. Matching: Match the definition in column II with the correct term in column I.

COLUMN I

_____ 1. Ambulate
_____ 2. Axilla
_____ 3. Balance
_____ 4. Flexibility
_____ 5. Gait
_____ 6. Mobility
_____ 7. Quad-base
_____ 8. Range-of-motion
_____ 9. Stabilize

COLUMN II

a. A type of cane
b. Manner of walking
c. Extent of movement
d. To walk
e. To hold secure
f. Area under arm
g. The ability to twist and bend
h. Equilibrium
i. Move about freely

10. Using the text, practice the range-of-motion exercises to become familiar with the movements. See text page 857.

11. Refer to the ABHES Course Content Requirements in Appendix C of the textbook. Within the area of *Medical Office Clinical Procedures,* which content requirement is discussed in this unit? _____

## ACHIEVING SKILL COMPETENCY

Reread the performance objective for each procedure and then practice the skills listed below, following the procedure in your textbook.

Procedure 19-1: Apply Arm Sling
Procedure 19-2: Use a Cane
Procedure 19-3: Use Crutches
Procedure 19-4: Use a Walker
Procedure 19-5: Assist Patient from Wheelchair to Examination Table
Procedure 19-6: Assist Patient from Examination Table to Wheelchair

When you feel you have mastered the performance of the skill, sign your name on the appropriate evaluation sheet and give it to your instructor to indicate you are prepared to perform the procedure for evaluation.

After your instructor has returned your work to you, make all necessary corrections and place in a three-ring notebook for future reference.

**ASSIGNMENT SHEET**

### Section 5:  BEHAVIORS AND HEALTH

### Chapter 20:  BEHAVIORS INFLUENCING HEALTH

Review the objectives and text for each unit before completing the assignment sheet for that unit. When you have completed all sheets for the chapter, remove them from this Workbook and give them to the instructor for evaluation.

### Unit 1:  NUTRITION, EXERCISE, AND WEIGHT CONTROL

**SUGGESTED RESPONSES TO CRITICAL THINKING CHALLENGE IN TEXTBOOK**

1. Why was Mrs. Fletcher so interested in those pamphlets? _____
_____

2. How did Darlene encourage the interest in the pamphlets without even knowing it? _____
_____

3. What should Darlene have done about Mrs. Fletcher's complaint of a stiff back? _____
_____
_____

4. Why did Mrs. Fletcher's back complaint disappear? _____

5. Did Mrs. Fletcher disclose another problem? What is it? _____
_____

6. What should Darlene have done in response to Mrs. Fletcher's request for her to explain each pamphlet?
_____
_____

7. What would you have done? _____
_____

### A.  Unscramble

1. _ _ _ _ _ _ _             LEACIRO
2. _ _ _ _ _ _ _ _           EPTVOIIS
3. _ _ _ _ _ _                YSRUCV
4. _ _ _ _ _ _ _ _           RAAIOXNE
5. _ _ _ _ _ _ _ _ _ _       IIANDTTI
6. _ _ _ _ _ _ _ _           KTRSCIE
7. _ _ _ _ _ _ _ _           ERBBIIRE
8. _ _ _ _ _ _                TONMOI
9. _ _ _ _ _                 NREGA
10. _ _ _ _ _ _               ETHALH
11. _ _ _ _ _ _ _ _ _         RIOUNTNTI
12. _ _ _ _ _ _ _ _ _ _       FNYMIIRTI
13. _ _ _ _ _ _ _ _ _ _ _ _    PHECUTATERI
14. _ _ _ _ _ _ _             LCEBMUI

**B. Brief Answer**

1. Explain the significance of diet and exercise to health. _____

_____

2. Name the food groups in the food guide pyramid and the amounts recommended daily for each. _____

_____

_____

_____

3. Name the fat-soluble vitamins. _____

4. Name the water-soluble vitamins. _____

5. Name the essential minerals that are most often missing from the average diet. _____

6. How might you encourage patients to comply in weight control? _____

_____

7. What is the purpose of flexibility or stretching exercises? _____

_____

8. List four things one can do to improve one's health. _____

_____

9. List the guidelines for promoting good health. _____

_____

_____

_____

10. Why is sleep and a positive outlook important to good health? _____

_____

11. Why is it helpful especially for weight reduction to eat slowly? _____

_____

12. What is the reason for eating several small meals a day instead of the traditional three meals a day? _____

_____

_____

13. What is anorexia nervosa? _____

_____

_____

14. Discuss health concerns in regard to adolescents in general. _____

_____

_____

**C. Labeling: Label this food guide pyramid. Refer to Figure 20-2 in the textbook.**

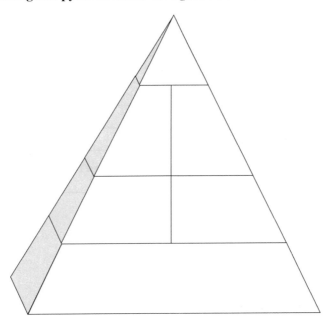

**D. Fill in the Blank**

1. A deficiency of vitamin A could cause _____
2. The main source of vitamin D is _____
3. Prothrombin formation and normal blood coagulation is the function of _____
4. Growth cessation and dermatosis is due to a deficiency of _____
5. Vegetable oil, wheat germ, leafy vegetables, egg yolk, margarine, and legumes are the principal sources of the _____
6. Carbohydrate metabolism, central and peripheral nerve cell function, and myocardial function are attributed to sufficient amounts of _____ or _____ in the diet.
7. Nicotinic acid and niacinamide are the other terms for the micronutrient, _____
8. The usual therapeutic dosage of folic acid is _____
9. Scurvy, hemorrhages, loose teeth, and gingivitis are caused by a deficiency of _____ or _____
10. Some sources of potassium include whole and skim milk, _____ prunes, and raisins.
11. Magnesium is necessary in bone and _____ formation.
12. One who is diagnosed as having anemia has a(n) _____
13. Simple goiter and cretinism are due to a deficiency of _____
14. A deficiency in _____ may cause growth retardation.
15. People who weigh more than _____ of their ideal body weight are considered to be _____
16. Generally, a _____ diet is recommended at least every 2 hours for the first 24 hours for patients who have diarrhea.
17. What do the letters of the BRAT diet stand for? _____
18. The _____ diet is recommended for patients who have tolerated the 24-hour clear liquid diet.
19. Those who have been sick and are just getting over an intestinal virus may find the _____ diet to be tolerated.
20. Patients who wish to reduce their weight should exercise at least _____ times a week and follow a _____ diet.

21. Patients who have special dietary needs should consult with a _____

22. _____ is a term used to describe not being able to sleep.

23. Lack of sleep is termed _____

24. Research shows that a person needs both REM and _____ stages of sleep.

25. People who sleep at least six hours at a time generally feel good because they benefit from the effects of the proper _____ of sleep.

**CRITICAL THINKING SCENARIOS: What would your response be in the following situations?**

1. A female patient in her late 20s calls to tell you that she just read about a diet plan in a new magazine that promises a weight loss of 20 pounds in two weeks. She wants to get the physician's permission for her to lose 20 pounds before her class reunion in three weeks. She has not been seen by the doctor for almost a year.

_____
_____

2. A male patient in his mid-40s is recovering from gall bladder surgery four weeks ago. He tells you that he's going to the health spa to work out because he's bored with sitting around. _____

_____
_____

3. A worried mother of three grade school children tells you as she is leaving the office that her children aren't eating well at dinner time anymore. She says that they eat so much junk food when they come home from school that they can't finish the meals she prepares. _____

_____
_____
_____

After your instructor has returned your work to you, make all necessary corrections and place in a three-ring notebook for future reference.

**ASSIGNMENT SHEET**

**Chapter 20: BEHAVIORS INFLUENCING HEALTH**

**Unit 2: HABIT-FORMING SUBSTANCES**

**A. Brief Answer**

1. List the most commonly abused major groups of drugs and give an example of each. _____

   _____

   _____

   _____

2. What are the effects of depressants? _____

   _____

3. What are the effects of hallucinogens? _____

   _____

4. What are the effects of narcotics? _____

5. What are the effects of stimulants? _____

   _____

6. List behaviors that are indicators of drug/alcohol abuse. _____

   _____

   _____

   _____

   _____

7. Describe the difference between an alcoholic-dependent drinker and an alcoholic. _____

   _____

   _____

8. Describe research efforts into the causes of alcoholism. _____

   _____

9. How can the medical assistant be influential in assisting the drug addict or the alcoholic toward rehabilitation?

   _____

10. List organizations and facilities that assist in the rehabilitation of drug addicts and alcoholics. _____

    _____

    _____

11. Describe the effects that tar, nicotine, and carbon monoxide have on the body. _____

    _____

    _____

    _____

    _____

    _____

12. List ways a person can stop smoking.

a. _____
b. _____
c. _____
d. _____
e. _____
f. _____
g. _____
h. _____
i. _____
j. _____
k. _____

13. Name the diseases that smokers are more likely to acquire. _____
_____

14. Describe the effects of passive or involuntary smoking. _____

15. What health problems do young children have as a result of being exposed to second-hand smoke of caretakers?
_____

**B. Matching: Match the definition in column II with the correct term in column I.**

COLUMN I

_____ 1. Euphoria
_____ 2. Synergism
_____ 3. Addiction
_____ 4. Bizarre
_____ 5. Narcolepsy
_____ 6. Al-Ateen
_____ 7. Barbiturate
_____ 8. Hallucinogen
_____ 9. Al-Anon
_____ 10. Depressant
_____ 11. Amphetamine
_____ 12. Alcoholic
_____ 13. Stimulant
_____ 14. Traumatic
_____ 15. Psychedelics

COLUMN II

a. The habitual use of drugs
b. Stimulates the central nervous system
c. Support group for adolescent family members of alcoholics
d. Induce sleep
e. Mixing two or more drugs
f. Refers to a painful emotional experience
g. Exaggerated good feeling
h. A drinker who has become totally dependent on alcohol
i. Referred to as mind-expanding chemicals
j. Support group for family members and close friends of alcoholics
k. Uncontrollable desire to sleep
l. Hallucinogens
m. Strange; odd in manner
n. Used in treatment of patients who need sedation
o. Comprehensive rehabilitation
p. Taken to stay awake, feel more energetic

**C. True or False:  Place a "T" for true or "F" for false in the space provided. For false statements, explain**
   **why they are false.**

_____  1. Men have a higher risk of premature death due to smoking cigarettes than women.

_____  2. Of the 2000 substances identified in tobacco smoke, most of the harm is done by tar, nicotine, and carbon monoxide.

_____  3. Nicotine stimulates the appetite.

_____  4. Approximately 10% of the blood supply in smokers is in the form of carboxyhemoglobin.

_____  5. Smokers need to become thoroughly educated on the facts about smoking before they can eliminate their habit.

_____  6. Tobacco contains poisons that could be fatal to toddlers and pets if swallowed.

_____  7. Cigarette smoking is dangerous to your health.

**CRITICAL THINKING SCENARIOS:  What would your response be in the following situations?**

1.  One of your high-school patients comes in, hanging on her mother's shoulder to help her stand up. Her speech is slurred and she is nauseated. The visit, of course, is unexpected. _____

   _____

   _____

2.  A concerned parent has found some strange pills in her son's room and calls to ask you what to do. She says her son's behavior has changed recently and she is worried about him. _____

   _____

   After your instructor has returned your work to you, make all necessary corrections and place in a three-ring notebook for future reference.

**ASSIGNMENT SHEET**

**Chapter 20: BEHAVIORS INFLUENCING HEALTH**

**Unit 3: STRESS AND TIME MANAGEMENT**

**A. Word Puzzle:** Use the list of *Words to Know* to spell out these terms.

1. __ __ __ __ P __ __ __ __ __ __ __
2. __ __ S __ __ __ __ __
3. __ __ Y __ __ __ __ __ __
4. __ __ C __ __ __ __ __ __
   H
5. __ __ __ O __ __ __ __ __ __
6. __ __ S __ __ __ __ __ __
7. __ O __ __ __ __ __
8. __ M __ __ __ __ __ __ __
9. A __ __ __ __ __ __ __
10. __ __ __ T __ __ __
11. I __ __ __ __ __ __ __ __
12. __ __ __ C __ __ __ __ __ __

**B. Brief Answer**

1. Describe the phenomenon of stress. _____
   _____
   _____
   _____

2. List the physical effects of stress. _____
   _____
   _____

3. What is "good stress"? _____
4. What is "bad stress"? _____
   _____

5. Describe the Type-A personality. _____
   _____

6. Describe the Type-B personality. _____
   _____

7. List the four basic human physical needs. _____
8. List the four basic human development needs. _____
9. What can be done to eliminate unnecessary stress? _____
   _____

10. List methods for dealing with stress. _____
    _____
    _____

11. List possible mental health resources for patient referrals. _____

12. List and discuss ways to relax and cope with daily stress. _____

_____

_____

13. What is the purpose of time management? _____
14. List some of the benefits of time management. _____

_____

## C. Matching: Match the definition in column II with the correct term in column I.

COLUMN I

_____ 1. Exercise
_____ 2. Perspective
_____ 3. Implement
_____ 4. Eustress
_____ 5. Psychosomatic
_____ 6. Psychosis
_____ 7. Prioritizing
_____ 8. Flexible
_____ 9. Conflict
_____ 10. Anxiety
_____ 11. Depression

COLUMN II

a. Low spirits; sadness
b. Impairment of normal intellectual and social functioning
c. Arranging in order of importance
d. Constant state of worry
e. Clash, be in opposition
f. To put into effect
g. Support group
h. Real symptoms, not imagined
i. Positive effect in reducing stress
j. Able to bend without breaking
k. Proper evaluation/consideration
l. Planned stress; it motivates

## D. Brief Answer

1. Make a list of the good and bad stress in your life.

_____

_____

_____

_____

## E. Use the following words in a complete sentence.

Anxiety _____

Discretion _____

Exemplify _____

Flexible _____

Nurture _____

Perspective _____

Prioritize _____

Name _____

After your instructor has returned your work to you, make all necessary corrections and place in a three-ring notebook for future reference.

**ASSIGNMENT SHEET**

**Chapter 20: BEHAVIORS INFLUENCING HEALTH**

**Unit 4: RELATED THERAPIES**

**SUGGESTED RESPONSES TO CRITICAL THINKING CHALLENGE IN TEXTBOOK**

1. Discuss how you think Renita felt during this situation. _____

_____

2. Who should she call? Why? _____

_____

_____

3. Should she call the doctor? _____

4. How should she speak to this patient? Why? _____

_____

_____

5. Should she continue the calls? _____

_____

6. Is there any potential legal problem here? _____

_____

_____

_____

7. What would you do in this situation? _____

_____

_____

**Mixed Quiz**

1. Define and give four examples of complementary therapy. _____

_____

2. Define and give three examples of alternative therapy. _____

_____

3. Why should a person using a related therapy inform her or his physician? _____

_____

4. List six guidelines to follow when using related therapies. _____

_____

_____

5. Identify nine specific goods with documented health benefits. _____

_____

6. Name the nine common herbal products that may have some benefits. _____

_____

7. Matching: Match the therapy in column I with its description in column II.

COLUMN I                           COLUMN II

_____ Accupuncture                 a. Uses the Low of Similiars
_____ Aromatherapy                 b. Uses a trance state
_____ Ayurvedic                    c. Uses laughter
_____ Biofeedback                  d. Used to treat neuropathy and pain
_____ Faith                        e. Stinulates points on the hand
_____ Homeopathy                   f. Uses thin, sterile needles inserted into the skin
_____ Humor                        g. Uses diet, rest, relaxation, exercise, and herbal products
_____ Hypnosis                     h. Uses brain activities to influence the nervous system
_____ Magnet therapy               i. Teaches how to control involuntary body functions
_____ Massage                      j. Uses a series of fluid movements
_____ Naturopathy                  k. Uses the power of prayer
_____ Reflexology                  l. Uses extracted plant oils for message and inhalation
_____ Visualization                m. Uses hands to manipulate muscles
_____ Yoga                         n. Uses brain control meditation, stretching and strengthening exercises
_____ Tai Chi                      o. Traditional healing system from India

8. Refer to the ABHES Course Content Requirements in Appendix C of the textbook. Within the area of *Psychology of Human Relations,* which content requirement is discussed in this unit? _____

   _____

9. Word Puzzle: Use the clues to spell out these terms.

   __ __ R __ __ __                    From plants

   __ __ __ E __ __ __ __ __           Dilute mixtures

   __ __ __ __ L __ __ __ __ __ __ __  Supplemental

   __ __ __ __ A __ __ __ __           Treatments

   __ __ T __ __ __ __ __ __ __        Instead of

   __ __ __ __ __ __ E __ __ __ __     Beneficial

   __ __ __ __ __ __ D __ __           Oldest medicine

Name _____

**CRITICAL THINKING SCENARIOS: What would your response be in the following situations?**

1. Your neighbor, Mrs. Slovosky, has just told you that she is probably dying. She said her doctor told her that her lung scan indicated she has a fairly large mass in her left upper lobe that appears to be malignant. He wants her to see a surgical oncologist as quickly as possible. She has heard people say that when they open up your body to do surgery it just makes the cancer spread. Because she is afraid, she has neglected to make arrangements to see the surgeon. However, she has been taking some pills she ordered over the Internet because the Web site had testimonials from a lot of cured people. She feels her chances are better with the medication than with surgery. _____

_____

_____

_____

_____

_____


2. Charlie Kantor has tried several times to quit smoking. He even chewed the gum and wore a patch for a while, but he couldn't break his habit. He has heard about hypnosis but is afraid the practitioner will make him do silly things while he's hypnotized, like he's seen on television. _____

_____

_____

_____

_____

_____


After your instructor has returned your work to you, make all necessary corrections and place in a three-ring notebook for future reference.

**ASSIGNMENT SHEET**

**Section 6: EMPLOYABILITY SKILLS**

**Chapter 21: ACHIEVING SATISFACTION IN EMPLOYMENT**

Review the objectives and text for each unit before completing the assignment sheet for that unit. When you have completed all sheets for the chapter, remove them from this Workbook and give them to the instructor for evaluation.

**Unit 1: THE JOB SEARCH**

**SUGGESTED RESPONSES TO CRITICAL THINKING CHALLENGE IN TEXTBOOK**

1. How do you think Anthony got the idea he had the job? _____
   _____

2. What should he do about this situation? _____
   _____

3. Does Anthony have a reason to seek legal counsel? _____
   _____

4. Why do you suppose Anthony wasn't hired? _____

5. What do you think of having a new person at the reception desk who is not qualified? _____
   _____
   _____

6. What would you do in this situation? _____
   _____
   _____
   _____
   _____

**A. Brief Answer**

1. What is the purpose of a resumé? _____

2. Why should a cover letter accompany a resumé? _____
   _____

3. List the different types of resumés and the purpose of each.
   a. _____
   b. _____
   c. _____
   d. _____
   e. _____

4. Describe the services of an employment agency. _____
   _____

5. List three contacts to assist the medical assistant in the job search. _____

_____

6. What is a classified ad? _____

_____

7. Where can the medical assistant find additional information abut job opportunities? _____

_____

## B. Fill in the Blank

1. The job search begins with the _____ to work.
2. The _____ should be complete, accurate, and neatly organized.
3. Preparation of a resumé requires you to list systematically experiences that show your valuable _____

4. In listing your educational background, you should note that a _____ can be furnished upon request.
5. Permission should be obtained from those persons listed as _____
6. Personal data are _____ on a resumé.
7. The resumé should be _____ and _____ as needed to document additional employment experience, educational achievements, awards, and personal development.
8. All states offer assistance in locating jobs through the state _____
9. Many potential jobs are _____ meaning that the employer pays the agency's fees.
10. The job search takes patience, persistence, and _____
11. _____ a resumé should be done only when an employer requests it.

## C. Matching: Match the acronym in column I with the correct term in column II.

| COLUMN I | | COLUMN II |
|---|---|---|
| _____ | 1. SAL | a. Position(s) |
| _____ | 2. PT | b. License |
| _____ | 3. INT | c. Beginning |
| _____ | 4. REQ | d. Necessary |
| _____ | 5. POS | e. Negotiable |
| _____ | 6. LIC | f. Education |
| _____ | 7. FB | g. Immediate |
| _____ | 8. BGN | h. Words per minute |
| _____ | 9. NEG | i. Experience |
| _____ | 10. COL | j. Required |
| _____ | 11. IMMED | k. Interview |
| _____ | 12. EDUC | l. Part-time |
| _____ | 13. NEC | m. Salary |
| _____ | 14. WPM | n. College |
| _____ | 15. EXP | o. Fringe benefits |

**D. Fill in the Blank:** **Grouped below are some of the qualities that employers expect from their employees. After the brief definition of each, place the appropriate quality on the line provided.**

initiative                dependability          courteous              responsible

reliability               cooperative            time management skill

punctuality               enthusiasm             interest

1. To excite the attention or curiosity of: _____
2. Trustworthy: _____
3. Answerable; accountable: _____
4. The ability to think and act without being urged: _____
5. Organization by priority: _____
6. Intense or eager interest: _____
7. Considerate toward others; well-mannered: _____
8. Working together for a common purpose: _____
9. Being on time: _____
10. Can be depended on: _____

**E. Ads/Cover Letter**

In the space below, paste a want ad from your local paper for a medical assistant position. Below it respond with the cover letter about yourself that you would send. Show it to your instructor to evaluate when you are finished.

_____
_____
_____
_____
_____
_____
_____
_____
_____
_____
_____
_____
_____
_____
_____

## F. Crossword Puzzle

ACROSS

2. A quality
5. It's said to be the best teacher
7. Words per minute (acronym)
10. A wish
11. Schooling
12. Salary (abbreviation)
14. High school (abbreviation)
15. Refers to form or _____ of resumé
16. Immediately (abbreviation)
17. Reference (abbreviation)
18. Type of letter sent with resumé
19. Outlined summary of your abilities and experience
21. Equal opportunity employer (acronym)
22. Strong ambition
24. College (abbreviation)
26. Capable for position

DOWN

1. Fringe benefit (abbreviation)
2. Appointment (abbreviation)
3. Aimed
4. To hire or _____
5. Work
6. Employment ads
7. Newspaper ad listings that say "help _____"
8. Skillful and precise
9. You may furnish on request
13. Payment for services
20. Secretary (abbreviation)
23. Required (abbreviation)
25. Advertisement (abbreviation)

**CRITICAL THINKING SCENARIOS:  What would your response be in the following situations?**

1. Planning ahead to allow spare time for traffic, you are on your way to an interview for a position you really want. Traffic is unusually congested because a truck is stalled on the freeway. You realize that you will most likely be late. _____

_____

_____

_____

2. During an interview, the employer asks you if you have ever been late to work. This employer also asks for references. _____

_____

After your instructor has returned your work to you, make all necessary corrections and place in a three-ring notebook for future reference.

**ASSIGNMENT SHEET**

**Chapter 21: ACHIEVING SATISFACTION IN EMPLOYMENT**

**Unit 2: GETTING THE JOB AND KEEPING IT**

**SUGGESTED RESPONSES TO CRITICAL THINKING CHALLENGE IN TEXTBOOK**

1.  What is the first thing that Juanita should have done? _____

_____

2.  Do you think Juanita will get a good reference from her former employer when she applies for a job?

_____

3.  What do you think of Juanita? Do you understand what she did? Why? _____

_____

4.  What do you think was the reaction of the office manager? the physician(s)? _____

_____

5.  What should Juanita have done? _____

_____

_____

6.  What would you tell Juanita? _____

_____

7.  What would you have done in her situation? _____

_____

**A.  Matching:  Match the definition in column II with the correct term in column I.**

COLUMN I

_____  1. Contemporary
_____  2. Negate
_____  3. Demeanor
_____  4. Competent
_____  5. Arbitrary
_____  6. Affiliate
_____  7. Apprise

COLUMN II

a.  Well-qualified
b.  To connect or associate
c.  To inform or notify
d.  To discriminate
e.  Modern
f.  Conduct; outward behavior
g.  To make ineffective
h.  Not fixed by rules; based on one's preference
i.  An attitude or system

**B.  Brief Answer**

1.  What information should you be prepared to provide on an application for employment? _____

_____

2.  What important factor must the medical assistant remember when completing a job application? _____

_____

3.  Why is appearance so important when interviewing for a job? _____

_____

4. What is the purpose of a job interview? _____

_____

5. Why must one be prompt and courteous at a job interview? _____

_____

6. Explain why it is a good idea to send a follow-up letter to the interviewer after the job interview. _____

_____

_____

7. What is the best way to close an interview. Why? _____

_____

8. How may a medical assistant demonstrate pride in the profession of medical assisting? _____

_____

9. How should you dress when applying for a job or when returning an application form? Why? _____

_____

_____

10. List areas of concern employers have regarding (prospective) employees. _____

_____

_____

_____

_____

11. What documents are employers required to ask for of prospective employees and why? _____

_____

_____

_____

12. How can time management skills be applied to the work day? _____

_____

_____

13. Explain what "work ethics" is and why it is important regarding employment. _____

_____

_____

14. What is the value of an employment evaluation review? _____

_____

_____

15. What are some of the subjects you should discuss with your employer during an evaluation review?

_____

_____

_____

_____

16. Discuss the purpose and advantages of a job description. _____

_____

_____

_____

17. Refer to ABHES Course Content Requirements in Appendix C of the textbook. Within the area of *Medical Office Clinical Procedures,* which four content requirements are discussed in this chapter? _____

_____

_____

## C. Fill in the Blank

1. An employer will expect you to perform with increasing _____ in your position as you continue to gain experience.
2. One particular quality that the medical assistant must keep in mind is _____
3. Your _____ will probably follow you throughout your working life.
4. Advancement will depend largely upon your _____ in performing administrative and clinical tasks.
5. In terminating employment, the employee has major responsibility of giving the employer at least a _____
6. The usual cause for termination initiated by the employer is _____ to perform job responsibilities.

## D. Letters

1. In the space below write a follow-up letter thanking an employer who interviewed you for a job. Show it to your instructor for evaluation.

_____
_____
_____
_____
_____
_____
_____
_____

2. Write a letter of resignation below and show it to your instructor for evaluation.

_____
_____
_____
_____
_____

**E. Word Search:  Find the following words hidden in the puzzle.**

| | |
|---|---|
| WORK | RELIABILITY |
| ON TIME | INITIATIVE |
| TACT | COOPERATION |
| VALUES | GRAMMAR |
| SMILE | COMMUNICATION |
| THANK | ADVANCEMENT |
| ACTIVE | OPPORTUNITY |
| ETHICS | COMPETENT |
| REVIEW | QUESTIONS |
| PROMPT | FORM |
| GOALS | SKILL |
| HONEST | MANNERS |
| RESPONSIBILITY | FOLLOW UP |
| ENTHUSIASM | |

```
Y T I L I B A I L E R L P T E V O J K T
T C A J N P U T A J E N T H U S I A S M
I A D H O N E S T S S M D A J B S D B R
N R R M I P B M N T P K C N N F L V K B
U T A C T F P K P Y O K I K C G O A L S
T N C Q A R V M S L N G C L K Z M N K M
R O T U R E O B J T S H J F L J S C S I
O C K H E R A G I N I T I A T I V E S L
P C F D P F G J D A B W J B N S M M D E
P R C F O C R C S T I G S C I H T E R Y
O H O R O S A A E C L M A D P S F N A P
J N M C C O M M U N I C A T I O N T M U
A Z P W L B M Y L O T M J N L C R L B W
F W E S C Z A F A I Y B O Y N S W F L O
B Q T A M G R E V I E W T N G E O K V L
J K E R D T L E F W K V Q R A I R I T L
C W N L L F Z I O Q U E S T I O N S V O
O N T I M E A W T W K I A L W R B M A F
```

**CRITICAL THINKING SCENARIOS: What would your response be in the following situations?**

1. You have just started to work on some reports, of which you are behind schedule in mailing, when your employer brings the new employee to you for a tour of the clinic. You are also asked to explain the office policy and duties to this person. _____

_____

_____

2. You have been employed at the clinic for almost three months. You know that your three-month (90-day) evaluation is scheduled for next week. Since you have done well, you feel you will be eligible for a promotion and raise. You have overheard that the supervisor is thinking about hiring a new person for the job. _____

_____

_____

After your instructor has returned your work to you, make all necessary corrections and place in a three-ring notebook for future reference.

# PERFORMANCE EVALUATION CHECKLIST

Name _____

Date _____ Score* _____

## PROCEDURE 5-1   Open the Office

*PERFORMANCE OBJECTIVE*—Follow all the steps in the procedure, role-play the actions necessary to prepare a medical office to see patients. Verbally describe actions while performing.

| PROCEDURE STEPS | STEP PERFORMED | POINTS POSSIBLE | COMMENTS |
|---|---|---|---|
| *EVALUATOR:* Place check mark in space following each step performed satisfactorily | | | |
| NOTE TIME BEGAN _____ | | | |
| 1. Unlocked the reception room door. | _____ | 10 | |
| 2. Adjusted heat or air conditioning for the comfort of the patients. | _____ | 5 | |
| 3. Checked for safety hazards in the office. | | | |
|    a. Checked electrical wires | _____ | 15 | |
|    b. Checked furniture condition | _____ | 15 | |
|    c. Checked floor | _____ | 15 | |
| 4. Checked magazines for condition and date. | _____ | 5 | |
| 5. Checked the telephone answering device or call the answering service for any messages. | _____ | 10 | |
| 6. Pulled the charts of patients to be seen. | _____ | 15 | |
| 7. Wrote or stamped today's date. | _____ | 15 | |
| 8. Checked for previously ordered studies and filed in chart. | _____ | 15 | |
| 9. Checked examining rooms to be sure they were clean and stocked with supplies. | _____ | 10 | |
| 10. If it is the policy of the office, prepared a list of the patients to be seen and the times of their appointments and placed this list on the physician's desk. | _____ | 5 | |
| *EVALUATOR:* NOTE TIME COMPLETED _____ | | | |

ADD POINTS OF STEPS CHECKED                                                           _____ EARNED

TOTAL POINTS POSSIBLE                                                                     135 POSSIBLE

Points assigned reflect importance of step to meeting objective: Important = (5)   Essential = (10)   Critical = (15)
Automatic failure results if any of the critical steps are omitted or performed incorrectly.

DETERMINE SCORE (divide points earned by total points possible, multiply results by 100)          _____ SCORE*

Evaluator's Name (print) _____ Signature _____

Comments _____

Name _____

Date _____ Score* _____

## PROCEDURE 5-2   Obtain New Patient Information

*PERFORMANCE OBJECTIVE*—In a simulated situation, clearly communicate instructions and complete the steps designated in the procedure within acceptable time limits.

| PROCEDURE STEPS | STEP PERFORMED | POINTS POSSIBLE | COMMENTS |
|---|---|---|---|
| *EVALUATOR:* Place check mark in space following each step performed satisfactorily | | | |
| NOTE TIME BEGAN _____ | | | |
| 1. Took new patient to private area to ask preliminary questions. | _____ | 10 | |
| 2. Instructed new patient to complete a data sheet. | _____ | 10 | |
|    a. Provided clipboard and pen | _____ | 10 | |
|    b. Requested return when completed | _____ | 10 | |
| 3. Checked form for completeness. | _____ | 15 | |
| 4. Prepared a patient folder by typing the patient's name on a label and attaching it to the tab of the folder. | _____ | 5 | |
| 5. Transferred information from the data sheet to the chart sheet. | _____ | 10 | |
| 6. Copied the insurance card and returned to patient. | _____ | 15 | |
| 7. Inserted the chart, data sheets, and insurance card copy in folder. | _____ | 15 | |
| 8. Placed any referral material in chart. | _____ | 15 | |
| 9. Prepared charge slip. | _____ | 10 | |
| 10. Placed the folder in the area reserved for charts of patients to be seen. | _____ | 5 | |
| 11. Completed within established time limit. | _____ | 15 | |
| *EVALUATOR:* NOTE TIME COMPLETED _____ | | | |

ADD POINTS OF STEPS CHECKED             _____ EARNED

TOTAL POINTS POSSIBLE             145 POSSIBLE

Points assigned reflect importance of step to meeting objective: Important = (5)   Essential = (10)   Critical = (15)
Automatic failure results if any of the critical steps are omitted or performed incorrectly.

DETERMINE SCORE (divide points earned by total points possible, multiply results by 100)       _____ SCORE*

Evaluator's Name (print) _____ Signature _____

Comments _____

Name _____

Date _____ Score* _____

## PROCEDURE 5-3   Close the Office

*PERFORMANCE OBJECTIVE*—Following all the steps in the procedure, role-play the actions required to close the office. Actions must be verbally described while performing the procedure.

| PROCEDURE STEPS | STEP PERFORMED | POINTS POSSIBLE | COMMENTS |
|---|---|---|---|
| *EVALUATOR:* Place check mark in space following each step performed satisfactorily | | | |
| NOTE TIME BEGAN _____ | | | |
| 1. Checked to see that records were collected and filed in locked cabinets. | _____ | 15 | |
| 2. Placed any money received in safe or took to the bank to be deposited. | _____ | 15 | |
| 3. Turned off all electrical appliances. | _____ | 15 | |
| 4. Checked that rooms were cleaned and supplied for the next day. | _____ | 10 | |
| 5. Straightened reception room if time allowed. | _____ | 5 | |
| 6. Pulled charts for the next day if time allowed. | _____ | 5 | |
| 7. Activated answering device on phone or called answering service with information about when the office would reopen. | _____ | 15 | |
| 8. Turned off lights. | _____ | 10 | |
| 9. Activated alarm system. | _____ | 15 | |
| 10. Securely locked doors. | _____ | 15 | |
| *EVALUATOR:* NOTE TIME COMPLETED _____ | | | |

ADD POINTS OF STEPS CHECKED                                         _____ EARNED
TOTAL POINTS POSSIBLE                                                      120 POSSIBLE

Points assigned reflect importance of step to meeting objective: Important  = (5)   Essential = (10)   Critical = (15)
Automatic failure results if any of the critical steps are omitted or performed incorrectly.

DETERMINE SCORE (divide points earned by total points possible, multiply results by 100)        _____ SCORE*

Evaluator's Name (print) _____ Signature _____

Comments _____

Name _____

Date _____ Score* _____

## PROCEDURE 6-1   Answer the Office Phone

*PERFORMANCE OBJECTIVE*—In a simulated (or actual) situation, using proper grammar, answer the telephone by the third ring, identifying the office and yourself.

| PROCEDURE STEPS | STEP PERFORMED | POINTS POSSIBLE | COMMENTS |
|---|---|---|---|
| *EVALUATOR:* Place check mark in space following each step performed satisfactorily | | | |
| NOTE TIME BEGAN _____ | | | |
| 1. Answered the phone promptly (by third ring) in a polite and pleasant manner. | _____ | 10 | |
| 2. Identified the office and self by name. | _____ | 15 | |
|    a. Voice clear, distinct, moderate rate of speaking | _____ | 10 | |
| 3. Listened to and recorded the name of the caller. | _____ | 15 | |
| 4. Recorded: | | | |
|    a. Date | _____ | 5 | |
|    b. Time | _____ | 5 | |
|    c. Reason for call | _____ | 5 | |
| 5. a. Spelled name correctly | _____ | 10 | |
|    b. Processed emergency call immediately | _____ | 15 | |
|    c. Waited for response before placing on hold | _____ | 15 | |
|    d. Checked with caller on hold once each minute | _____ | 5 | |
|    e. Completed interrupted on-hold calls | _____ | 5 | |
| 6. Screened and completed as many calls as possible before adding to the physician's call-back list. | _____ | 10 | |
| 7. Responded to an untimely request to speak to physician by taking a message. | _____ | 10 | |
| *EVALUATOR:* NOTE TIME COMPLETED _____ | | | |

ADD POINTS OF STEPS CHECKED                                                    _____ EARNED
TOTAL POINTS POSSIBLE                                                               135 POSSIBLE

Points assigned reflect importance of step to meeting objective: Important = (5)   Essential = (10)   Critical = (15)
Automatic failure results if any of the critical steps are omitted or performed incorrectly.

DETERMINE SCORE (divide points earned by total points possible, multiply results by 100)         _____ SCORE*

Evaluator's Name (print) _____ Signature _____

Comments _____

## PROCEDURE 6-2   Process Phone Message

*PERFORMANCE OBJECTIVE*—In a simulated situation (or actual situation) receive, evaluate, and document a phone message.

| PROCEDURE STEPS | STEP PERFORMED | POINTS POSSIBLE | COMMENTS |
|---|---|---|---|
| *EVALUATOR:* Place check mark in space following each step performed satisfactorily | | | |
| NOTE TIME BEGAN _____ | | | |
| 1. Answered the phone properly. | _____ | 10 | |
| 2. Listened carefully and determined caller's needs. | _____ | 15 | |
| 3. Documented information regarding message (including date/time) on message pad/phone call log—included: | | | |
|   a. Whom the request was for | _____ | 15 | |
|   b. What it concerned | _____ | 15 | |
|   c. When information was needed | _____ | 15 | |
|   d. Where to return call | _____ | 15 | |
| 4. Repeated message to caller to verify the contents. | _____ | 10 | |
| 5. Closed conversation politely. | _____ | 5 | |
| 6. Allowed caller to hang up first. | _____ | 5 | |
| 7. Signed initials after the message. | _____ | 5 | |
| 8. Pulled patient's chart and recorded or attached message. | _____ | 10 | |
| *EVALUATOR:* NOTE TIME COMPLETED _____ | | | |

ADD POINTS OF STEPS CHECKED                                                                 _____ EARNED
TOTAL POINTS POSSIBLE                                                                              120 POSSIBLE

Points assigned reflect importance of step to meeting objective: Important = (5)   Essential = (10)   Critical = (15)
Automatic failure results if any of the critical steps are omitted or performed incorrectly.

DETERMINE SCORE (divide points earned by total points possible, multiply results by 100)          _____ SCORE*

Evaluator's Name (print) _____ Signature _____

Comments _____

## PROCEDURE 6-3   Record Telephone Message on Recording Device

*PERFORMANCE OBJECTIVE*—In a simulated situation (or actual situation) procedure, with all necessary information in a pleasant
tone of voice, a clear, accurate, and precise phone message on the telephone message device.

| PROCEDURE STEPS | STEP PERFORMED | POINTS POSSIBLE | COMMENTS |
|---|---|---|---|
| *EVALUATOR:* Place check mark in space following each step performed satisfactorily | | | |
| NOTE TIME BEGAN _____ | | | |
| 1. Assembled necessary items away from noise and distractions. | _____ | 10 | |
|   a. Determined amount of time allowed on recording device for message before beginning | _____ | 10 | |
| 2. Wrote out appropriate message. | | | |
|   a. Checked for completeness and accuracy | _____ | 10 | |
|   b. Read and determined the amount of time of message | _____ | 10 | |
| 3. Recorded message following directions of answering device. | _____ | 15 | |
|   a. Spoke in a pleasant, clear, and articulate tone of voice | _____ | 5 | |
|   b. Sat up straight and projected voice into the speaker | _____ | 5 | |
|   c. Identified the office | _____ | 10 | |
|   d. Was not too wordy or overly friendly | _____ | 5 | |
|   e. Complete and accurate information | _____ | 10 | |
| 4. Played message back and evaluated quality of message. | _____ | 5 | |
|   a. Listened and determined if the message was of good quality | _____ | 5 | |
|   b. Appropriate for all callers | _____ | 5 | |
| 5. Set the device to play messages when unavailable to answer phone. | _____ | 15 | |
| *EVALUATOR:* NOTE TIME COMPLETED _____ | | | |

ADD POINTS OF STEPS CHECKED                                         _____ EARNED

TOTAL POINTS POSSIBLE                                                  120 POSSIBLE

Points assigned reflect importance of step to meeting objective: Important = (5)   Essential = (10)   Critical = (15)
Automatic failure results if any of the critical steps are omitted or performed incorrectly.

DETERMINE SCORE (divide points earned by total points possible, multiply results by 100)        _____ SCORE*

Evaluator's Name (print) _____ Signature _____

Comments _____

## PROCEDURE 6-4  Obtain Telephone Message from Phone Recording Device

*PERFORMANCE OBJECTIVE*—In a simulated situation (or actual situation), obtain necessary and pertinent information from all phone messages from the phone message recording device.

| PROCEDURE STEPS | STEP PERFORMED | POINTS POSSIBLE | COMMENTS |
|---|---|---|---|
| *EVALUATOR:* Place check mark in space following each step performed satisfactorily | | | |
| NOTE TIME BEGAN _____ | | | |
| 1. Assembled necessary items in an area away from noise and distractions. | _____ | 5 | |
| 2. Listened to recordings and wrote message(s) accurately. | _____ | 15 | |
| 3. Repeated listening to difficult messages to obtain complete information. | _____ | 5 | |
| 4. Signed initials after message(s). | _____ | 5 | |
| 5. Noted date and time of the message(s). | _____ | 10 | |
| 6. Listed all patients who left messages and pulled their charts. | _____ | 15 | |
| 7. Prioritized messages according to their seriousness. | _____ | 15 | |
| 8. Distributed messages to appropriate staff member/ department to be processed. | _____ | 10 | |
| *EVALUATOR:* NOTE TIME COMPLETED _____ | | | |

ADD POINTS OF STEPS CHECKED                                                    _____ EARNED

TOTAL POINTS POSSIBLE                                                              80 POSSIBLE

Points assigned reflect importance of step to meeting objective: Important = (5)   Essential = (10)   Critical = (15)
Automatic failure results if any of the critical steps are omitted or performed incorrectly.

DETERMINE SCORE (divide points earned by total points possible, multiply results by 100)    _____ SCORE*

Evaluator's Name (print) _____ Signature _____

Comments _____

# PERFORMANCE EVALUATION CHECKLIST

Name _____

Date _____ Score* _____

## PROCEDURE 6-5   Schedule Appointments

*PERFORMANCE OBJECTIVE*—In a simulated situation, schedule an appointment for a patient according to accepted medical standards with consideration for the physician, staff, and needs of the patient.

| PROCEDURE STEPS | STEP PERFORMED | POINTS POSSIBLE | COMMENTS |
|---|---|---|---|
| *EVALUATOR:* Place check mark in space following each step performed satisfactorily | | | |
| NOTE TIME BEGAN _____ | | | |
| 1. Determined the means of scheduling: appointment book or computer entry. | _____ | 10 | |
| 2. Marked off hours when the physician was unable to see patients. | _____ | 15 | |
| 3. Attempted to give patients two appointment choices. | _____ | 5 | |
| 4. Recorded names in black ink with phone number(s). | _____ | 10 | |
| 5. Asked patient(s) to schedule next appointment before leaving office. | _____ | 5 | |
| 6. Wrote patients' names in the schedule book. | _____ | 10 | |
| 7. Recorded appointment first in appointment book and then on appointment card. | _____ | 15 | |
| 8. Completed appointment card and gave to patient. | _____ | 15 | |
| 9. Left sufficient time for work-ins in appointment book. | _____ | 10 | |
| 10. Allowed time for return phone calls to be made by the doctor. | _____ | 5 | |
| *EVALUATOR:* NOTE TIME COMPLETED _____ | | | |

ADD POINTS OF STEPS CHECKED                                                        _____ EARNED
TOTAL POINTS POSSIBLE                                                                   100 POSSIBLE

Points assigned reflect importance of step to meeting objective:  Important  = (5)   Essential = (10)   Critical = (15)
Automatic failure results if any of the critical steps are omitted or performed incorrectly.

DETERMINE SCORE (divide points earned by total points possible, multiply results by 100)   _____ SCORE*

Evaluator's Name (print) _____ Signature _____

Comments _____

## PROCEDURE 6-6   Arrange Referral Appointment

*PERFORMANCE OBJECTIVE*—In a simulated situation, schedule a referral appointment for a patient by phoning the requested medical facility according to accepted medical standards with consideration for the physician, staff, and needs of the patient.

| PROCEDURE STEPS | STEP PERFORMED | POINTS POSSIBLE | COMMENTS |
|---|---|---|---|
| *EVALUATOR:* Place check mark in space following each step performed satisfactorily | | | |
| NOTE TIME BEGAN _____ | | | |
| 1. Obtained patient's chart with request for referral to another facility. | _____ | 15 | |
| 2. Used phone directory to obtain phone number and address of referral office. | _____ | 10 | |
| 3. Placed the call to referral office and provided receptionist with: | | | |
|   a. Your name/physician's name and address | _____ | 15 | |
|   b. Patient's name, address, etc., and reason for appointment | _____ | 15 | |
|   c. Indicated that confirmation letter will be mailed/faxed | _____ | 5 | |
|   d. Recorded appointment information on patient's chart | _____ | 10 | |
|   e. Gave complete information to patient (time, day, date, name, address, etc.) | _____ | 10 | |
| 4. Gave patient printed instructions regarding appointment as appropriate. | _____ | 5 | |
|   a. Initialed patient's chart signifying completion of request | _____ | 5 | |
| *EVALUATOR:* NOTE TIME COMPLETED _____ | | | |

ADD POINTS OF STEPS CHECKED                  _____ EARNED

TOTAL POINTS POSSIBLE                              90 POSSIBLE

Points assigned reflect importance of step to meeting objective: Important = (5)   Essential = (10)   Critical = (15)
Automatic failure results if any of the critical steps are omitted or performed incorrectly.

DETERMINE SCORE (divide points earned by total points possible, multiply results by 100)     _____ SCORE*

Evaluator's Name (print) _____ Signature _____

Comments _____

## PROCEDURE 6-7   Compose a Business Letter

*PERFORMANCE OBJECTIVE*—Given access to equipment and supplies, complete a mailable letter following the steps in the procedure within the number of attempts and time frame specified by the instructor. The final copy must meet mailable standards described in the text.

| PROCEDURE STEPS | STEP PERFORMED | POINTS POSSIBLE | COMMENTS |
|---|---|---|---|
| *EVALUATOR:* Place check mark in space following each step performed satisfactorily | | | |
| NOTE TIME BEGAN _____ | | | |
| 1. Moved cursor down at least three lines below letterhead. | _____ | 5 | |
| 2. Entered the date in appropriate location for letter style. | _____ | 10 | |
| 3. Moved to the fifth line below the date. | _____ | 5 | |
| 4. Entered the inside address in appropriate location for letter style. | _____ | 5 | |
| a. Entered name as received on letter or listed in a directory | _____ | 15 | |
| 5. Double spaced after the last line of the address. | _____ | 5 | |
| 6. Entered the appropriate salutation followed by a colon. | _____ | 10 | |
| 7. Double spaced. | _____ | 5 | |
| 8. a. Entered the reference line in the location appropriate for letter style | _____ | 5 | |
| b. Entered RE: Entered patient's name or person about whom the letter was written | _____ | 10 | |
| 9. Double spaced. | _____ | 5 | |
| 10. Prepared the body of letter. | | | |
| a. Paragraph style appropriate to the style of the letter | _____ | 5 | |
| b. Double spaced between paragraphs | _____ | 5 | |
| 11. (When second page)— | | | |
| a. Entered second page heading at 7th line | _____ | — | |
| b. Entered name, page number, date | _____ | — | |
| c. At least two lines of paragraph were on first page | _____ | — | |
| d. Last word on first page not divided | _____ | — | |
| (Note: Subtract 10 points for each step a–e if omitted) | | | |
| 12. Continued body of letter | _____ | — | |

| PROCEDURE STEPS | STEP PERFORMED | POINTS POSSIBLE | COMMENTS |
|---|---|---|---|
| 13. Complimentary closing entered in letter style format. | _____ | 10 | |
| 14. Four spaces entered. | _____ | 5 | |
| 15. Sender's name entered in letter style format exactly as printed on letterhead; | _____ | 15 | |
| a. Title followed name after comma or | | | |
| b. Title entered below name | | | |
| 16. Double space. | _____ | 5 | |
| 17. Entered reference initials to indicate typist. | _____ | 15 | |
| 18. Single or double spaced if enclosed materials. | _____ | — | |
| 19. "cc" and recipient's name entered | _____ | — | |
| a. Numbered and identified if more than one. | _____ | — | |
| 20. Double spaced (if needed) | _____ | — | |
| (Subtract 10 points if omitted in error) | | | |
| 21. PS for postscript if applicable | _____ | — | |
| (Subtract 10 points if omitted in error) | | | |
| EVALUATOR: NOTE TIME COMPLETED _____ | | | |
| Completed within specified time | | 15 | |
| Meets mailable standard | | 15 | |

ADD POINTS OF STEPS CHECKED                                            _____ EARNED
TOTAL POINTS POSSIBLE                                                      170 POSSIBLE

Points assigned reflect importance of step to meeting objective:  Important = (5)   Essential = (10)   Critical = (15)
Automatic failure results if any of the critical steps are omitted or performed incorrectly.

DETERMINE SCORE (divide points earned by total points possible, multiply results by 100)        _____ SCORE*

Evaluator's Name (print) _____ Signature _____

Comments _____

Name _____

Date _____ Score* _____

## PROCEDURE 6-8   Total Charges on Calculator

*PERFORMANCE OBJECTIVE*—Provided with necessary equipment and materials, calculate a list of 20 charges, performing any necessary mathematical functions, and correctly determine the total amount. The same correct answer must be obtained twice within a maximum of three attempts.

| PROCEDURE STEPS | STEP PERFORMED | POINTS POSSIBLE | COMMENTS |
|---|---|---|---|
| *EVALUATOR:* Place check mark in space following each step performed satisfactorily | | | |
| NOTE TIME BEGAN _____ | | | |
| 1. Turned on calculator. | _____ | 5 | |
| 2. Cleared machine. | _____ | 15 | |
| 3. Accurately entered figures from list. | _____ | 15 | |
| 4. Totaled fees. | _____ | 10 | |
| 5. Refigured to see if the same answer was obtained twice. | _____ | 15 | |
| 6. Recorded correct total. _____ | _____ | 15 | |
| *EVALUATOR:* NOTE TIME COMPLETED _____ | | | |

ADD POINTS OF STEPS CHECKED                                                    _____ EARNED
TOTAL POINTS POSSIBLE                                                              75 POSSIBLE

Points assigned reflect importance of step to meeting objective: Important = (5)   Essential = (10)   Critical = (15)
Automatic failure results if any of the critical steps are omitted or performed incorrectly.

DETERMINE SCORE (divide points earned by total points possible, multiply results by 100)        _____ SCORE*

Evaluator's Name (print) _____ Signature _____

Comments _____

Name _____

Date _____ Score* _____

## PROCEDURE 6-9   Operate Copy Machine

*PERFORMANCE OBJECTIVE*—Given access to necessary equipment and supplies, demonstrate adjustment of settings in order to produce the specified copy or copies, while operating the copy machine accurately following the steps in the procedure.

| PROCEDURE STEPS | STEP PERFORMED | POINTS POSSIBLE | COMMENTS |
|---|---|---|---|
| *EVALUATOR:* Place check mark in space following each step performed satisfactorily | | | |
| NOTE TIME BEGAN _____ | | | |
| 1. Assembled material to be copied. | _____ | 10 | |
| 2. Determined number of copies needed. | _____ | 10 | |
| 3. Turned on copy machine. | _____ | 5 | |
| 4. Adjusted settings to produce desired copy. | | | |
| a. Paper size | _____ | 15 | |
| b. One/two sided | _____ | 15 | |
| c. Regular/reduced/enlarged size | _____ | 15 | |
| d. Number of copies | _____ | 15 | |
| 5. Checked paper supply. | _____ | 15 | |
| 6. Raised lid and placed material to be copied, one sheet at a time, face down on glass, or in feeder. | _____ | 10 | |
| 7. Closed lid, if appropriate. | _____ | — | |
| 8. Pressed button or key pad to activate copier. | _____ | 5 | |
| 9. Removed original(s) and copy/copies. | _____ | 10 | |
| 10. Removed special paper, if used, from supply. | _____ | 10 | |
| 11. Returned machine to "standard" settings if changed. | _____ | 5 | |
| 12. Turned off machine (if policy). | _____ | 5 | |

*EVALUATOR:* NOTE TIME COMPLETED _____

ADD POINTS OF STEPS CHECKED                                   _____ EARNED

TOTAL POINTS POSSIBLE                                               145 POSSIBLE

Points assigned reflect importance of step to meeting objective: Important = (5)   Essential = (10)   Critical = (15)

Automatic failure results if any of the critical steps are omitted or performed incorrectly.

DETERMINE SCORE (divide points earned by total points possible, multiply results by 100)          _____ SCORE*

Evaluator's Name (print) _____   Signature _____

Comments _____

Name _____

Date _____ Score* _____

## PROCEDURE 6-10   Operate Transcriber

*PERFORMANCE OBJECTIVE*—Given access to equipment and supplies, operate the transcriber, correctly following all steps in the procedure. Complete an accurate transcription within a specified time period.

| PROCEDURE STEPS | STEP PERFORMED | POINTS POSSIBLE | COMMENTS |
|---|---|---|---|
| *EVALUATOR:* Place check mark in space following each step performed satisfactorily | | | |
| NOTE TIME BEGAN _____ | | | |
| 1. Turned on the transcriber. | _____ | 5 | |
| 2. Attached headset with earphones and the foot control to the unit. | _____ | 10 | |
| 3. Selected tape; chose rush reports or oldest dictation first. | _____ | 10 | |
| 4. Adjusted headset with earphones. | _____ | 5 | |
| 5. Inserted tape. Pressed play tab or the pedal to listen for the beginning of the dictation. | _____ | 10 | |
| 6. Adjusted volume, tone, and speed controls for clearest communication reception. | _____ | 10 | |
| 7. Listened for physician's instructions. | _____ | 15 | |
| 8. Set word processor or computer margins and tabulator stops. | _____ | 10 | |
| 9. Selected appropriate paper for transcription. | _____ | 10 | |
| 10. Brought up blank screen on computer. | _____ | 5 | |
| 11. Alternately pressed and released foot pedal to listen and transcribe the recorded message. | _____ | 10 | |
| 12. Turned off the machine and placed accessory items in proper storage space. | _____ | 5 | |
| 13. Completed transcript is accurate copy of recorded message, on appropriate paper, within specified time period. | _____ | 15 | |
| *EVALUATOR:* NOTE TIME COMPLETED _____ | | | |

ADD POINTS OF STEPS CHECKED                                              _____ EARNED
TOTAL POINTS POSSIBLE                                                    120 POSSIBLE

Points assigned reflect importance of step to meeting objective: Important = (5)   Essential = (10)   Critical = (15)
Automatic failure results if any of the critical steps are omitted or performed incorrectly.

DETERMINE SCORE (divide points earned by total points possible, multiply results by 100)   _____ SCORE*

Evaluator's Name (print) _____ Signature _____

Comments _____

# PERFORMANCE EVALUATION CHECKLIST

Name _____

Date _____ Score* _____

## PROCEDURE 6-11    Operate Office Computer

*PERFORMANCE OBJECTIVE*—Given access to equipment and material to be entered, operate system following steps in the procedure to produce an accurate print copy of a schedule.

| PROCEDURE STEPS | STEP PERFORMED | POINTS POSSIBLE | COMMENTS |
|---|---|---|---|
| *EVALUATOR:* Place check mark in space following each step performed satisfactorily | | | |
| NOTE TIME BEGAN _____ | | | |
| 1. Turned on power to computer. | _____ | 5 | |
| 2. Positioned cursor on appropriate program on main menu, keyed "ENTER" or clicked mouse. | _____ | 5 | |
| 3. Positioned cursor on scheduling software program, keyed "ENTER" or clicked mouse. | _____ | 5 | |
| 4. Positioned cursor or clicked on first cell to be completed. | _____ | 5 | |
| 5. Entered 1:00 P.M. appointment for first patient on list. | _____ | 10 | |
| 6. Entered remaining names at 15-minute intervals. | _____ | 15 | |
| 7. Saved data. | _____ | 15 | |
| 8. Exited scheduling program to main menu. | _____ | 10 | |
| 9. Exited from main menu. | _____ | 10 | |
| 10. Re-entered main menu. | _____ | 10 | |
| 11. Brought up scheduling software. | _____ | 10 | |
| 12. Located cursor at 2:30, entered patient as work-in who was currently scheduled for 1:30. | _____ | 10 | |
| 13. Located cursor at 1:30, canceled appointment. | _____ | 5 | |
| 14. Scrolled through schedule to view and proofread. | _____ | 10 | |
| 15. Turned on printer. | _____ | 5 | |
| 16. Allowed time for test sheet. (If appropriate; subtract 10 points if omitted) | _____ | — | |
| 17. Checked paper supply. | _____ | 5 | |
| 18. Keyed or clicked on print. | _____ | 10 | |
| 19. Selected from options. | _____ | 10 | |
| 20. Printed document. | _____ | 15 | |
| 21. Exited program. | _____ | 10 | |

## PROCEDURE 6-11   Operate Office Computer—continued

| PROCEDURE STEPS | STEP PERFORMED | POINTS POSSIBLE | COMMENTS |
|---|---|---|---|
| 22. Exited main menu. | _____ | 10 | |
| 23. Turned off power to printer. | _____ | 5 | |
| 24. Turned off power to computer. | _____ | 5 | |
| *EVALUATOR:* NOTE TIME COMPLETED _____ | | | |

ADD POINTS OF STEPS CHECKED                                              _____ EARNED
TOTAL POINTS POSSIBLE                                                    200 POSSIBLE

Points assigned reflect importance of step to meeting objective: Important = (5)   Essential = (10)   Critical = (15)
Automatic failure results if any of the critical steps are omitted or performed incorrectly.

DETERMINE SCORE (divide points earned by total points possible, multiply results by 100)      _____ SCORE*

Evaluator's Name (print) _____ Signature _____

Comments _____

Name _____

Date _____ Score* _____

## PROCEDURE 7-1  File Item(s) Alphabetically

*PERFORMANCE OBJECTIVE*—In a simulated situation, given the patient's file or other items, accurately file and store the file(s) and/or other items within acceptable time limit according to acceptable medical standards.

| PROCEDURE STEPS | STEP PERFORMED | POINTS POSSIBLE | COMMENTS |
|---|---|---|---|
| *EVALUATOR:* Place check mark in space following each step performed satisfactorily | | | |
| NOTE TIME BEGAN _____ | | | |
| 1. Used rules for filing items alphabetically. | _____ | 10 | |
|    a. Double-checked spelling of name for accuracy when using cross-reference file | _____ | 15 | |
| 2. Determined appropriate storage file. | _____ | 10 | |
| 3. For new material, scanned guides for area nearest to letters of name(s) on items to file. | _____ | 10 | |
| 4. Placed folder in correct alphabetical order between two files. | _____ | 15 | |
|    a. Inserted new file *between* two other folders and *not* within another folder, where it could be lost | _____ | 15 | |
| 5. In filing material previously in file, scanned for the OUTguide. | | | |
|    a. Removed OUTguide after removing file | _____ | 5 | |
|    b. Checked to be sure it was marking the space for the file just returned and not another | _____ | 5 | |
| *EVALUATOR:* NOTE TIME COMPLETED _____ | | | |

ADD POINTS OF STEPS CHECKED                  _____ EARNED

TOTAL POINTS POSSIBLE                                    85 POSSIBLE

Points assigned reflect importance of step to meeting objective: Important = (5)   Essential = (10)   Critical = (15)

Automatic failure results if any of the critical steps are omitted or performed incorrectly.

DETERMINE SCORE (divide points earned by total points possible, multiply results by 100)        _____ SCORE*

Evaluator's Name (print) _____ Signature _____

Comments _____

## PROCEDURE 7-2   Pull File Folder from Alphabetic Files

*PERFORMANCE OBJECTIVE*—In a simulated situation, given the patient's name, accurately prepare the OUTguide and pull the file, replacing the file with the OUTguide within acceptable time limit according to accepted medical standards.

| PROCEDURE STEPS | STEP PERFORMED | POINTS POSSIBLE | COMMENTS |
|---|---|---|---|
| *EVALUATOR:* Place check mark in space following each step performed satisfactorily | | | |
| NOTE TIME BEGAN _____ | | | |
| 1. Found name of patient in alphabetic file. | _____ | 15 | |
| a. Double-checked the spelling of the name for accuracy | _____ | 15 | |
| 2. Completed OUTguide with date and name. | _____ | 5 | |
| 3. Pulled file(s) needed and replaced with OUTguide(s). | _____ | 5 | |
| *EVALUATOR:* NOTE TIME COMPLETED _____ | | | |

ADD POINTS OF STEPS CHECKED                                                _____ EARNED
TOTAL POINTS POSSIBLE                                                        40  POSSIBLE

Points assigned reflect importance of step to meeting objective: Important = (5)   Essential = (10)   Critical = (15)
Automatic failure results if any of the critical steps are omitted or performed incorrectly.

DETERMINE SCORE (divide points earned by total points possible, multiply results by 100)        _____ SCORE*

Evaluator's Name (print) _____ Signature _____

Comments _____

# PERFORMANCE EVALUATION CHECKLIST

Name _____

Date _____ Score* _____

## PROCEDURE 7-3   File Item(s) Numerically

*PERFORMANCE OBJECTIVE*—In a simulated situation, given the patient's file or other items, accurately file and store the file(s) and/or other items within acceptable time limit according to accepted medical standards.

| PROCEDURE STEPS | STEP PERFORMED | POINTS POSSIBLE | COMMENTS |
|---|---|---|---|
| *EVALUATOR:* Place check mark in space following each step performed satisfactorily | | | |
| NOTE TIME BEGAN _____ | | | |
| 1. Used rules for numerical filing. | _____ | 15 | |
|    a. Double-checked spelling of name for accuracy using cross-reference file | _____ | 15 | |
| 2. Determined appropriate storage file. | _____ | 5 | |
| 3. Matched the first two or three numbers with those already in the file. | _____ | 15 | |
| 4. Matched remaining numbers with those in the file. | _____ | 15 | |

*EVALUATOR:* NOTE TIME COMPLETED _____

ADD POINTS OF STEPS CHECKED          _____ EARNED
TOTAL POINTS POSSIBLE          35 POSSIBLE

Points assigned reflect importance of step to meeting objective: Important = (5)   Essential = (10)   Critical = (15)
Automatic failure results if any of the critical steps are omitted or performed incorrectly.

DETERMINE SCORE (divide points earned by total points possible, multiply results by 100)   _____ SCORE*

Evaluator's Name (print) _____ Signature _____

Comments _____

413

## PROCEDURE 7-4   Pull File Folder from Numeric Files

*PERFORMANCE OBJECTIVE*—In a simulated situation, given the patient's name or account number, accurately prepare the OUTguide and pull the file, replacing the file with the OUTguide within acceptable time limit according to accepted medical standards.

| PROCEDURE STEPS | STEP PERFORMED | POINTS POSSIBLE | COMMENTS |
|---|---|---|---|
| *EVALUATOR:* Place check mark in space following each step performed satisfactorily | | | |
| NOTE TIME BEGAN _____ | | | |
| 1. Found name of patient in card file and obtained account number. | _____ | 10 | |
|    a. Double-checked the spelling of name for accuracy | _____ | 10 | |
| 2. Completed OUTguide with date and name. | _____ | 5 | |
| 3. Located corresponding section of numeric file. | _____ | 10 | |
| 4. Scanned the files for the number. | _____ | 15 | |
| 5. Pulled requested file and replaced with prepared OUTguide. | _____ | 15 | |
| *EVALUATOR:* NOTE TIME COMPLETED _____ | | | |

ADD POINTS OF STEPS CHECKED                                           _____ EARNED

TOTAL POINTS POSSIBLE                                                   65 POSSIBLE

Points assigned reflect importance of step to meeting objective: Important = (5)   Essential = (10)   Critical = (15)
Automatic failure results if any of the critical steps are omitted or performed incorrectly.

DETERMINE SCORE (divide points earned by total points possible, multiply results by 100)      _____ SCORE*

Evaluator's Name (print) _____ Signature _____

Comments _____

Name _____

Date _____ Score* _____

## PROCEDURE 8-1   Prepare Patient Ledger Card

*PERFORMANCE OBJECTIVE*—In a simulated medical office situation, prepare a patient ledger card following the steps in the procedure.

| PROCEDURE STEPS | STEP PERFORMED | POINTS POSSIBLE | COMMENTS |
|---|---|---|---|
| *EVALUATOR:* Place check mark in space following each step performed satisfactorily | | | |
| NOTE TIME BEGAN _____ | | | |
| 1. Typed the name of patient, last name first. | _____ | 15 | |
| 2. Typed complete address with zip code. | _____ | 10 | |
| 3. Typed name and address of person responsible for charges if different from patient. | _____ | 5 | |
| 4. Typed telephone number of patient. | _____ | 10 | |
| 5. Typed name of insurance company. | _____ | 15 | |
| 6. Typed referring individual. | _____ | 5 | |
| 7. Typed balance due amount. | _____ | 10 | |
| *EVALUATOR:* NOTE TIME COMPLETED _____ | | | |

ADD POINTS OF STEPS CHECKED                                          _____ EARNED
TOTAL POINTS POSSIBLE                                                        70 POSSIBLE

Points assigned reflect importance of step to meeting objective: Important = (5)   Essential = (10)   Critical = (15)
Automatic failure results if any of the critical steps are omitted or performed incorrectly.

DETERMINE SCORE (divide points earned by total points possible, multiply results by 100)          _____ SCORE*

Evaluator's Name (print) _____ Signature _____

Comments _____

# PERFORMANCE EVALUATION CHECKLIST

Name _____

Date _____ Score* _____

## PROCEDURE 8-2   Record Charges and Credits

*PERFORMANCE OBJECTIVE*—In a simulated medical office situation, record charges and credits following the steps in the procedure.

| PROCEDURE STEPS | STEP PERFORMED | POINTS POSSIBLE | COMMENTS |
|---|---|---|---|
| *EVALUATOR:* Place check mark in space following each step performed satisfactorily | | | |
| NOTE TIME BEGAN _____ | | | |
| 1. Pulled patients' ledger cards. | _____ | 10 | |
| 2. Posted charges and credits on ledger cards. | _____ | 15 | |
|    a. Used small, neat figures | _____ | 5 | |
| 3. Checked each off on day sheet | _____ | 5 | |
| 4. Posted charges in debit column | _____ | 15 | |
|    a. Added balance and new debit for new balance | _____ | 10 | |
| 5. Posted payments in credit column | _____ | 15 | |
|    a. Subtracted payments from balance due | _____ | 10 | |
|    b. Showed credits in red | _____ | 5 | |
| *EVALUATOR:* NOTE TIME COMPLETED _____ | | | |

ADD POINTS OF STEPS CHECKED                               _____ EARNED

TOTAL POINTS POSSIBLE                                                     90 POSSIBLE

Points assigned reflect importance of step to meeting objective: Important = (5)   Essential = (10)   Critical = (15)
Automatic failure results if any of the critical steps are omitted or performed incorrectly.

DETERMINE SCORE (divide points earned by total points possible, multiply results by 100)     _____ SCORE*

Evaluator's Name (print) _____ Signature _____

Comments _____

Name _____

Date _____ Score* _____

## PROCEDURE 8-3    Generate Itemized Statement

*PERFORMANCE OBJECTIVE*—In a simulated medical office situation, type itemized statement(s) with 100 percent accuracy following the steps in the procedure.

| PROCEDURE STEPS | STEP PERFORMED | POINTS POSSIBLE | COMMENTS |
|---|---|---|---|
| *EVALUATOR:* Place check mark in space following each step performed satisfactorily | | | |
| NOTE TIME BEGAN _____ | | | |
| 1. Stacked ledger cards beside typewriter. | _____ | 5 | |
| 2. Assembled statement forms and window envelopes. | _____ | 5 | |
| 3. Stamped ledger card on line below last entry with date stamp. | _____ | 5 | |
| 4. Typed name and complete address in area that shows in window of envelope. | _____ | 15 | |
| 5. Listed balance first under services. | _____ | 10 | |
| 6. Typed each service charge and payment for current month. | _____ | 15 | |
| 7. Folded and placed form in envelope | _____ | 5 | |
| a. Address shown in window | _____ | 15 | |
| b. Only one form in envelope | _____ | 15 | |
| 8. Fanned and exposed several envelope flaps. | _____ | 5 | |
| 9. Dampened flaps sufficiently. | _____ | 5 | |
| 10. Folded flaps of envelopes down to seal. | _____ | 10 | |
| *EVALUATOR:* NOTE TIME COMPLETED _____ | | | |

ADD POINTS OF STEPS CHECKED                                                          _____ EARNED
TOTAL POINTS POSSIBLE                                                                            110 POSSIBLE

Points assigned reflect importance of step to meeting objective:  Important  = (5)   Essential = (10)   Critical = (15)
Automatic failure results if any of the critical steps are omitted or performed incorrectly.

DETERMINE SCORE (divide points earned by total points possible, multiply results by 100)        _____ SCORE*

Evaluator's Name (print) _____ Signature _____

Comments _____

## PROCEDURE 8-4   Compose Collection Letter

*PERFORMANCE OBJECTIVE*—In a simulated medical office situation, compose and type appropriate collection letters for assigned accounts to be collected following the procedure.

| PROCEDURE STEPS | STEP PERFORMED | POINTS POSSIBLE | COMMENTS |
|---|---|---|---|
| *EVALUATOR:* Place check mark in space following each step performed satisfactorily | | | |
| NOTE TIME BEGAN _____ | | | |
| 1. Identified patients to whom an initial collection letter should be sent. | _____ | 10 | |
| 2. Composed a rough draft | _____ | 10 | |
|   a. First paragraph stated reason for letter | _____ | 10 | |
| 3. Second paragraph indicated expected response. | _____ | 10 | |
| 4. Reread rough draft | _____ | 5 | |
|   a. Had clear message | _____ | 10 | |
|   b. Contained correctly spelled words | _____ | 5 | |
|   c. Had correct punctuation | _____ | 5 | |
| 5. Typed letter according to standard form. | _____ | 5 | |
|   a. Proofread letter | _____ | 10 | |
|   b. Signed letter | _____ | 10 | |
| 6. Typed envelope. | _____ | 5 | |
| 7. Folded letter properly. | _____ | 5 | |
|   a. Sealed envelope | _____ | 5 | |
|   b. Stamped and mailed letter | _____ | 10 | |
| *EVALUATOR:* NOTE TIME COMPLETED _____ | | | |

ADD POINTS OF STEPS CHECKED _____ EARNED

TOTAL POINTS POSSIBLE 115 POSSIBLE

Points assigned reflect importance of step to meeting objective: Important = (5)   Essential = (10)   Critical = (15)
Automatic failure results if any of the critical steps are omitted or performed incorrectly.

DETERMINE SCORE (divide points earned by total points possible, multiply results by 100) _____ SCORE*

Evaluator's Name (print) _____ Signature _____

Comments _____

## PROCEDURE 9-1   Complete a Claim Form

*PERFORMANCE OBJECTIVE*—Given access to all necessary equipment and information, follow the procedure to complete the HCFA-approved claim form without error within the instructor's prescribed time limit.

| PROCEDURE STEPS | STEP PERFORMED | POINTS POSSIBLE | COMMENTS |
|---|---|---|---|
| *EVALUATOR:* Place check mark in space following each step performed satisfactorily | | | |
| NOTE TIME BEGAN _____ | | | |
| 1. Checked for a photocopy of the patient's insurance card. | _____ | 10 | |
| 2. Checked the chart to see if the patient signature was on file for release of information and assignment of benefits. | _____ | 15 | |
| 3. Explained procedure to obtain signature when not on file. | _____ | 10 | |
| 4. Using Figure 9–6 as an example, completed the HCFA claim form. | | | |
|   a. Checked appropriate box at top of form | _____ | 5 | |
|   b. Entered name of patient | _____ | 10 | |
|   c. Entered birthdate using digits | _____ | 10 | |
|   d. Checked box for male or female | | | |
| 5. Entered insured's name. | _____ | 5 | |
| 6. Entered patient's full address and telephone number. | _____ | 5 | |
| 7. Entered patient's relationship to insured. | _____ | 5 | |
| 8. Entered insured's full address and telephone number. | _____ | 5 | |
| 9. Entered patient's status. | _____ | 5 | |
| 10. Entered other insured's name, if applicable. | _____ | — | |
|   a. Other insured's policy or group number | _____ | — | |
|   b. Other insured's birthdate and box for male or female | _____ | — | |
|   c. Employer's name or school name | _____ | — | |
|   d. Insurance plan name or program name | _____ | — | |
| 11. Checked appropriate box regarding employment and/or accident. | _____ | 5 | |
| 12. Entered insured's policy number | | | |
|   a. Insured's birthdate and box for male or female | _____ | 5 | |
|   b. Employer or school name | _____ | 5 | |
|   c. Insurance plan name or program name | _____ | 5 | |
|   d. Was there another health benefit plan? | _____ | 5 | |
| 13. Obtained signature or indicated "on file." | _____ | 15 | |

## PROCEDURE 9-1 Complete a Claim Form—continued

| PROCEDURE STEPS | STEP PERFORMED | POINTS POSSIBLE | COMMENTS |
|---|---|---|---|
| 14. Obtained insured's or authorized signature. | _____ | 10 | |
| 15. Entered current illness date, accident, or pregnancy. | _____ | 10 | |
| 16. Entered date patient first treated for same or similar illness. | _____ | 5 | |
| 17. Entered dates unable to work or stated N/A. | _____ | — | |
| 18. Entered referring physician or other. | _____ | 5 | |
|    a. Physician's ID number | _____ | 5 | |
| 19. Entered hospital dates or stated N/A. | _____ | — | |
| 20. Left blank. | _____ | — | |
| 21. Completed outside lab as appropriate. | _____ | — | |
| 22. Entered ICN codes. | _____ | 15 | |
| 23. Completed Medicaid resubmission if applicable. | _____ | — | |
| 24. Entered prior authorization number. | _____ | — | |
| 25. Completed Section 24 A–E with dates, appropriate codes, and charges for services. | _____ | 15 | |
| 26. Entered physician's Social Security number or practice tax identification number. | _____ | 10 | |
| 27. Entered patient's account number if applicable. | _____ | — | |
| 28. Checked appropriate box for assignment. | _____ | 10 | |
| 29. Totaled charges. | _____ | 15 | |
| 30. Entered amount paid. | _____ | 15 | |
| 31. Entered balance due. | _____ | 15 | |
| 32. Obtained physician's signature and date. | _____ | 15 | |
| 33. Completed name and address where services given. | _____ | 5 | |
| 34. Completed physician's information. | _____ | 5 | |
| 35. Completed within time specified. | _____ | 15 | |

*EVALUATOR:* NOTE TIME COMPLETED _____

Note: Subtract 10 points each for steps 9, 16, 18, 19, 20, 23, and 26 if applicable and not entered.

ADD POINTS OF STEPS CHECKED                _____ EARNED
TOTAL POINTS POSSIBLE                295 POSSIBLE

Points assigned reflect importance of step to meeting objective: Important = (5)   Essential = (10)   Critical = (15)
Automatic failure results if any of the critical steps are omitted or performed incorrectly.

DETERMINE SCORE (divide points earned by total points possible, multiply results by 100)     _____ SCORE*

Evaluator's Name (print) _____ Signature _____

Comments _____

Name _____

Date _____ Score* _____

## PROCEDURE 10-1    Prepare a Check

*PERFORMANCE OBJECTIVE*—Prepare a check following the steps of the procedure. The check must be dated, accurately identify the payer, have the correct numeric and written amount, and have appropriate signature. The register must accurately reflect the check.

| PROCEDURE STEPS | STEP PERFORMED | POINTS POSSIBLE | COMMENTS |
|---|---|---|---|
| *EVALUATOR:* Place check mark in space following each step performed satisfactorily | | | |
| NOTE TIME BEGAN _____ | | | |
| 1. Filled out check register using black or blue ink. | | | |
|    a. Check number | _____ | 5 | |
|    b. Date | _____ | 10 | |
|    c. Payee information | _____ | 10 | |
|    d. Amount | _____ | 15 | |
|    e. Previous balance | _____ | 10 | |
|    f. Entered new balance | _____ | 10 | |
| 2. Entered date on check. | _____ | 5 | |
| 3. Entered payee. | _____ | 15 | |
| 4. Entered numerically the amount of check. | _____ | 10 | |
| 5. Wrote out amount of check. | | | |
|    a. Began as far left as possible | _____ | 10 | |
|    b. Wrote out amount correctly | _____ | 15 | |
|    c. Made straight line to fill space | _____ | 10 | |
| 6. Obtained signature; must agree with authorization card. | _____ | 15 | |
| *EVALUATOR:* NOTE TIME COMPLETED _____ | | | |

ADD POINTS OF STEPS CHECKED                                                      _____ EARNED
TOTAL POINTS POSSIBLE                                                                      140 POSSIBLE

Points assigned reflect importance of step to meeting objective:  Important = (5)   Essential = (10)   Critical = (15)
Automatic failure results if any of the critical steps are omitted or performed incorrectly.

DETERMINE SCORE (divide points earned by total points possible, multiply results by 100)        _____ SCORE*

Evaluator's Name (print) _____ Signature _____

Comments _____

**PERFORMANCE EVALUATION CHECKLIST**

Name _____

Date _____ Score* _____

## PROCEDURE 10-2   Prepare a Deposit Slip

*PERFORMANCE OBJECTIVE*—Prepare a bank deposit slip following the steps in the procedure. The slip will correctly reflect the currency, coin, and checks to be deposited, and be totaled accurately.

| PROCEDURE STEPS | STEP PERFORMED | POINTS POSSIBLE | COMMENTS |
|---|---|---|---|
| *EVALUATOR:* Place check mark in space following each step performed satisfactorily | | | |
| NOTE TIME BEGAN _____ | | | |
| 1. Separated money to be deposited, by check, currency, and coin. | _____ | 5 | |
| 2. Listed currency. | | | |
|    a. Sorted bills by denomination | _____ | 5 | |
|    b. Portrait side up | _____ | 5 | |
|    c. Highest denomination to lowest | _____ | 5 | |
|    d. Totaled currency accurately | _____ | 15 | |
|    e. Recorded accurately on deposit slip | _____ | 10 | |
| 3. Listed coin. | | | |
|    a. Sorted by denomination | _____ | 5 | |
|    b. Totaled coin accurately | _____ | 15 | |
|    c. Recorded accurately on deposit slip | _____ | 10 | |
| 4. Listed checks. | | | |
|    a. Checked for endorsement | _____ | 10 | |
|    b. Listed by number, maker, amount | _____ | 5 | |
|    c. Listed from largest to smallest amount | _____ | 5 | |
|    d. Listed money orders with MO and name | _____ | 5 | |
|    e. Accurately totaled and entered on slip | _____ | 15 | |
| 5. Accurately totaled currency, coin, and checks to be deposited. | _____ | 15 | |
| 6. Made copy of deposit slip for files. | _____ | 5 | |
| 7. Entered deposit total in checkbook. | _____ | 10 | |
| 8. Made deposit at bank and kept record for files. | _____ | 10 | |
| *EVALUATOR:* NOTE TIME COMPLETED _____ | | | |

ADD POINTS OF STEPS CHECKED                                                 _____ EARNED

TOTAL POINTS POSSIBLE                                                  155 POSSIBLE

Points assigned reflect importance of step to meeting objective: Important = (5)  Essential = (10)  Critical = (15)

Automatic failure results if any of the critical steps are omitted or performed incorrectly.

DETERMINE SCORE (divide points earned by total points possible, multiply results by 100)     _____ SCORE*

Evaluator's Name (print) _____ Signature _____

Comments _____

# PERFORMANCE EVALUATION CHECKLIST

Name _____

Date _____ Score* _____

## PROCEDURE 10-3    Reconcile a Bank Statement

*PERFORMANCE OBJECTIVE*—Follow the steps in the procedure "Reconcile a Bank Statement;" after performing mathematical calculations, the checkbook and bank statement balance should agree.

| PROCEDURE STEPS | STEP PERFORMED | POINTS POSSIBLE | COMMENTS |
|---|---|---|---|
| *EVALUATOR:* Place check mark in space following each step performed satisfactorily | | | |
| NOTE TIME BEGAN _____ | | | |
| 1. Compared the opening balance on the new statement with the closing balance on the previous statement. | _____ | 10 | |
| 2. Listed the bank balance in the appropriate space on the reconciliation worksheet. | _____ | 5 | |
| 3. Compared the check entries on the statement with the returned checks. | _____ | 10 | |
| 4. Determined if any outstanding checks. | | | |
|    a. Marked stub or entry on register if check returned | _____ | 5 | |
|    b. Listed ones not checked on worksheet | _____ | 15 | |
|    c. Totaled outstanding checks | _____ | 10 | |
| 5. Subtracted from checkbook balance items such as withdrawals, automatic payments or service charges that appeared on the statement but not in the checkbook. | _____ | 15 | |
| 6. Added to checkbook any interest earned as indicated on statement. | _____ | 15 | |
| 7. Added to the bank statement balance any deposits not shown on the bank statement. | _____ | 15 | |
| 8. The balance in the checkbook and the bank statement agreed. | _____ | 15 | |
| *EVALUATOR:* NOTE TIME COMPLETED _____ | | | |

ADD POINTS OF STEPS CHECKED _____ EARNED

TOTAL POINTS POSSIBLE 115 POSSIBLE

Points assigned reflect importance of step to meeting objective: Important = (5)   Essential = (10)   Critical = (15)
Automatic failure results if any of the critical steps are omitted or performed incorrectly.

DETERMINE SCORE (divide points earned by total points possible, multiply results by 100) _____ SCORE*

Evaluator's Name (print) _____ Signature _____

Comments _____

# PERFORMANCE EVALUATION CHECKLIST

Name _____

Date _____ Score* _____

## PROCEDURE 12-1   Handwashing

*PERFORMANCE OBJECTIVE*—Provided with liquid hand soap in a dispenser, cuticle stick, nail brush, paper towels, and a waste receptacle, the student will stand at a sink with hot and cold faucets and demonstrate each step in the handwashing procedure as specified in the procedure sheet.

| PROCEDURE STEPS | STEP PERFORMED | POINTS POSSIBLE | COMMENTS |
|---|---|---|---|
| *EVALUATOR:* Place check mark in space following each step performed satisfactorily | | | |
| NOTE TIME BEGAN _____ | | | |
| 1.  Removed jewelry. | _____ | 5 | |
| 2.  a.  Stood, not touching sink | _____ | 10 | |
|     b.  Used paper towel to turn on faucets | _____ | 5 | |
|     c.  Adjusted water temperature | _____ | 5 | |
|     d.  Discarded paper towel | _____ | 5 | |
| 3.  a.  Wet hands | _____ | 10 | |
|     b.  Dispensed 1 tsp soap into palm | _____ | 10 | |
|     c.  Distributed soap into lather on both hands | _____ | 15 | |
|     d.  Washed, in circular motion, for two minutes | _____ | 15 | |
| 4.  a.  Used nail brush/1 dozen circular motions | _____ | 5 | |
|     b.  Used cuticle stick under nails | _____ | 5 | |
| 5.  a.  Rinsed thoroughly | _____ | 10 | |
|     b.  Wet arms to elbow | _____ | 5 | |
|     c.  Re-applied soap (1 tsp) to palm | _____ | 5 | |
|     d.  Did not touch inside of sink or faucets | _____ | 10 | |
|     e.  Used brush in one dozen circular motions to elbow | _____ | 5 | |
|     f.  Rinsed thoroughly | _____ | 5 | |
| 6  a.  Let water continue to run | _____ | 5 | |
|     b.  Got paper towels | _____ | 5 | |
|     c.  Dried hands and arms to elbow | _____ | 5 | |
|     d.  Turned water off with paper towel | _____ | 5 | |
|     e.  Discarded paper towel in proper receptacle | | | |
| *EVALUATOR:* NOTE TIME COMPLETED _____ | | | |

ADD POINTS OF STEPS CHECKED                     _____ EARNED

TOTAL POINTS POSSIBLE                                155 POSSIBLE

Points assigned reflect importance of step to meeting objective:  Important = (5)   Essential = (10)   Critical = (15)

Automatic failure results if any of the critical steps are omitted or performed incorrectly.

DETERMINE SCORE (divide points earned by total points possible, multiply results by 100)    _____ SCORE*

Evaluator's Name (print) _____ Signature _____

Comments _____

# PERFORMANCE EVALUATION CHECKLIST

Name _____

Date _____ Score* _____

## PROCEDURE 12-2  Wrap Items for Autoclave

*PERFORMANCE OBJECTIVE*—Provided with several items to be autoclaved or sterilized, the student will wrap each in autoclave paper in preparation for the sterilization process. Each item must be wrapped neatly and snugly but not too tightly. After the paper wrapping procedure is demonstrated and checked, the paper should be removed and discarded. This procedure should be performed with both paper and muslin wrap.

| PROCEDURE STEPS | STEP PERFORMED | POINTS POSSIBLE | COMMENTS |
|---|---|---|---|
| *EVALUATOR:* Place check mark in space following each step performed satisfactorily | | | |
| NOTE TIME BEGAN _____ | | | |
| Wrapping Items | | | |
| 1. Washed hands. | _____ | 10 | |
| a. Assembled all necessary items | _____ | 10 | |
| b. Worked in a clean area | _____ | 5 | |
| c. Allowed for sufficient work space | _____ | 5 | |
| 2. Checked items for flaws. | _____ | 15 | |
| a. Checked items for proper functioning | _____ | 15 | |
| b. Made sure items were sanitized before wrapping | _____ | 15 | |
| 3. Wrapped items in double thickness paper wrap. | _____ | 10 | |
| a. Made sure of no opening | _____ | 10 | |
| b. Sealed with autoclave tape | _____ | 5 | |
| c. Wrapped items snugly | _____ | 10 | |
| d. Did not wrap items too tight | _____ | 10 | |
| 4. Made tab with tape for ease in opening following sterilization. | _____ | 5 | |
| 5. Labeled contents. | _____ | 15 | |
| a. Wrote date on package | _____ | 10 | |
| b. Wrote your initials on package | _____ | 5 | _____ EARNED |
| 6. Returned all items to proper storage. | _____ | 5 | 160 POSSIBLE |
| Envelope Type | | | |
| Repeated steps 1–2 | _____ | 65 | |
| 3. Placed item in envelope and | _____ | 15 | |
| a. Sealed | _____ | 5 | |
| b. Labeled contents | _____ | 15 | |
| c. Dated label | _____ | 10 | |
| d. Initialed label | _____ | 5 | _____ EARNED |
| 4. Returned items to proper storage. | _____ | 5 | 120 POSSIBLE |

| PROCEDURE STEPS | STEP PERFORMED | POINTS POSSIBLE | COMMENTS |
|---|---|---|---|
| Spinal needle(s), small items | | | |
| Repeated steps 1–2. | _____ | 65 | |
| 3. Placed cotton/gauze in bottom of glass test tube. | _____ | 10 | |
| 4. Wrapped autoclave tape around top of test tube to seal. | _____ | 15 | |
| a. Made pull tab with tape | _____ | 5 | |
| 5. Labeled contents on piece of tape, secured to glass and | _____ | 15 | |
| a. Dated label | _____ | 15 | |
| b. Initialed | _____ | 5 | |
| 6. Returned items to storage. | _____ | 5 | |

EVALUATOR: NOTE TIME COMPLETED _____

_____ EARNED

135 POSSIBLE

ADD POINTS OF STEPS CHECKED
TOTAL POINTS POSSIBLE

Points assigned reflect importance of step to meeting objective: Important = (5) Essential = (10) Critical = (15)
Automatic failure results if any of the critical steps are omitted or performed incorrectly.

DETERMINE SCORE (divide points earned by total points possible, multiply results by 100) _____ SCORE*

Evaluator's Name (print) _____ Signature _____

Comments _____

## PROCEDURE 13-1   Interview Patient to Complete Medical History Form

*PERFORMANCE OBJECTIVE*—Using copies of the medical history forms included in the textbook and a blue or black pen, obtain and record a medical history from a patient within a set time specified by the instructor.

| PROCEDURE STEPS | STEP PERFORMED | POINTS POSSIBLE | COMMENTS |
|---|---|---|---|
| *EVALUATOR:* Place check mark in space following each step performed satisfactorily | | | |
| NOTE TIME BEGAN _____ | | | |
| 1. Assembled necessary items. | _____ | 15 | |
| 2. Courteously escorted patient to private area. | _____ | 5 | |
| 3. Sat opposite patient. | _____ | 5 | |
| 4. Explained procedure to patient and put them at ease. | _____ | 15 | |
| 5. Maintained eye contact with patient throughout procedure. | _____ | 10 | |
| 6. Asked questions clearly and distinctly. | _____ | 15 | |
| 7. Gave patient sufficient time to answer. | _____ | 10 | |
| 8. Recorded information neatly and accurately. | _____ | 15 | |
| 9. Avoided getting off subject. | _____ | 5 | |
| 10. Made necessary comments. | _____ | 5 | |
| 11. Highlighted in red ink when necessary (example: allergies). | _____ | 10 | |
| 12. Clearly stated patient's chief complaint. | _____ | 15 | |
| 13. Thanked patient for cooperation. | _____ | 5 | |
| 14. Explained next procedure to patient. | _____ | 5 | |
| 15. Made patient comfortable. | _____ | 5 | |
| 16. Placed patient's history form in chart. | _____ | 10 | |
| 17. Placed chart in appropriate area for physician. | _____ | 10 | |
| *EVALUATOR:* NOTE TIME COMPLETED _____ | | | |

ADD POINTS OF STEPS CHECKED                                                    _____ EARNED
TOTAL POINTS POSSIBLE                                                                  160 POSSIBLE

Points assigned reflect importance of step to meeting objective: Important = (5)   Essential = (10)   Critical = (15)
Automatic failure results if any of the critical steps are omitted or performed incorrectly.

DETERMINE SCORE (divide points earned by total points possible, multiply results by 100)     _____ SCORE*

Evaluator's Name (print) _____ Signature _____

Comments _____

Name _____

Date _____ Score* _____

## PROCEDURE 13-2   Measure Height

*PERFORMANCE OBJECTIVE*—Demonstrate each step of the height measurement procedure to determine the precise height of five
students who have been measured previously by the instructor. Measurements should be recorded and agree with instructor by
± ⅛ inch.

| PROCEDURE STEPS | STEP PERFORMED | POINTS POSSIBLE | COMMENTS |
|---|---|---|---|
| *EVALUATOR:* Place check mark in space following each step performed satisfactorily | | | |
| NOTE TIME BEGAN _____ | | | |
| 1. Raised measuring bar higher than patient. | _____ | 15 | |
| 2. Aware of patient's safety. | _____ | 10 | |
| 3. Asked patient to remove shoes. | _____ | 5 | |
| 4. Placed paper towel on platform. | _____ | 5 | |
| 5. Helped patient onto scale. | _____ | 10 | |
| 6. Moved measuring bar slowly and carefully to rest on top of patient's head. | _____ | 10 | |
| 7. Gently compressed hair. | _____ | 15 | |
| 8. Read measurement correctly. | _____ | 15 | |
| 9. Told patient the reading. | _____ | 5 | |
| 10. Helped patient down from scale. | _____ | 10 | |
| 11. Asked patient to put shoes back on. | _____ | 5 | |
| 12. Placed measuring extension bar back. | _____ | 5 | |
| 13. Discarded paper towel. | _____ | 5 | |
| 14. Recorded measurement accurately on patient's chart. | _____ | 15 | |
| *EVALUATOR:* NOTE TIME COMPLETED _____ | | | |

ADD POINTS OF STEPS CHECKED                                                              _____ EARNED

TOTAL POINTS POSSIBLE                                                                          130 POSSIBLE

Points assigned reflect importance of step to meeting objective: Important = (5)   Essential = (10)   Critical = (15)
Automatic failure results if any of the critical steps are omitted or performed incorrectly.

DETERMINE SCORE (divide points earned by total points possible, multiply results by 100)          _____ SCORE*

Evaluator's Name (print) _____ Signature _____

Comments _____

# DOCUMENTATION

Chart the procedure in the patient's medical record.

Date: _____

Charting: _____

_____

_____

_____

Student's Name: _____         Physician's Initials: _( ___ )_

## PROCEDURE 13-3   Weigh Patient on Upright Scale

*PERFORMANCE OBJECTIVE*—Demonstrate each step of the procedure of weighing a patient on an upright scale and record; weight measurement should agree with instructor's by ± ¼ lb.

| PROCEDURE STEPS | STEP PERFORMED | POINTS POSSIBLE | COMMENTS |
|---|---|---|---|
| *EVALUATOR:* Place check mark in space following each step performed satisfactorily | | | |
| NOTE TIME BEGAN _____ | | | |
| 1. Washed hands. | _____ | 5 | |
| 2. Balanced scales. | _____ | 15 | |
| 3. Asked patient to remove shoes. | _____ | 5 | |
| 4. Placed paper towel on scale. | _____ | 5 | |
| 5. Helped patient onto scale. | _____ | 5 | |
| 6. Asked patient to stand in center of platform. | _____ | 10 | |
| 7. Asked patient to stand still. | _____ | 10 | |
| 8. Adjusted balance. | _____ | 10 | |
| 9. Read weight accurately. | _____ | 15 | |
| 10. Told patient the reading. | _____ | 5 | |
| 11. Helped patient from scales. | _____ | 5 | |
| 12. Discarded paper towel. | _____ | 5 | |
| 13. Recorded weight accurately on patient's chart. | _____ | 15 | |
|    a. Noted what patient was wearing | _____ | 10 | |
| 14. Returned scales to balance at zero. | _____ | 5 | |

*EVALUATOR:* NOTE TIME COMPLETED _____

ADD POINTS OF STEPS CHECKED            _____ EARNED

TOTAL POINTS POSSIBLE                 125 POSSIBLE

Points assigned reflect importance of step to meeting objective: Important = (5)   Essential = (10)   Critical = (15)
Automatic failure results if any of the critical steps are omitted or performed incorrectly.

DETERMINE SCORE (divide points earned by total points possible, multiply results by 100)    _____ SCORE*

Evaluator's Name (print) _____ Signature _____

Comments _____

## DOCUMENTATION

Chart the procedure in the patient's medical record.

Date: _____

Charting: _____

_____

_____

_____

Student's Name: _____         Physician's Initials: __(_____)__

## PROCEDURE 13-4   Clean and Store Mercury Thermometers

*PERFORMANCE OBJECTIVE*—Given soiled mercury thermometers and access to all necessary equipment and supplies, clean, inspect, disinfect, and store the thermometers aseptically, in accordance with procedure technique and observing aseptic and safety precautions.

| PROCEDURE STEPS | STEP PERFORMED | POINTS POSSIBLE | COMMENTS |
|---|---|---|---|
| *EVALUATOR:* Place check mark in space following each step performed satisfactorily. Check to see if oral and rectal are separated. Subtract 15 pts if not. | | | |
| NOTE TIME BEGAN _____ | | | |
| 1. Washed hands, assembled equipment, and put on gloves. | _____ | 15 | |
| 2. Took soiled thermometers to sink. | _____ | — | |
| 3. Applied soap or other cleanser to cotton ball and added water to make solution. | _____ | 10 | |
| 4. While holding thermometer by stem, rotated and wiped it from stem to bulb with soapy solution. | _____ | 5 | |
| 5. Discarded cotton ball in biohazardous waste container. | _____ | 5 | |
| 6. While holding by stem with bulb pointed downward, rinsed thermometer in cool running water. | _____ | 5 | |
| 7. Inspected for cleanliness and condition, discarded damaged thermometer in a sharps biohazardous waste container. | _____ | 15 | |
| 8. Grasped stem firmly between thumb and index finger. | _____ | 5 | |
| 9. Shook mercury down to 95.0°F or below. | _____ | 15 | |
| 10. Placed thermometers in gauze-lined container filled with disinfectant. | _____ | 10 | |
| 11. Using correct procedure, removed and discarded gloves. | _____ | 10 | |
| 12. Washed hands. | _____ | 5 | |
| 13. Noted time or set timer for at least 20 minutes. | _____ | 15 | |
| 14. After allowing time for disinfection, washed hands. | _____ | 5 | |
| 15. Rinsed, inspected, and placed clean thermometers in individual envelopes, individual dry holders, or storage container. | _____ | 15 | |

| PROCEDURE STEPS | STEP PERFORMED | POINTS POSSIBLE | COMMENTS |
|---|---|---|---|
| 16. Cleaned area and equipment. Returned thermometers to appropriate locations. | _____ | 5 | |
| *EVALUATOR:* NOTE TIME COMPLETED _____ | | | |

ADD POINTS OF STEPS CHECKED                                    _____ EARNED
TOTAL POINTS POSSIBLE                                                      140 POSSIBLE

Points assigned reflect importance of step to meeting objective:  Important  = (5)    Essential = (10)    Critical = (15)
Automatic failure results if any of the critical steps are omitted or performed incorrectly.

DETERMINE SCORE (divide points earned by total points possible, multiply results by 100)        _____ SCORE*

Evaluator's Name (print) _____ Signature _____

Comments _____

## PROCEDURE 13-5   Measure Oral Temperature with Mercury Thermometer

*PERFORMANCE OBJECTIVE*—In a simulated or actual situation and given access to all necessary equipment and supplies, measure and record a patient's oral temperature. The procedure will be done within six minutes, following correct procedural technique and observing aseptic and safety precautions. The recorded findings must agree with the instructor's reading.

| PROCEDURE STEPS | STEP PERFORMED | POINTS POSSIBLE | COMMENTS |
|---|---|---|---|
| *EVALUATOR:* Place check mark in space following each step performed satisfactorily | | | |
| NOTE TIME BEGAN _____ | | | |
| 1. Washed hands, assembled equipment, and put on gloves. | _____ | 15 | |
| 2. Identified patient. | _____ | 5 | |
| 3. Explained procedure. | _____ | 5 | |
| 4. Determined if patient had recently had a hot or cold drink or smoked. | _____ | 15 | |
| 5. Removed thermometer from holder or envelope. Avoided touching bulb end with fingers. | _____ | 5 | |
| 6. Inspected thermometer. Discarded a chipped or cracked thermometer in a sharps biohazardous waste container. | _____ | 15 | |
| 7. Read thermometer and shook down to 95°F or below if necessary. | _____ | 15 | |
| 8. Put plastic sheath on thermometer and ensured it is intact. | _____ | 10 | |
| 9. Placed bulb sublingually in patient's mouth. | _____ | 10 | |
| 10. Told patient how to maintain proper position of thermometer: to keep lips closed, breathe through nose, and avoid biting. | _____ | 5 | |
| 11. Left thermometer in position a minimum of three minutes. | _____ | 15 | |
| 12. Removed and read thermometer. Reinserted for one minute if less than 97°F. | _____ | 10 | |
| 13. Reread thermometer, if appropriate. | _____ | — | |
| 14. Holding by stem, pulled off plastic sheath and discarded in biohazardous waste container. | _____ | 5 | |
| *EVALUATOR:* NOTE TIME COMPLETED _____ | | | |
| Completed within six minutes | _____ | 15 | |
| *EVALUATOR:* Read thermometer and record temperature: _____ | | | |

| PROCEDURE STEPS | STEP PERFORMED | POINTS POSSIBLE | COMMENTS |
|---|---|---|---|
| 15. Followed procedure for soiled thermometers. | _____ | 5 | |
| 16. Removed gloves and discarded in biohazardous waste container. | _____ | 5 | |
| 17. Washed hands. | _____ | 5 | |
| 18. Accurately noted temperature. | _____ | 15 | |
| 19. Recorded and signed procedure on patient's chart. | _____ | 10 | |

ADD POINTS OF STEPS CHECKED          _____ EARNED
TOTAL POINTS POSSIBLE                              185 POSSIBLE

Points assigned reflect importance of step to meeting objective:  Important  = (5)   Essential = (10)   Critical = (15)
Automatic failure results if any of the critical steps are omitted or performed incorrectly.

DETERMINE SCORE (divide points earned by total points possible, multiply results by 100)          _____ SCORE*

Evaluator's Name (print) _____ Signature _____

Comments _____

---

## DOCUMENTATION

Chart the procedure in the patient's medical record.

Date: _____

Charting: _____

_____

_____

_____

Student's Name: _____          Physician's Initials:  _(   )_

## PROCEDURE 13-6   Measure Rectal Temperature with Mercury Thermometer

*PERFORMANCE OBJECTIVE*—In a simulated or actual situation and given access to all necessary equipment and supplies, measure and record a patient's rectal temperature within eight minutes, following correct procedural technique and observing aseptic and safety precautions. The recorded findings must agree with the instructor's reading.

| PROCEDURE STEPS | STEP PERFORMED | POINTS POSSIBLE | COMMENTS |
|---|---|---|---|
| *EVALUATOR:* Place check mark in space following each step performed satisfactorily | | | |
| NOTE TIME BEGAN _____ | | | |
| 1. Washed hands, assembled equipment, and put on gloves. | _____ | 15 | |
| 2. Identified patient. | _____ | 5 | |
| 3. Explained procedure. | _____ | 5 | |
| 4. Placed a small amount of lubricant on a tissue. | _____ | 5 | |
| 5. Removed thermometer from holder or envelope. | _____ | 5 | |
| 6. Inspected thermometer. Discarded a chipped or cracked thermometer in a sharps biohazardous waste container. | _____ | 15 | |
| 7. Read thermometer and shook down to 95°F, or below. | _____ | 15 | |
| 8. Placed thermometer in plastic sheath. Checked that sheath is intact. | _____ | 15 | |
| 9. Rotated thermometer bulb in lubricant on tissue and placed in convenient location. | _____ | 5 | |
| 10. Instructed patient to remove appropriate clothing, assisting as needed. | _____ | 5 | |
| 11. Provided privacy. | _____ | 5 | |
| 12. Assisted adult patient onto examining table and covered with drape. Avoided overexposure. | _____ | 5 | |
| 13. Positioned patient on side. Ensured patient's comfort and safety. | _____ | 5 | |
| 14. Arranged drape to expose buttocks. | _____ | 5 | |
| 15. With one hand raised upper buttock to expose anus. | _____ | 5 | |
| 16. With other hand, carefully inserted lubricated thermometer into anal canal approximately 1½ ″. | _____ | 5 | |
| a. Did not force thermometer. Rotated if necessary to facilitate insertion | _____ | 10 | |
| b. If opening was not apparent, requested patient to bear down slightly | _____ | 5 | |
| 17. Held thermometer in place for a minimum of three minutes. | _____ | 15 | |

| PROCEDURE STEPS | STEP PERFORMED | POINTS POSSIBLE | COMMENTS |
|---|---|---|---|
| 18. Withdrew thermometer. Carefully removed plastic sheath and discarded it in biohazardous waste container. | _____ | 10 | |
| 19. Read thermometer. | _____ | 5 | |
| 20. Reread to check temperature. | _____ | 5 | |
| 21. Placed thermometer on tissue. | _____ | 5 | |
| *EVALUATOR:* NOTE TIME COMPLETED _____ | | | |
| Completed within eight minutes | _____ | 15 | |
| *EVALUATOR:* Read thermometer and record temperature: _____ | | | |
| 22. Removed any excess lubricant from anal area with tissue; wiped from front to back. | _____ | 5 | |
| 23. Assisted adult patient from examining table and instructed to redress. | _____ | 5 | |
| 24. Followed procedure for soiled thermometer. | _____ | 5 | |
| 25. Removed and discarded gloves in biohazardous waste container. | _____ | 5 | |
| 26. Accurately noted temperature. | _____ | 15 | |
| 27. Recorded and signed procedure on patient's chart. | _____ | 10 | |

ADD POINTS OF STEPS CHECKED                                                      _____ EARNED
TOTAL POINTS POSSIBLE                                                                 235 POSSIBLE

Points assigned reflect importance of step to meeting objective:  Important = (5)   Essential = (10)   Critical = (15)
Automatic failure results if any of the critical steps are omitted or performed incorrectly.

DETERMINE SCORE (divide points earned by total points possible, multiply results by 100)        _____ SCORE*

Evaluator's Name (print) _____ Signature _____

Comments _____

**DOCUMENTATION**

Chart the procedure in the patient's medical record.

Date: _____

Charting: _____

_____

_____

_____

Student's Name: _____         Physician's Initials: __(      )__

## PROCEDURE 13-7   Measure Axillary Temperature with Mercury Thermometer

*PERFORMANCE OBJECTIVE*—In a simulated or actual situation and given access to all necessary equipment and supplies, measure and record axillary temperature within 14 minutes, following correct procedural technique and observing aseptic and safety precautions. Recorded findings must agree with the instructor's reading.

| PROCEDURE STEPS | STEP PERFORMED | POINTS POSSIBLE | COMMENTS |
|---|---|---|---|
| *EVALUATOR:* Place check mark in space following each step performed satisfactorily | | | |
| NOTE TIME BEGAN _____ | | | |
| 1. Washed hands, assembled equipment. | _____ | 5 | |
| 2. Identified patient. | _____ | 5 | |
| 3. Explained procedure. | _____ | 5 | |
| 4. Removed thermometer from holder or envelope. | _____ | 5 | |
| 5. Inspected thermometer. Discarded a chipped or cracked thermometer in a sharps biohazardous waste container. | _____ | 15 | |
| 6. Read thermometer and shook down to 95° F or below. | _____ | 15 | |
| 7. Placed thermometer on tissue or in envelope in convenient location. | _____ | 5 | |
| 8. Assisted patient, as necessary, to expose axilla, provided privacy. | _____ | 5 | |
| 9. Patted axillary space with tissue to remove perspiration. | _____ | 10 | |
| 10. Placed thermometer deep in the axillary space. | _____ | 10 | |
|    a. Bulb at top of axillary space | _____ | 5 | |
|    b. Stem projecting anteriorly or posteriorly | _____ | 5 | |
| 11. Instructed patient to hold arm tightly against body and to maintain position for a minimum of ten minutes. | _____ | 15 | |
| 12. Removed thermometer and wiped with tissue from stem to bulb. | _____ | 5 | |
| 13. Read and noted findings accurately. | _____ | 15 | |
| 14. Reread and checked recording. | _____ | 5 | |
| *EVALUATOR:* NOTE TIME COMPLETED _____ Completed within fourteen minutes. | | 15 | |
| *EVALUATOR:* Read thermometer and record temperature: _____ | | | |

| PROCEDURE STEPS | STEP PERFORMED | POINTS POSSIBLE | COMMENTS |
|---|---|---|---|
| 15. Helped patient replace clothing. | _____ | 5 | |
| 16. Followed procedure for soiled thermometer. | _____ | 5 | |
| 17. Washed hands. | _____ | 5 | |
| 18. Recorded and signed procedure on patient's chart. | _____ | 10 | |

ADD POINTS OF STEPS CHECKED

TOTAL POINTS POSSIBLE

_____ EARNED

170  POSSIBLE

Points assigned reflect importance of step to meeting objective:  Important  = (5)   Essential = (10)   Critical = (15)
Automatic failure results if any of the critical steps are omitted or performed incorrectly.

DETERMINE SCORE (divide points earned by total points possible, multiply results by 100)     _____ SCORE*

Evaluator's Name (print) _____ Signature _____

Comments _____

---

## DOCUMENTATION

Chart the procedure in the patient's medical record.

Date: _____

Charting: _____

_____

_____

_____

Student's Name: _____        Physician's Initials:  __(_____)__

## PROCEDURE 13-8   Measure Oral Temperature with Disposable Plastic Thermometer

*PERFORMANCE OBJECTIVE*—In a simulated or actual situation and given access to all necessary equipment and supplies, measure and record oral temperature within four minutes, following correct procedural technique and observing aseptic and safety precautions. Recorded findings must agree with the instructor's reading.

| PROCEDURE STEPS | STEP PERFORMED | POINTS POSSIBLE | COMMENTS |
|---|---|---|---|
| *EVALUATOR:* Place check mark in space following each step performed satisfactorily | | | |
| NOTE TIME BEGAN _____ | | | |
| 1. Washed hands, assembled equipment, put on gloves. | _____ | 5 | |
| 2. Identified patient. | _____ | 5 | |
| 3. Explained procedure. | _____ | 5 | |
| 4. Determined if patient had recently had a hot or cold drink or smoked. | _____ | 15 | |
| 5. Opened package by peeling back top of wrapper to expose handle end of thermometer. | _____ | 5 | |
| 6. Grasped handle and removed from wrapper without touching matrix section. | _____ | 15 | |
| 7. Inserted thermometer into patient's mouth as far back as possible into one of the heat pockets. | _____ | 10 | |
| 8. Instructed patient to press tongue down on thermometer and keep mouth closed. | _____ | 10 | |
| 9. Instructed patient to maintain position for sixty seconds; timed by watch. | _____ | 15 | |
| 10. Removed thermometer and waited ten seconds for dots to stabilize. Did not touch dots. | _____ | 15 | |
| 11. Read thermometer. | _____ | — | |
| *EVALUATOR:* NOTE TIME COMPLETED _____ | | | |
| Completed within four minutes. | | 15 | |
| *EVALUATOR:* Read thermometer and record temperature: _____ | | | |
| 12. Discarded thermometer in biohazardous waste container. | _____ | 10 | |
| 13. Washed hands. | _____ | 5 | |
| 14. Accurately noted temperature. | _____ | 15 | |
| 15. Recorded and signed procedure on patient's chart. | _____ | 10 | |

ADD POINTS OF STEPS CHECKED                                    _____ EARNED
TOTAL POINTS POSSIBLE                                                     155 POSSIBLE

Points assigned reflect importance of step to meeting objective: Important = (5)   Essential = (10)   Critical = (15)
Automatic failure results if any of the critical steps are omitted or performed incorrectly.

DETERMINE SCORE (divide points earned by total points possible, multiply results by 100)     _____ SCORE*

Evaluator's Name (print) _____ Signature _____

Comments _____

## DOCUMENTATION

Chart the procedure in the patient's medical record.

Date: _____

Charting: _____

_____

_____

_____

Student's Name: _____          Physician's Initials: __(____)__

Name _____

Date _____ Score* _____

## PROCEDURE 13-9   Measure Oral Temperature Electronically

*PERFORMANCE OBJECTIVE*—In a simulated or actual situation and given access to all necessary equipment and supplies, measure the patient's temperature electronically. The temperature will be read and recorded in two minutes, following correct procedural technique and observing aseptic and safety precautions. Recorded findings must agree with instructor's reading.

| PROCEDURE STEPS | STEP PERFORMED | POINTS POSSIBLE | COMMENTS |
|---|---|---|---|
| *EVALUATOR:* Place check mark in space following each step performed satisfactorily | | | |
| NOTE TIME BEGAN _____ | | | |
| 1. Washed hands, assembled equipment. | _____ | 5 | |
| 2. Identified patient. | _____ | 5 | |
| 3. Explained procedure. | _____ | 5 | |
| 4. Placed probe connector in receptacle of unit base and checked to make sure it was properly seated. | _____ | 10 | |
| 5. Holding it by the collar, removed appropriate probe from stored position. | _____ | 5 | |
| 6. Inserted probe firmly into probe cover to ensure that it was properly seated. | _____ | 5 | |
| 7. Inserted covered probe into mouth, and provided support. | _____ | 15 | |
| 8. Maintained covered probe in position until unit signals. | _____ | 10 | |
| 9. Removed probe; avoided touching cover. | _____ | 15 | |
| 10. Accurately read and noted temperature measurement. | _____ | 15 | |
| 11. Rechecked reading and recording. | _____ | 5 | |
| 12. Pressed the eject button and discarded used probe cover into biohazardous waste container. | _____ | 10 | |
| 13. Returned probe to stored position in unit. Thermometer display read zero and shut off. | _____ | 5 | |
| 14. Stored unit in charging stand. | _____ | 5 | |
| 15. Recorded and signed procedure on patient's chart. | _____ | 10 | |
| *EVALUATOR:* NOTE TIME COMPLETED _____ | | | |
| Completed within two minutes | _____ | 15 | |
| *EVALUATOR:* Read thermometer and record temperature: _____ | | | |

ADD POINTS OF STEPS CHECKED _____ EARNED
TOTAL POINTS POSSIBLE 140 POSSIBLE

Points assigned reflect importance of step to meeting objective:  Important = (5)   Essential = (10)   Critical = (15)
Automatic failure results if any of the critical steps are omitted or performed incorrectly.

DETERMINE SCORE (divide points earned by total points possible, multiply results by 100) _____ SCORE*

Evaluator's Name (print) _____ Signature _____

Comments _____

## DOCUMENTATION

Chart the procedure in the patient's medical record.

Date: _____

Charting: _____

_____

_____

_____

Student's Name: _____     Physician's Initials: __(_____)__

## PROCEDURE 13-10   Measure Core Body Temperature
## with an Infrared Tympanic Thermometer

*PERFORMANCE OBJECTIVE*—In a simulated or actual situation and given access to all necessary equipment and supplies, measure and record core temperature within three minutes, following correct procedural technique and observing aseptic and safety precautions. Recorded findings must agree with the instructor's reading.

| PROCEDURE STEPS | STEP PERFORMED | POINTS POSSIBLE | COMMENTS |
|---|---|---|---|
| *EVALUATOR:* Place check mark in space following each step performed satisfactorily | | | |
| NOTE TIME BEGAN _____ | | | |
| 1. Washed hands, assembled equipment. | _____ | 5 | |
| 2. Identified patient. | _____ | 5 | |
| 3. Explained procedure. | _____ | 5 | |
| 4. Removed thermometer from base. | _____ | 5 | |
| 5. Attached a disposable probe cover to the earpiece. | _____ | 10 | |
| 6. Inserted covered probe into ear canal, sealing opening. | _____ | 15 | |
| 7. Pressed the scan button to activate the thermometer. | _____ | 5 | |
| 8. Withdrew the thermometer. | _____ | — | |
| 9. Observed the display window, noting the temperature. | _____ | 5 | |
| 10. Pressed the release button on the thermometer and ejected probe cover into a biohazardous waste container. | _____ | 5 | |
| 11. Accurately read and noted temperature. | _____ | 15 | |
| 12. Returned thermometer to base. | _____ | 5 | |
| 13. Recorded and signed procedure on patient's chart. | _____ | 10 | |
| *EVALUATOR:* NOTE TIME COMPLETED _____ | | | |
| Completed within three minutes. | _____ | 15 | |
| *EVALUATOR:* Read thermometer and record temperature: _____ | | | |

ADD POINTS OF STEPS CHECKED                                             _____ EARNED
TOTAL POINTS POSSIBLE                                                              105 POSSIBLE

Points assigned reflect importance of step to meeting objective: Important = (5)   Essential = (10)   Critical = (15)
Automatic failure results if any of the critical steps are omitted or performed incorrectly.

DETERMINE SCORE (divide points earned by total points possible, multiply results by 100)          _____ SCORE*

Evaluator's Name (print) _____ Signature _____

Comments _____

## DOCUMENTATION

Chart the procedure in the patient's medical record.

Date: _____

Charting: _____

_____

_____

_____

Student's Name: _____          Physician's Initials: __( ___ )__

## PROCEDURE 13-11   Measure Radial Pulse

*PERFORMANCE OBJECTIVE*—In a simulated or actual situation and given access to all necessary equipment and supplies, within four minutes, assess and record the quality and measure and record the rate of a patient's radial pulse following correct procedural technique. Recorded rate findings must be within two beats per minute of instructor's measurement and agree as to rhythm and quality characteristics.

| PROCEDURE STEPS | STEP PERFORMED | POINTS POSSIBLE | COMMENTS |
|---|---|---|---|
| *EVALUATOR:* Place check mark in space following each step performed satisfactorily | | | |
| NOTE TIME BEGAN _____ | | | |
| 1. Washed hands, assembled equipment. | _____ | 5 | |
| 2. Identified patient. | _____ | 5 | |
| 3. Explained procedure. | _____ | 5 | |
| 4. Determined patient's recent activity. | _____ | 10 | |
| 5. Had patient assume a comfortable position. | _____ | 5 | |
| 6. Located radial artery. | _____ | 15 | |
| 7. Observed quality of pulse before beginning to count. | _____ | 15 | |
| 8. Counted pulse. | _____ | 15 | |
| a. Regular for 30 seconds—*or*— | | | |
| b. Irregular for one minute | | | |
| 9. Accurately recorded pulse rate. | _____ | 15 | |
| 10. Described characteristics. | _____ | 15 | |
| 11. Recorded and signed procedure on patient's chart. | _____ | 10 | |
| *EVALUATOR:* NOTE TIME COMPLETED _____ | | | |
| Completed within four minutes. | _____ | 15 | |
| *EVALUATOR:* Record pulse rate _____ | | | |
| Characteristics _____ | | | |
| _____ | | | |
| _____ | | | |

ADD POINTS OF STEPS CHECKED                                          _____ EARNED
TOTAL POINTS POSSIBLE                                                    130 POSSIBLE

Points assigned reflect importance of step to meeting objective: Important = (5)   Essential = (10)   Critical = (15)
Automatic failure results if any of the critical steps are omitted or performed incorrectly.

DETERMINE SCORE (divide points earned by total points possible, multiply results by 100)         _____ SCORE*

Evaluator's Name (print) _____ Signature _____

Comments _____

## DOCUMENTATION

Chart the procedure in the patient's medical record.

Date: _____

Charting: _____

_____

_____

_____

Student's Name: _____          Physician's Initials: __(___)__

Name _____

Date _____ Score* _____

## PROCEDURE 13-12   Measure Apical Pulse

*PERFORMANCE OBJECTIVE*—In a simulated or actual situation and given access to all necessary equipment and supplies, within five minutes, locate the apex of the heart, assess and record the quality and measure and record the rate of a patient's apical pulse following correct technique and observing aseptic precautions. Recorded rate findings must be within one beat per minute of instructor's measurement and agree as to rhythm and quality characteristics.

| PROCEDURE STEPS | STEP PERFORMED | POINTS POSSIBLE | COMMENTS |
|---|---|---|---|
| *EVALUATOR:* Place check mark in space following each step performed satisfactorily | | | |
| NOTE TIME BEGAN _____ | | | |
| 1. Washed hands, assembled equipment. | _____ | 5 | |
| 2. Prepared stethoscope by wiping earpieces and chestpiece with germicidal solution to prevent transfer of organisms. | _____ | 10 | |
| 3. Identified patient. | _____ | 5 | |
| 4. Explained procedure. If infant or small child, explained to parent. | _____ | 5 | |
| 5. Provided privacy and a gown or drape if indicated. | _____ | 5 | |
| 6. Uncovered left side of chest. | _____ | 10 | |
| 7. Placed earpieces in ears. Openings in tips should be forward, entering auditory canal: held chestpiece in hand. | _____ | 10 | |
| 8. Located apex. | _____ | 15 | |
| 9. Placed chestpiece of stethoscope at apex. | _____ | 5 | |
| 10. Determined quality of heart sounds. | _____ | 15 | |
| 11. Counted beats for a full minute. | _____ | 15 | |
| 12. Removed earpieces from ears. | _____ | 5 | |
| 13. Accurately noted rate of heart sounds. | _____ | 15 | |
| 14. Accurately noted quality of heart sounds. | _____ | 15 | |
| 15. Assisted patient as necessary to redress. | _____ | — | |
| 16. Wiped earpieces and chestpiece of stethoscope with disinfectant. Returned to storage. | _____ | 5 | |
| 17. Washed hands. | _____ | 5 | |
| 18. Recorded and signed procedure on patient's chart. | _____ | 10 | |
| *EVALUATOR:* NOTE TIME COMPLETED _____ | | | |
| Completed within five minutes. | _____ | 15 | |
| *EVALUATOR:* Record rate _____ | | | |
| Characteristics _____ | | | |

ADD POINTS OF STEPS CHECKED                         _____ EARNED
TOTAL POINTS POSSIBLE                                          170  POSSIBLE

Points assigned reflect importance of step to meeting objective: Important = (5)   Essential = (10)   Critical = (15)
Automatic failure results if any of the critical steps are omitted or performed incorrectly.

DETERMINE SCORE (divide points earned by total points possible, multiply results by 100)        _____ SCORE*

Evaluator's Name (print) _____ Signature _____

Comments _____

## DOCUMENTATION

Chart the procedure in the patient's medical record.

Date: _____

Charting: _____

_____

_____

_____

Student's Name: _____          Physician's Initials: __(____)__

Name _____

Date _____ Score* _____

## PROCEDURE 13-13   Measure Respirations

*PERFORMANCE OBJECTIVE*—In a simulated or actual situation and given access to all necessary equipment and supplies, assess and record the quality and rate of a patient's respirations within three minutes, following correct procedural technique. Recorded rate findings must be within two breaths per minute of instructor's measurement and agree as to rhythm, sound, and depth quality characteristics.

| PROCEDURE STEPS | STEP PERFORMED | POINTS POSSIBLE | COMMENTS |
|---|---|---|---|
| *EVALUATOR:* Place check mark in space following each step performed satisfactorily | | | |
| NOTE TIME BEGAN _____ | | | |
| 1. Washed hands, assembled equipment. | _____ | 5 | |
| 2. Identified patient. | _____ | 5 | |
| 3. Asked about recent activity level. | _____ | 10 | |
| 4. Avoided identifying respiration evaluation. | _____ | 10 | |
| 5. Placed patient in comfortable position. | _____ | 5 | |
| 6. Assumed pulse measurement position. | _____ | 10 | |
| 7. Assessed respiration quality. | _____ | 15 | |
| 8. Accurately counted respirations for thirty seconds. | _____ | 15 | |
| 9. Accurately noted rate. | _____ | 15 | |
| 10. Recorded characteristics. | _____ | 15 | |
| 11. Recorded and signed procedure on patient's chart. | _____ | 10 | |
| *EVALUATOR:* NOTE TIME COMPLETED _____ | | | |
| Completed within three minutes. | _____ | 15 | |
| *EVALUATOR:* Record rate _____ | | | |
| Characteristics _____ | | | |

ADD POINTS OF STEPS CHECKED                                          _____ EARNED
TOTAL POINTS POSSIBLE                                                    130 POSSIBLE

Points assigned reflect importance of step to meeting objective: Important = (5)   Essential = (10)   Critical = (15)
Automatic failure results if any of the critical steps are omitted or performed incorrectly.

DETERMINE SCORE (divide points earned by total points possible, multiply results by 100)        _____ SCORE*

Evaluator's Name (print) _____ Signature _____

Comments _____

## DOCUMENTATION

Chart the procedure in the patient's medical record.

Date: _____

Charting: _____

_____

_____

_____

Student's Name: _____          Physician's Initials: __(_____)__

Name _____

Date _____ Score* _____

## PROCEDURE 13-14   Measure Blood Pressure

*PERFORMANCE OBJECTIVE*—In a simulated or actual situation and given access to all necessary equipment and supplies, within
a four-minute period of time, measure palpatory and auscultatory blood pressure and record findings, following correct
procedural technique and observing safety and aseptic precautions. Recorded rate findings must be within 4 mmHg of
instructor's measurement using teaching stethoscope.

| PROCEDURE STEPS | STEP PERFORMED | POINTS POSSIBLE | COMMENTS |
|---|---|---|---|
| *EVALUATOR:* Place check mark in space following each step performed satisfactorily | | | |
| NOTE TIME BEGAN _____ | | | |
| 1. Washed hands. | _____ | 5 | |
| 2. Assembled equipment. | _____ | 5 | |
| 3. Cleaned earpieces and head of stethoscope with antiseptic. | _____ | 5 | |
| 4. Identified patient. | _____ | 5 | |
| 5. Explained procedure. | _____ | 5 | |
| 6. Placed a mercury manometer on a flat, level surface near patient. Put aneroid type within easy reach. | _____ | 5 | |
| 7. Placed patient in a relaxed and comfortable sitting or lying position. | _____ | 5 | |
| 8. a. Positioned arm, palm up | _____ | 5 | |
| b. Clothing appropriately managed | _____ | 10 | |
| 9. a. Opened valve, deflated bladder completely | _____ | 5 | |
| b. Located center of bladder; assured adequate cuff size | _____ | 15 | |
| c. Applied cuff to upper arm, bladder centered over brachial artery; 1″ to 2″ above elbow | _____ | 15 | |
| d. Attached tubing if disconnected | _____ | — | |
| 10. Assured manometer in proper view. | _____ | 5 | |
| 11. Closed valve with one hand. | _____ | 5 | |
| 12. Positioned other hand to palpate radial pulse. | _____ | 5 | |
| 13. Observing manometer, rapidly inflated cuff to 30 mm above level where radial pulse disappears. | _____ | 10 | |
| 14. Opened valve, slowly releasing air until radial pulse was detected. | _____ | 10 | |
| 15. Observed mercury or dial reading. | _____ | 10 | |
| 16. Deflated cuff rapidly and completely. Squeezed cuff with hands to empty **air.** | _____ | 5 | |
| 17. Positioned earpieces of stethoscope in ears with openings entering ear canal; held head of scope in one hand. | _____ | 5 | |
| 18. Palpated brachial artery at medial antecubital space with fingertips. | _____ | 15 | |
| 19. Placed head of stethoscope directly over palpated pulse. | _____ | 5 | |
| 20. Closed valve on bulb and rapidly inflated cuff to 30 mm above palpated systolic pressure. | _____ | 10 | |

| PROCEDURE STEPS | STEP PERFORMED | POINTS POSSIBLE | COMMENTS |
|---|---|---|---|
| 21. Opened valve, slowly deflating cuff. | _____ | 10 | |
| 22. With eyes at level of descending meniscus or directly in line with dial, noted reading at which systolic pressure heard. | _____ | 10 | |
| 23. Allowed pressure to lower steadily. | _____ | 5 | |
| 24. Continued to release pressure until all sound disappears. | _____ | 5 | |
| 25. Released remaining air. Squeezed cuff between hands. | _____ | 5 | |
| 26. Recorded accurate systolic and whichever diastolic instructed to read. | _____ | 15 | |
| 27. Reevaluated if indicated after a minimum of fifteen seconds. | _____ | — | |
| 28. Removed stethoscope from ears. | _____ | — | |
| 29. Removed cuff from patient's arm. | _____ | — | |
| *EVALUATOR:* NOTE TIME COMPLETED _____ | | | |
| Completed within four minutes. | _____ | 15 | |
| *EVALUATOR:* Record B/P _____ | | | |
| 30. Assisted patient with clothing, if necessary. | _____ | — | |
| 31. Cleaned tips and head of stethoscope with alcohol to disinfect. | _____ | 10 | |
| 32. Folded cuff properly and placed with manometer and stethoscope in storage. | _____ | 5 | |
| 33. Washed hands. | _____ | 5 | |
| 34. Recorded and signed procedure on patient's chart. | _____ | 10 | |

ADD POINTS OF STEPS CHECKED                    _____ EARNED
TOTAL POINTS POSSIBLE                                        265 POSSIBLE

Points assigned reflect importance of step to meeting objective:  Important = (5)   Essential = (10)   Critical = (15)
Automatic failure results if any of the critical steps are omitted or performed incorrectly.

DETERMINE SCORE (divide points earned by total points possible, multiply results by 100)    _____ SCORE*

Evaluator's Name (print) _____ Signature _____

Comments _____

## DOCUMENTATION
Chart the procedure in the patient's medical record.

Date: _____

Charting: _____

_____

_____

_____

Student's Name: _____        Physician's Initials: __(____)__

Name _____

Date _____ Score* _____

## PROCEDURE 14-1  Irrigate the Eye

*PERFORMANCE OBJECTIVE*—Provided with a mannequin and all equipment required for eye irrigation, demonstrate the steps of the procedure in proper order.

| PROCEDURE STEPS | STEP PERFORMED | POINTS POSSIBLE | COMMENTS |
|---|---|---|---|
| *EVALUATOR:* Place check mark in space following each step performed satisfactorily | | | |
| NOTE TIME BEGAN _____ | | | |
| 1. Assembled necessary items. | _____ | 10 | |
| 2. Washed hands and put on gloves. | _____ | 15 | |
| 3. Prepared solution. | _____ | 10 | |
| 4. Identified patient, called by name. | _____ | 5 | |
| 5. Explained procedure to patient. | _____ | 5 | |
| 6. Positioned patient comfortably. | _____ | 5 | |
| 7. Draped patient. | _____ | 5 | |
| 8. Asked patient to turn head to side then back. | _____ | 10 | |
| 9. Placed emesis basin against head to catch solution, gave tissues. | _____ | 10 | |
| 10. Wiped eye with gauze square from bridge of nose out. | _____ | 10 | |
| 11. Filled bulb syringe with solution. | _____ | 10 | |
| 12. Held eye open with thumb and index finger. | _____ | 15 | |
| 13. Released solution over eye gently from inner canthus to outer canthus. | _____ | 15 | |
| 14. Used sterile gauze square to blot area dry. | _____ | 5 | |
| 15. Attended to patient's comfort. | _____ | 5 | |
| 16. Removed gloves and washed hands. | _____ | 10 | |
| 17. Provided patient education. | _____ | 5 | |
| 18. Recorded procedure in patient's chart. | _____ | 10 | |
| 19. Initialed procedure. | _____ | 5 | |
| 20. Noted observations during procedure. | _____ | 5 | |
| 21. Washed items and returned to storage. | _____ | 5 | |
| *EVALUATOR:* NOTE TIME COMPLETED _____ | | | |

ADD POINTS OF STEPS CHECKED                                          _____ EARNED

TOTAL POINTS POSSIBLE                                                        175 POSSIBLE

Points assigned reflect importance of step to meeting objective: Important = (5)   Essential = (10)   Critical = (15)
Automatic failure results if any of the critical steps are omitted or performed incorrectly.

DETERMINE SCORE (divide points earned by total points possible, multiply results by 100)        _____ SCORE*

Evaluator's Name (print) _____ Signature _____

Comments _____

## DOCUMENTATION

Chart the procedure in the patient's medical record.

Date: _____

Charting: _____

_____

_____

_____

Student's Name: _____        Physician's Initials: __( )__

Name _____

Date _____ Score* _____

## PROCEDURE 14-2   Irrigate the Ear

*PERFORMANCE OBJECTIVE*—Provided with anatomical model of the ear and all equipment required for ear irrigation, demonstrate the steps of the procedure in proper order.

| PROCEDURE STEPS | STEP PERFORMED | POINTS POSSIBLE | COMMENTS |
|---|---|---|---|
| *EVALUATOR:* Place check mark in space following each step performed satisfactorily | | | |
| NOTE TIME BEGAN _____ | | | |
| 1. Washed hands and put on gloves. | _____ | 10 | |
| 2. Assembled necessary items. | _____ | 15 | |
| 3. Prepared solution between 100°F and 105°F as directed by the physician. | _____ | 15 | |
| 4. a. Identified patient, called by name | _____ | 10 | |
| b. Explained procedure to patient | _____ | 5 | |
| 5. Viewed affected area with otoscope. | _____ | 10 | |
| 6. Asked patient to turn head to side and back. | _____ | 10 | |
| 7. Placed ear basin under ear. | _____ | 5 | |
| 8. Placed towel over patient's shoulder. | _____ | 5 | |
| 9. Used gauze square to wipe ear. | _____ | 5 | |
| 10. Filled syringe with solution. | _____ | 10 | |
| 11. Pulled auricle up and back for adult or down and back for child. | _____ | 15 | |
| 12. Placed tip of syringe into side of ear canal. | _____ | 5 | |
| 13. Irrigated ear with solution to desired results. | _____ | 15 | |
| 14. Used gauze square to wipe excess solution from outside of patient's ear. | _____ | 5 | |
| 15. Instructed patient to tilt head to allow drainage, give tissues. | _____ | 5 | |
| 16. Inspected ear canal with otoscope to determine results of irrigation. Repeat irrigation PRN. | _____ | 5 | |
| 17. Provided patient education. | _____ | 5 | |
| 18. a. Recorded procedure in patient's chart | _____ | 10 | |
| b. Initialed chart | _____ | 5 | |
| c. Wrote observations | _____ | 5 | |

## PROCEDURE 14-2    Irrigate the Ear—continued

| PROCEDURE STEPS | STEP PERFORMED | POINTS POSSIBLE | COMMENTS |
|---|---|---|---|
| 19. Washed equipment. | _____ | 5 | |
| 20. Removed gloves and washed hands. | _____ | 5 | |
| 21. Returned equipment to proper storage area. | _____ | 5 | |
| *EVALUATOR:* NOTE TIME COMPLETED _____ | | | |

ADD POINTS OF STEPS CHECKED                                                                                          _____ EARNED

TOTAL POINTS POSSIBLE                                                                                                           190 POSSIBLE

Points assigned reflect importance of step to meeting objective:  Important = (5)   Essential = (10)   Critical = (15)
Automatic failure results if any of the critical steps are omitted or performed incorrectly.

DETERMINE SCORE (divide points earned by total points possible, multiply results by 100)          _____ SCORE*

Evaluator's Name (print) _____ Signature _____

Comments _____

---

# DOCUMENTATION

Chart the procedure in the patient's medical record.

Date: _____

Charting: _____

_____

_____

_____

Student's Name: _____          Physician's Initials: _( _____ )_

Name _____

Date _____ Score* _____

## PROCEDURE 14-3   Instill Eardrops

*PERFORMANCE OBJECTIVE*—Provided with a mannequin or anatomical model of the ear and all necessary equipment, demonstrate each step of the procedure for instilling eardrops in proper order.

| PROCEDURE STEPS | STEP PERFORMED | POINTS POSSIBLE | COMMENTS |
|---|---|---|---|
| *EVALUATOR:* Place check mark in space following each step performed satisfactorily | | | |
| NOTE TIME BEGAN _____ | | | |
| 1. Verified medication ordered. | _____ | 15 | |
|   a. Assembled items | _____ | 5 | |
| 2. Washed hands and put on gloves. | _____ | 10 | |
| 3. Called patient by name. | _____ | 10 | |
|   a. Explained procedure | _____ | 10 | |
| 4. Opened medication container/drew up ordered amount in dropper. | _____ | 15 | |
| 5. Positioned patient/tilt head to instill left for right ear (right for left). | _____ | 10 | |
| 6. Asked for assistance if necessary. | _____ | 5 | |
| 7. Gave patient tissues. | _____ | 5 | |
| 8. Instilled drops in ear (without touching ear tissues). | _____ | 15 | |
| 9. Advised patient to remain in position for drops to settle in ear. | _____ | 10 | |
| 10. Provided patient education. | _____ | 5 | |
| 11. Repeated for other ear if ordered. | _____ | 10 | |
| 12. Closed medication container without touching outside of the container. | _____ | 15 | |
| 13. Removed gloves and washed hands. | _____ | 10 | |
| 14. Recorded procedure on patient's chart. | _____ | 5 | |
|   a. Noted observations | _____ | 5 | |
|   b. Initialed | _____ | 10 | |
| 15. Returned items to proper storage area. | _____ | 5 | |
| *EVALUATOR:* NOTE TIME COMPLETED _____ | | | |

ADD POINTS OF STEPS CHECKED                                     _____ EARNED

TOTAL POINTS POSSIBLE                                                    175 POSSIBLE

Points assigned reflect importance of step to meeting objective:  Important = (5)   Essential = (10)   Critical = (15)
Automatic failure results if any of the critical steps are omitted or performed incorrectly.

DETERMINE SCORE (divide points earned by total points possible, multiply results by 100)        _____ SCORE*

Evaluator's Name (print) _____ Signature _____

Comments _____

## DOCUMENTATION

Chart the procedure in the patient's medical record.

Date: _____

Charting: _____

_____

_____

_____

Student's Name: _____         Physician's Initials: __(____)__

Name _____

Date _____ Score* _____

## PROCEDURE 14-4   Instill Eyedrops

*PERFORMANCE OBJECTIVE*—Provided with a mannequin or anatomical model of the eye and all necessary equipment, demonstrate each step of the procedure for instilling eyedrops in proper order.

| PROCEDURE STEPS | STEP PERFORMED | POINTS POSSIBLE | COMMENTS |
|---|---|---|---|
| *EVALUATOR:* Place check mark in space following each step performed satisfactorily | | | |
| NOTE TIME BEGAN _____ | | | |
| 1. Verified medication ordered. | _____ | 15 | |
|    a. Assembled items | _____ | 5 | |
| 2. Washed hands and put on gloves. | _____ | 10 | |
| 3. Called patient by name. | _____ | 10 | |
|    a. Explained procedure | _____ | 10 | |
| 4. Opened medication container/drew up ordered amount in dropper. | _____ | 15 | |
| 5. Positioned patient/asked for assistance if necessary. | _____ | 10 | |
| 6. Used gauze to touch area just under eyelid to form pocket. | _____ | 10 | |
| 7. Instilled drops into pocket of eye **without** touching tissues. | _____ | 15 | |
| 8. Asked patient to blink to distribute medication. | _____ | 15 | |
|    a. Repeated for other eye | _____ | 10 | |
| 9. Advised patient **not** to rub eyes. | _____ | 10 | |
| 10. Offered patient tissues to blot excess medication gently. | _____ | 5 | |
| 11. Provided patient education. | _____ | 5 | |
| 12. Closed medication container without touching cap to the outside of the container. | _____ | 10 | |
| 13. Removed gloves and washed hands. | _____ | 5 | |
| 14. Recorded procedure on patient's chart. | _____ | 10 | |
|    a. Noted observations | _____ | 5 | |
|    b. Initialed | _____ | 5 | |
| 15. Returned items to proper storage area. | _____ | 5 | |
| *EVALUATOR:* NOTE TIME COMPLETED _____ | | | |

ADD POINTS OF STEPS CHECKED          _____ EARNED
TOTAL POINTS POSSIBLE          185 POSSIBLE

Points assigned reflect importance of step to meeting objective:  Important = (5)   Essential = (10)   Critical = (15)
Automatic failure results if any of the critical steps are omitted or performed incorrectly.

DETERMINE SCORE (divide points earned by total points possible, multiply results by 100)    _____ SCORE*

Evaluator's Name (print) _____ Signature _____

Comments _____

# DOCUMENTATION

Chart the procedure in the patient's medical record.

Date: _____

Charting: _____

_____

_____

_____

Student's Name: _____          Physician's Initials: __( )__

Name _____

Date _____ Score* _____

## PROCEDURE 14-5   Screen Visual Acuity with Snellen Chart

*PERFORMANCE OBJECTIVE*—Measure the visual acuity of a patient by demonstrating each step of the vision screening procedure using the Snellen chart; record the results accurately on the patient's chart.

| PROCEDURE STEPS | STEP PERFORMED | POINTS POSSIBLE | COMMENTS |
|---|---|---|---|
| *EVALUATOR:* Place check mark in space following each step performed satisfactorily | | | |
| NOTE TIME BEGAN _____ | | | |
| 1. Identified patient. | _____ | 10 | |
| 2. Explained the procedure to the patient. | _____ | 10 | |
| 3. Instructed patient to stand 20 feet from chart. | _____ | 10 | |
| a. Adjusted eye chart to patient's eye level | _____ | 10 | |
| 4. Told patient to keep both eyes open. | _____ | 10 | |
| a. Instructed patient to keep corrective lenses on/in during the first part of the screening | _____ | 10 | |
| 5. Instructed patient to read lines as you point to them. | _____ | 5 | |
| 6. Asked patient to read chart with both eyes. | _____ | 5 | |
| 7. Recorded smallest line patient could read (without making a mistake). | _____ | 15 | |
| 8. Asked patient to cover left eye. | _____ | 10 | |
| a. Instructed patient to leave both eyes open | _____ | 10 | |
| b. Recorded smallest line patient could read (without making a mistake) | _____ | 15 | |
| 9. Asked patient to cover right eye. | _____ | 10 | |
| a. Instructed patient to leave both eyes open | _____ | 10 | |
| 10. Recorded smallest line patient could read (without making a mistake). | _____ | 15 | |
| 11. Recorded observations of patient during screening. | _____ | 5 | |
| *EVALUATOR:* NOTE TIME COMPLETED _____ | | | |

ADD POINTS OF STEPS CHECKED                                                                                   _____ EARNED

TOTAL POINTS POSSIBLE                                                                                                       160 POSSIBLE

Points assigned reflect importance of step to meeting objective: Important = (5)   Essential = (10)   Critical = (15)
Automatic failure results if any of the critical steps are omitted or performed incorrectly.

DETERMINE SCORE (divide points earned by total points possible, multiply results by 100)          _____ SCORE*

Evaluator's Name (print) _____   Signature _____

Comments _____

## DOCUMENTATION

Chart the procedure in the patient's medical record.

Date: _____

Charting: _____

_____

_____

_____

Student's Name: _____          Physician's Initials: __(____)__

## PROCEDURE 14-6   Screen Visual Acuity with Jaeger System

*PERFORMANCE OBJECTIVE*—Determine the near distance visual acuity of a patient using the Jaeger near vision acuity chart by demonstrating each step of the visual acuity procedure; record results accurately in patient's chart.

| PROCEDURE STEPS | STEP PERFORMED | POINTS POSSIBLE | COMMENTS |
|---|---|---|---|
| *EVALUATOR:* Place check mark in space following each step performed satisfactorily | | | |
| NOTE TIME BEGAN _____ | | | |
| 1. Identified patient. | _____ | 10 | |
| 2. Positioned patient for procedure. | _____ | 10 | |
| 3. Instructed patient to hold Jaeger chart between 14″ and 16″ from eyes. | _____ | 15 | |
| 4. Instructed patient to read various paragraphs/both eyes open first without corrective lenses. | _____ | 10 | |
|    a. With corrective lenses | _____ | 10 | |
| 5. Instructed patient to cover left eye and read. | _____ | 10 | |
| 6. Instructed patient to cover right eye and read. | _____ | 10 | |
| 7. Observed patient during procedure. | _____ | 5 | |
| 8. Listened to remarks made by patient during procedure. | _____ | 5 | |
| 9. Recorded results on patient's chart listing the smallest print patient could read (without making a mistake). | _____ | 15 | |
| 10. Initialed patient's chart. | _____ | 5 | |
| 11. Thanked patient for cooperation. | _____ | 5 | |
| 12. Answered patient's questions. | _____ | 5 | |
| 13. Returned Jaeger chart to proper storage. | _____ | 5 | |
| *EVALUATOR:* NOTE TIME COMPLETED _____ | | | |

ADD POINTS OF STEPS CHECKED                                              _____ EARNED
TOTAL POINTS POSSIBLE                                                          120 POSSIBLE

Points assigned reflect importance of step to meeting objective: Important = (5)   Essential = (10)   Critical = (15)
Automatic failure results if any of the critical steps are omitted or performed incorrectly.

DETERMINE SCORE (divide points earned by total points possible, multiply results by 100)       _____ SCORE*

Evaluator's Name (print) _____ Signature _____

Comments _____

# DOCUMENTATION

Chart the procedure in the patient's medical record.

Date: _____

Charting: _____

_____

_____

_____

Student's Name: _____          Physician's Initials: __(____)__

# PERFORMANCE EVALUATION CHECKLIST

Name _____

Date _____ Score* _____

## PROCEDURE 14-7   Determine Color Vision Acuity by Ishihara Method

*PERFORMANCE OBJECTIVE*—In a well-lighted area, determine the color vision acuity of a patient using the Ishihara method demonstrating each step of the procedure and accurately recording the results in the patient's chart.

| PROCEDURE STEPS | STEP PERFORMED | POINTS POSSIBLE | COMMENTS |
|---|---|---|---|
| *EVALUATOR:* Place check mark in space following each step performed satisfactorily | | | |
| NOTE TIME BEGAN _____ | | | |
| 1. Identified patient. | _____ | 10 | |
| a. Explained procedure to patient | _____ | 10 | |
| 2. Obtained chart from back of Ishihara book. | _____ | 10 | |
| a. Worked in well-lighted area | _____ | 10 | |
| 3. Instructed patient to wear corrective lenses during procedure. | _____ | 10 | |
| 4. Asked patient to read plates with both eyes. | _____ | 10 | |
| 5. Instructed patient to trace the letters/numbers, etc. with finger. | _____ | 5 | |
| 6. Asked patient to cover left eye. | _____ | 5 | |
| a. Repeated steps 3–5 | _____ | 25 | |
| 7. Asked patient to cover right eye. | _____ | 5 | |
| a. Repeated steps 3–5 | _____ | 25 | |
| 8. Recorded any difficulty/complaints on patient's chart. | _____ | 5 | |
| 9. Compared answers of patient with Ishihara chart. | _____ | 10 | |
| 10. Recorded frames patient missed. | _____ | 10 | |
| 11. Recorded what patient reports. | _____ | 5 | |
| 12. Initialed procedure on patient's chart. | _____ | 5 | |

*EVALUATOR:* NOTE TIME COMPLETED _____

ADD POINTS OF STEPS CHECKED                                         _____ EARNED
TOTAL POINTS POSSIBLE                                                     160 POSSIBLE

Points assigned reflect importance of step to meeting objective: Important = (5)   Essential = (10)   Critical = (15)
Automatic failure results if any of the critical steps are omitted or performed incorrectly.

DETERMINE SCORE (divide points earned by total points possible, multiply results by 100)          _____ SCORE*

Evaluator's Name (print) _____ Signature _____

Comments _____

## DOCUMENTATION

Chart the procedure in the patient's medical record.

Date: _____

Charting: _____

_____

_____

_____

Student's Name: _____      Physician's Initials: __(_____)__

Name _____

Date _____ Score* _____

---

## PROCEDURE 14-8   Assist Patient to Horizontal Recumbent Position

*PERFORMANCE OBJECTIVE*—Assist patient to assume the horizontal recumbent position while providing for safety and privacy according to the standards identified in the procedure.

| PROCEDURE STEPS | STEP PERFORMED | POINTS POSSIBLE | COMMENTS |
|---|---|---|---|
| *EVALUATOR:* Place check mark in space following each step performed satisfactorily | | | |
| NOTE TIME BEGAN _____ | | | |
| 1. Checked examination room for cleanliness. | _____ | 5 | |
|   a. Provided clean table paper | _____ | 5 | |
|   b. Provided clean pillow cover | _____ | 5 | |
| 2. Identified patient. | _____ | 15 | |
| 3. Instructed patient to remove appropriate clothing. | _____ | 10 | |
|   a. Instructed patient where to put belongings | _____ | 5 | |
| 4. Instructed patient in putting on gown. | _____ | 5 | |
| 5. Assisted patient as necessary. | _____ | 5 | |
| 6. Instructed patient to sit on side of exam table. | _____ | 5 | |
| 7. Instructed patient to lie flat on table with legs together. | _____ | 15 | |
| 8. Pulled out extension of table for leg support. | _____ | 5 | |
| 9. Provided pillow under patient's head. | _____ | 5 | |
| 10. Asked patient to put arms at side or crossed over chest. | _____ | 5 | |
| 11. Placed drape sheet over patient. | _____ | 5 | |
| 12. Assisted with examination as necessary. | _____ | 5 | |
| 13. Assisted patient from table as necessary. | _____ | 5 | |
| 14. Cleaned up examination room as needed. | _____ | 5 | |
|   a. Replaced supplies as needed (Gloves PRN) | _____ | 5 | |

*EVALUATOR:* NOTE TIME COMPLETED _____

ADD POINTS OF STEPS CHECKED                 _____ EARNED

TOTAL POINTS POSSIBLE                             115 POSSIBLE

Points assigned reflect importance of step to meeting objective: Important = (5)   Essential = (10)   Critical = (15)
Automatic failure results if any of the critical steps are omitted or performed incorrectly.

DETERMINE SCORE (divide points earned by total points possible, multiply results by 100)     _____ SCORE*

Evaluator's Name (print) _____ Signature _____

Comments _____

Name _____

Date _____ Score* _____

## PROCEDURE 14-9   Assist Patient to Prone Position

*PERFORMANCE OBJECTIVE*—Assist patient to assume the prone position while providing for safety and privacy according to the standards identified in the procedure.

| PROCEDURE STEPS | STEP PERFORMED | POINTS POSSIBLE | COMMENTS |
|---|---|---|---|
| *EVALUATOR:* Place check mark in space following each step performed satisfactorily | | | |
| NOTE TIME BEGAN _____ | | | |
| 1. Checked examination room for cleanliness. | _____ | 5 | |
| a. Provided clean table paper | _____ | 5 | |
| b. Provided clean pillow cover | _____ | 5 | |
| 2. Identified patient. | _____ | 15 | |
| 3. Instructed patient to remove appropriate clothing. | _____ | 10 | |
| a. Instructed patient where to put belongings | _____ | 5 | |
| 4. Instructed patient in putting on gown. | _____ | 5 | |
| 5. Assisted patient as necessary. | _____ | 5 | |
| 6. Instructed patient to sit on side of exam table. | _____ | 5 | |
| 7. Instructed patient to lie flat on table with legs together. | _____ | 10 | |
| 8. Pulled out extension of table for leg support. | _____ | 5 | |
| 9. Placed drape sheet over patient. | _____ | 5 | |
| 10. Asked patient to turn toward you onto her stomach. | _____ | 15 | |
| a. Cautioned patient to stay in center of table to avoid falling | _____ | 5 | |
| 11. Instructed patient to turn her head to one side. | _____ | 5 | |
| 12. Instructed patient to flex arms at elbows with her hands at side or under head. | _____ | 5 | |
| 13. Adjusted drape sheet evenly and loosely on all sides. | _____ | 5 | |
| 14. Assisted with examination as necessary. | _____ | 5 | |
| 15. Instructed patient to turn on back. | _____ | 5 | |
| a. Reminded her to stay in center of table | _____ | 5 | |
| 16. Assisted patient in sitting up. | _____ | 5 | |
| 17. Advised patient to regain balance before standing. | _____ | 5 | |

## PROCEDURE 14-9   Assist Patient to Prone Position—continued

| PROCEDURE STEPS | STEP PERFORMED | POINTS POSSIBLE | COMMENTS |
|---|---|---|---|
| 18. Assisted patient from table as necessary. | _____ | 5 | |
| 19. Cleaned up examination room as needed. | _____ | 5 | |
|    a. Replaced supplies as needed  (Gloves PRN) | _____ | 5 | |
| *EVALUATOR:* NOTE TIME COMPLETED _____ | | | |

ADD POINTS OF STEPS CHECKED                                             _____ EARNED
TOTAL POINTS POSSIBLE                                                         155 POSSIBLE

Points assigned reflect importance of step to meeting objective: Important = (5)   Essential = (10)   Critical = (15)
Automatic failure results if any of the critical steps are omitted or performed incorrectly.

DETERMINE SCORE (divide points earned by total points possible, multiply results by 100)     _____ SCORE*

Evaluator's Name (print) _____ Signature _____

Comments _____

Name _____

Date _____ Score* _____

## PROCEDURE 14-10   Assist Patient to Sims' Position

*PERFORMANCE OBJECTIVE*—Assist patient to assume the Sims' position while providing for safety and privacy according to the standards identified in the procedure.

| PROCEDURE STEPS | STEP PERFORMED | POINTS POSSIBLE | COMMENTS |
|---|---|---|---|
| *EVALUATOR:* Place check mark in space following each step performed satisfactorily | | | |
| NOTE TIME BEGAN _____ | | | |
| 1. Checked examination room for cleanliness. | _____ | 5 | |
| a. Provided clean table paper | _____ | 5 | |
| b. Provided clean pillow cover | _____ | 5 | |
| 2. Identified patient. | _____ | 15 | |
| 3. Instructed patient to remove appropriate clothing. | _____ | 10 | |
| a. Instructed patient where to put belongings | _____ | 5 | |
| 4. Instructed patient in putting on gown. | _____ | 5 | |
| 5. Assisted patient as necessary. | _____ | 5 | |
| 6. Instructed patient to sit on side of exam table. | _____ | 5 | |
| 7. Instructed patient to lie on left side. | _____ | 10 | |
| 8. Provided pillow under patient's head. | _____ | 5 | |
| 9. Asked patient to put left arm and shoulder behind body. | _____ | 5 | |
| 10. Asked patient to flex right arm with hand toward head. | _____ | 5 | |
| 11. Asked patient to flex left leg slightly. | _____ | 5 | |
| 12. Asked patient to move buttocks near side of table. | _____ | 5 | |
| 13. Instruct patient to flex right leg sharply toward chest. | _____ | 15 | |
| 14. Placed fenestrated drape sheet over patient. | _____ | 5 | |
| 15. Assisted with examination as necessary. | _____ | 5 | |
| 16. Assisted patient from table as necessary. | _____ | 5 | |
| 17. Cleaned up examination room as needed. | _____ | 5 | |
| a. Replaced supplies as needed (Gloves PRN) | _____ | 5 | |

*EVALUATOR:* NOTE TIME COMPLETED _____

ADD POINTS OF STEPS CHECKED                                   _____ EARNED
TOTAL POINTS POSSIBLE                                              135 POSSIBLE

Points assigned reflect importance of step to meeting objective: Important = (5)   Essential = (10)   Critical = (15)
Automatic failure results if any of the critical steps are omitted or performed incorrectly.

DETERMINE SCORE (divide points earned by total points possible, multiply results by 100)        _____ SCORE*

Evaluator's Name (print) _____ Signature _____

Comments _____

Name _____

Date _____ Score* _____

## PROCEDURE 14-11   Assist Patient to Knee-Chest Position

*PERFORMANCE OBJECTIVE*—Assist patient to assume the knee-chest position while providing for safety and privacy according to the standards identified in the procedure.

| PROCEDURE STEPS | STEP PERFORMED | POINTS POSSIBLE | COMMENTS |
|---|---|---|---|
| *EVALUATOR:* Place check mark in space following each step performed satisfactorily | | | |
| NOTE TIME BEGAN _____ | | | |
| 1. Checked examination room for cleanliness. | _____ | 5 | |
|    a. Provided clean table paper | _____ | 5 | |
|    b. Provided clean pillow cover | _____ | 5 | |
| 2. Prepared examination equipment on tray. | _____ | 5 | |
| 3. Identified patient. | _____ | 15 | |
| 4. Instructed patient to remove appropriate clothing. | _____ | 15 | |
|    a. Instructed patient where to put belongings | _____ | 5 | |
| 5. Instructed patient in putting on gown. | _____ | 5 | |
| 6. Assisted patient as necessary. | _____ | 5 | |
| 7. Instructed patient to sit on side of exam table. | _____ | 5 | |
| 8. Instructed patient to lie down on table. | _____ | 5 | |
| 9. Placed drape sheet over patient. | _____ | 5 | |
| 10. Instructed patient to turn toward you onto stomach. | _____ | 5 | |
|    a. Guided patient to center of table | _____ | 5 | |
| 11. Instructed patient to get on hands and knees. | _____ | 10 | |
| 12. Instructed patient to flex arms and fold under head. | _____ | 5 | |
| 13. Asked patient to separate knees slightly and keep thighs at right angle to table. | _____ | 15 | |
| 14. Adjusted drape sheet as needed. | _____ | 5 | |
| 15. Called physician to begin exam. | _____ | 5 | |
| 16. Assisted with examination as necessary. | _____ | 5 | |
| 17. Instructed patient to lie flat on stomach. | _____ | 5 | |
|    a. Assisted patient to turn over on back | _____ | 5 | |

# PROCEDURE 14-11    Assist Patient to Knee-Chest Position—continued

| PROCEDURE STEPS | STEP PERFORMED | POINTS POSSIBLE | COMMENTS |
|---|---|---|---|
| 18. Assisted patient to sit up. | _____ | 5 | |
| 19. Assisted patient from table as necessary. | _____ | 5 | |
| 20. Cleaned up examination room as needed. | _____ | 5 | |
|    a. Replaced supplies as needed (Gloves PRN) | _____ | 5 | |

*EVALUATOR:* NOTE TIME COMPLETED _____

ADD POINTS OF STEPS CHECKED                                                          _____ EARNED
TOTAL POINTS POSSIBLE                                                                      165  POSSIBLE

Points assigned reflect importance of step to meeting objective:  Important = (5)    Essential = (10)    Critical = (15)
Automatic failure results if any of the critical steps are omitted or performed incorrectly.

DETERMINE SCORE (divide points earned by total points possible, multiply results by 100)          _____ SCORE*

Evaluator's Name (print) _____ Signature _____

Comments _____

---

## PROCEDURE 14-12   Assist Patient to Semi-Fowler's Position

---

*PERFORMANCE OBJECTIVE*—Assist patient to assume the semi-Fowler's position while providing for safety and privacy according to the standards identified in the procedure.

| PROCEDURE STEPS | STEP PERFORMED | POINTS POSSIBLE | COMMENTS |
|---|---|---|---|
| *EVALUATOR:* Place check mark in space following each step performed satisfactorily | | | |
| NOTE TIME BEGAN _____ | | | |
| 1. Checked examination room for cleanliness. | _____ | 5 | |
| a. Provided clean table paper | _____ | 5 | |
| b. Provided clean pillow cover | _____ | 5 | |
| 2. Identified patient. | _____ | 15 | |
| 3. Instructed patient to remove appropriate clothing. | _____ | 15 | |
| a. Instructed patient where to put belongings | _____ | 5 | |
| 4. Instructed patient in putting on gown. | _____ | 5 | |
| 5. Assisted patient as necessary. | _____ | 5 | |
| 6. Instructed patient to sit at end of exam table. | _____ | 10 | |
| a. Asked patient to scoot back toward center of table | _____ | 10 | |
| 7. Raised head of table to desired height—45° angle for semi-Fowler's (90° angle for Fowler's) | _____ | 15 | |
| 8. Instructed patient to lie flat on table with legs together. | _____ | 5 | |
| 9. Asked patient to lean back for comfort. | _____ | 5 | |
| 10. Pulled out extension of table for leg support. | _____ | 5 | |
| 11. Placed drape sheet over patient. | _____ | 5 | |
| 12. Assisted patient as necessary. | _____ | 5 | |
| 13. Assisted patient in sitting up. | _____ | 5 | |
| 14. Advised patient to regain balance before standing. | _____ | 5 | |
| 15. Assisted patient from table as necessary. | _____ | 5 | |
| 16. Cleaned up examination room as needed. | _____ | 5 | |
| a. Replaced supplies as needed (Gloves PRN) | _____ | 5 | |
| *EVALUATOR:* NOTE TIME COMPLETED _____ | | | |

ADD POINTS OF STEPS CHECKED                                              _____ EARNED
TOTAL POINTS POSSIBLE                                                         145 POSSIBLE

Points assigned reflect importance of step to meeting objective:  Important = (5)   Essential = (10)   Critical = (15)
Automatic failure results if any of the critical steps are omitted or performed incorrectly.

DETERMINE SCORE (divide points earned by total points possible, multiply results by 100)          _____ SCORE*

Evaluator's Name (print) _____ Signature _____

Comments _____

## PROCEDURE 14-13   Assist Patient to Lithotomy Position

*PERFORMANCE OBJECTIVE*—Assist patient to assume the lithotomy position while providing for safety and privacy according to the standards identified in the procedure.

| PROCEDURE STEPS | STEP PERFORMED | POINTS POSSIBLE | COMMENTS |
|---|---|---|---|
| *EVALUATOR:* Place check mark in space following each step performed satisfactorily | | | |
| NOTE TIME BEGAN _____ | | | |
| 1. Checked examination room for cleanliness. | _____ | 5 | |
|   a. Provided clean table paper | _____ | 5 | |
|   b. Provided clean pillow cover | _____ | 5 | |
| 2. Assembled necessary equipment. | _____ | 5 | |
| 3. Identified patient. | _____ | 15 | |
| 4. Instructed patient to remove appropriate clothing. | _____ | 10 | |
|   a. Instructed patient where to put belongings | _____ | 5 | |
| 5. Instructed patient in putting on gown. | _____ | 5 | |
| 6. Assisted patient as necessary. | _____ | 5 | |
| 7. Instructed patient to sit at end of exam table. | _____ | 10 | |
| 8. Instructed patient to lie back on table. | _____ | 10 | |
| 9. Pulled out extension of table for leg support. | _____ | 5 | |
| 10. Positioned stirrups away from table. | _____ | 5 | |
|   a. Adjusted height of stirrups | _____ | 5 | |
|   b. Secured stirrups in place | _____ | 5 | |
| 11. Asked patient to move buttocks toward end of table. | _____ | 10 | |
|   a. Placed the back of your hand at end of table to guide patient | _____ | 5 | |
|   b. Assisted patient's feet into stirrups | _____ | 15 | |
| 12. Pushed table extension in. | _____ | 5 | |
|   a. Positioned examination stool for physician | _____ | 5 | |
|   b. Positioned examination light for physician | _____ | 5 | |
| 13. Placed drape sheet over patient. | _____ | 5 | |
| 14. Assisted with examination as necessary. | _____ | 5 | |

| PROCEDURE STEPS | STEP PERFORMED | POINTS POSSIBLE | COMMENTS |
|---|---|---|---|
| 15. Assisted patient from table as necessary. | _____ | 5 | |
| 16. Cleaned up examination room as needed. | _____ | 5 | |
|    a. Replaced supplies as needed (Gloves PRN) | _____ | 5 | |
| *EVALUATOR:* NOTE TIME COMPLETED _____ | | | |

ADD POINTS OF STEPS CHECKED                                              _____ EARNED
TOTAL POINTS POSSIBLE                                                 170 POSSIBLE

Points assigned reflect importance of step to meeting objective:  Important = (5)   Essential = (10)   Critical = (15)
Automatic failure results if any of the critical steps are omitted or performed incorrectly.

DETERMINE SCORE (divide points earned by total points possible, multiply results by 100)         _____ SCORE*

Evaluator's Name (print) _____ Signature _____

Comments _____

---

## PROCEDURE 14-14    Assist with a Gynecological Examination and Pap Test

*PERFORMANCE OBJECTIVE*—Demonstrate each of the steps required in assisting with he gynecological (GYN) examination and Pap test.

| PROCEDURE STEPS | STEP PERFORMED | POINTS POSSIBLE | COMMENTS |
|---|---|---|---|
| *EVALUATOR:* Place check mark in space following each step performed satisfactorily | | | |
| NOTE TIME BEGAN _____ | | | |
| 1. Stated purpose of procedure. | _____ | 10 | |
| 2. Washed hands. | _____ | 5 | |
| 3. Assembled all needed items on Mayo table. | _____ | 10 | |
| 4. Asked patient to empty her bladder. | _____ | 5 | |
| (Instructed patient to leave urine specimen if ordered by physician). | _____ | — | |
| 5. Printed patient's name in pencil on frosted end of slide(s). | _____ | 10 | |
| 6. Explained procedure to patient. | _____ | 5 | |
| 7. Gave gown/drape sheet to patient and instructed her how to put it on. | _____ | 10 | |
| a. Assisted patient PRN | _____ | 5 | |
| b. Instructed patient to sit at end of table when ready and left door unlocked | _____ | 5 | |
| 8. Assisted patient to horizontal recumbent position. | _____ | 10 | |
| 9. Assisted patient into lithotomy position and draped. | _____ | 15 | |
| 10. Encouraged patient to breathe slowly and deeply through the mouth during exam. | _____ | 10 | |
| 11. Put on gloves. | _____ | 5 | |
| 12. Warmed vaginal speculum with warm water. | _____ | 5 | |
| 13. Handed speculum and spatula to physician. | _____ | 10 | |
| 14. Held slide for physician to apply smear. | _____ | 10 | |
| 15. Marked smear(s) accordingly. | _____ | 15 | |
| 16. Applied fixative or placed in alcohol-ether solution bottle. | _____ | 10 | |
| 17. Placed lubricant on physician's fingers for bimanual exam. | _____ | 5 | |
| 18. Discarded disposables in biohazardous container. | _____ | 10 | |
| 19. Removed gloves and washed hands. | _____ | 5 | |

| PROCEDURE STEPS | STEP PERFORMED | POINTS POSSIBLE | COMMENTS |
|---|---|---|---|
| 20. Helped patient to sit up. | _____ | 5 | |
| a. Pushed foot rest in | _____ | 5 | |
| 21. Helped patient down from exam table. | _____ | 5 | |
| 22. Returned items to proper storage area. | _____ | 5 | |
| a. If metal speculum was used—placed in cool water to soak | _____ | 5 | |
| 23. Regloved PRN. | _____ | 5 | |
| 24. Instructed patient to dress. | _____ | 5 | |
| 25. Placed Pap smear slide(s) with completed request form in lab pick-up area. | _____ | 10 | |

*EVALUATOR:* NOTE TIME COMPLETED _____

ADD POINTS OF STEPS CHECKED                                    _____ EARNED

TOTAL POINTS POSSIBLE                                          220 POSSIBLE

Points assigned reflect importance of step to meeting objective:  Important = (5)   Essential = (10)   Critical = (15)
Automatic failure results if any of the critical steps are omitted or performed incorrectly.

DETERMINE SCORE (divide points earned by total points possible, multiply results by 100)      _____ SCORE*

Evaluator's Name (print) _____ Signature _____

Comments _____

## DOCUMENTATION

Chart the procedure in the patient's medical record.

Date: _____

Charting: _____
_____
_____
_____

Student's Name: _____          Physician's Initials:  __(____)__

Name _____

Date _____ Score* _____

## PROCEDURE 14-15   Measure Recumbent Length of Infant

*PERFORMANCE OBJECTIVE*—Demonstrate each step required in measuring the recumbent length of an infant and record; measurement should agree with instructor's by ± ⅙ inch.

| PROCEDURE STEPS | STEP PERFORMED | POINTS POSSIBLE | COMMENTS |
|---|---|---|---|
| *EVALUATOR:* Place check mark in space following each step performed satisfactorily | | | |
| NOTE TIME BEGAN _____ | | | |
| 1. Washed hands. | _____ | 15 | |
| 2. Asked parent to place infant on exam table and explained procedure. | _____ | 5 | |
| 3. Instructed parent to remove shoes, socks/booties from infant. | _____ | 5 | |
| 4. Moved infant to end of table so that infant's head was at the zero mark of the ruler. | _____ | 15 | |
| 5. Asked parent to hold infant's head against the end of the table. | _____ | 15 | |
| 6. Straightened (gently) infant's back and legs to line up along ruler. | _____ | 10 | |
| 7. Placed infant's heels against footboard. | _____ | 10 | |
| 8. Read length of infant in inches or centimeters from ruler accurately. | _____ | 15 | |
| 9. Returned infant to parent. | _____ | 5 | |
| 10. Recorded measurement on | | | |
| a. Growth chart | _____ | 10 | |
| b. Patient's chart | _____ | 10 | |
| c. Parent's booklet | _____ | 5 | |
| d. Initialed all | _____ | 5 | |
| *EVALUATOR:* NOTE TIME COMPLETED _____ | | | |

ADD POINTS OF STEPS CHECKED                                   _____ EARNED
TOTAL POINTS POSSIBLE                                                     125 POSSIBLE

Points assigned reflect importance of step to meeting objective: Important = (5)   Essential = (10)   Critical = (15)
Automatic failure results if any of the critical steps are omitted or performed incorrectly.

DETERMINE SCORE (divide points earned by total points possible, multiply results by 100)          _____ SCORE*

Evaluator's Name (print) _____ Signature _____

Comments _____

## DOCUMENTATION

Chart the procedure in the patient's medical record.

Date: _____

Charting: _____

_____

_____

_____

Student's Name: _____        Physician's Initials: __(____)__

## PROCEDURE 14-17   Weigh Infant

*PERFORMANCE OBJECTIVE*—Demonstrate each step of the procedure of weighing infants and record; weight must agree with instructor's by ± ⅛ lb.

| PROCEDURE STEPS | STEP PERFORMED | POINTS POSSIBLE | COMMENTS |
|---|---|---|---|
| *EVALUATOR:* Place check mark in space following each step performed satisfactorily | | | |
| NOTE TIME BEGAN _____ | | | |
| 1. Washed hands. | _____ | 15 | |
| 2. Asked parent to remove infant's clothes. | _____ | 5 | |
| 3. Placed towel on scale. | _____ | 5 | |
| 4. Balanced scale at zero with towel in place. | _____ | 15 | |
| 5. Placed infant gently on scale. | _____ | 5 | |
| 6. Held hand over infant—not touching. | _____ | 5 | |
| 7. Talked to infant in quiet tone. | _____ | 5 | |
| 8. Kept diaper over genital area. | _____ | 5 | |
| 9. Slid weight easily. | _____ | 10 | |
| 10. Returned infant to parent. | _____ | 5 | |
| 11. Read weight accurately. | _____ | 15 | |
| 12. Removed towel from scale. | _____ | 5 | |
| 13. Placed towel in proper receptacle. | _____ | 5 | |
| 14. Balanced scale at zero. | _____ | 10 | |
| 15. Recorded weight accurately on: | | | |
| a. Growth chart | _____ | 15 | |
| b. Patient's chart | _____ | 15 | |
| c. Parent's booklet | _____ | 5 | |
| d. Initialed all | _____ | 5 | |
| *EVALUATOR:* NOTE TIME COMPLETED _____ | | | |

ADD POINTS OF STEPS CHECKED _____ EARNED

TOTAL POINTS POSSIBLE 150 POSSIBLE

Points assigned reflect importance of step to meeting objective: Important = (5)   Essential = (10)   Critical = (15)
Automatic failure results if any of the critical steps are omitted or performed incorrectly.

DETERMINE SCORE (divide points earned by total points possible, multiply results by 100) _____ SCORE*

Evaluator's Name (print) _____ Signature _____

Comments _____

## DOCUMENTATION

Chart the procedure in the patient's medical record.

Date: _____

Charting: _____

_____

_____

_____

Student's Name: _____          Physician's Initials: __( )__

## PROCEDURE 14-18   Measure Head Circumference

*PERFORMANCE OBJECTIVE*—Demonstrate each step of the procedure for measuring head circumference of infants and record; measurement must agree with instructor's by ± ½ inch or 0.1 cm.

| PROCEDURE STEPS | STEP PERFORMED | POINTS POSSIBLE | COMMENTS |
|---|---|---|---|
| *EVALUATOR:* Place check mark in space following each step performed satisfactorily | | | |
| NOTE TIME BEGAN _____ | | | |
| 1. Washed hands. | _____ | 15 | |
| 2. Talked to infant. | _____ | 5 | |
| 3. Asked parent for assistance. | _____ | 5 | |
| 4. Used thumb to hold tape measure at zero mark against forehead over the eyebrows. | _____ | 15 | |
| 5. Brought tape measure around infant's head over the ears to meet in front. | _____ | 15 | |
| 6. Pulled tape measure snugly to compress hair. | _____ | 10 | |
| 7. Read measurement to nearest 0.1 cm or 0.5 inch. | _____ | 15 | |
| 8. Recorded measurement accurately on: | | | |
|    a. Growth chart | _____ | 15 | |
|    b. Patient's chart | _____ | 15 | |
|    c. Parent's booklet | _____ | 5 | |
|    d. Initialed all | _____ | 5 | |
| *EVALUATOR:* NOTE TIME COMPLETED _____ | | | |

ADD POINTS OF STEPS CHECKED                                          _____ EARNED

TOTAL POINTS POSSIBLE                                                      120 POSSIBLE

Points assigned reflect importance of step to meeting objective: Important = (5)   Essential = (10)   Critical = (15)
Automatic failure results if any of the critical steps are omitted or performed incorrectly.

DETERMINE SCORE (divide points earned by total points possible, multiply results by 100)          _____ SCORE*

Evaluator's Name (print) _____ Signature _____

Comments _____

**DOCUMENTATION**

Chart the procedure in the patient's medical record.

Date: _____

Charting: _____

_____

_____

_____

Student's Name: _____          Physician's Initials: __( ___ )__

Name _____

Date _____ Score* _____

## PROCEDURE 14-19   Measure Infant's Chest

*PERFORMANCE OBJECTIVE*—Provided with a lifelike clinical infant doll and a flexible tape measure, demonstrate each step required in obtaining the chest measurement and record; the chest measurement must agree with instructor's by ± ⅛ inch (0.3 cm).

| PROCEDURE STEPS | STEP PERFORMED | POINTS POSSIBLE | COMMENTS |
|---|---|---|---|
| *EVALUATOR:* Place check mark in space following each step performed satisfactorily | | | |
| NOTE TIME BEGAN _____ | | | |
| 1. Washed hands. | _____ | 15 | |
| 2. Talked to infant/gained cooperation. | _____ | 5 | |
| 3. Asked parent for assistance. | _____ | 5 | |
| 4. Held tape at zero with thumb at mid-sternal area of chest. | _____ | 15 | |
| 5. Brought tape around child's back to meet in front at zero mark under axillary region. | _____ | 15 | |
| 6. Made tape snug against chest. | _____ | 10 | |
| 7. Read measurement to nearest 0.1 cm or ½ inch. | _____ | 15 | |
| 8. Recorded measurement accurately on: | | | |
| a. Patient's chart | _____ | 15 | |
| b. Parent's booklet | _____ | 15 | |
| c. Initialed both | _____ | 5 | |
| *EVALUATOR:* NOTE TIME COMPLETED _____ | | | |

ADD POINTS OF STEPS CHECKED           _____ EARNED
TOTAL POINTS POSSIBLE           115 POSSIBLE

Points assigned reflect importance of step to meeting objective:  Important = (5)   Essential = (10)   Critical = (15)
Automatic failure results if any of the critical steps are omitted or performed incorrectly.

DETERMINE SCORE (divide points earned by total points possible, multiply results by 100)      _____ SCORE*

Evaluator's Name (print) _____ Signature _____

Comments _____

# DOCUMENTATION

Chart the procedure in the patient's medical record.

Date: _____

Charting: _____

_____

_____

_____

Student's Name: _____          Physician's Initials: __(____)__

Name _____

Date _____ Score* _____

## PROCEDURE 14-20   Assist with Sigmoidoscopy

*PERFORMANCE OBJECTIVE*—Demonstrate each of the steps required in assisting with the sigmoidoscopy procedure.

| PROCEDURE STEPS | STEP PERFORMED | POINTS POSSIBLE | COMMENTS |
|---|---|---|---|
| *EVALUATOR:* Place check mark in space following each step performed satisfactorily | | | |
| NOTE TIME BEGAN _____ | | | |
| 1. Stated purpose of procedure. | _____ | 10 | |
| 2. Explained procedure to patient. | _____ | 5 | |
| 3. Asked patient to empty bladder. | _____ | 10 | |
| 4. Assembled all needed items on Mayo table at end of exam table. | _____ | 10 | |
|   a. Completed lab request form for biopsy if requested; labeled container | _____ | 10 | |
| 5. Checked light source. | _____ | 5 | |
| 6. Instructed patient to disrobe from waist down. | _____ | 5 | |
|   a. Assisted patient to sit at end of exam table | _____ | 5 | |
|   b. Covered patient with drape | _____ | 5 | |
| 7. Assisted patient with knee-chest or Sims' position just before exam. | _____ | 15 | |
| 8. Applied approximately two tablespoons of lubricant on gauze square for physician to use during exam. | _____ | 5 | |
| 9. Plugged in light source of sigmoidoscope. | _____ | 5 | |
|   a. Secured air inflation tubing | _____ | 5 | |
| 10. Washed hands and put on gloves. | _____ | 10 | |
| 11. Handed sigmoidoscope to physician. | _____ | 10 | |
|   a. Assisted as needed | _____ | 5 | |
| 12. Cleaned patient's anal area with tissues. | _____ | 5 | |
| 13. Removed gloves and washed hands. | _____ | 5 | |
| 14. Assisted patient to resting prone position. | _____ | 5 | |
| 15. Assisted patient to sitting position. | _____ | 5 | |
|   a. Then from table to dress | _____ | 5 | |
| 16. Regloved. | _____ | 5 | |
| 17. Cleaned up exam area. | _____ | 5 | |
|   a. Placed used instruments in basin of detergent solution to soak | _____ | 5 | |

| PROCEDURE STEPS | STEP PERFORMED | POINTS POSSIBLE | COMMENTS |
|---|---|---|---|
| 18. Removed gloves and washed hands. | _____ | 5 | |
| 19. Scheduled patient for further appointment(s). | _____ | 5 | |
| 20. Recorded procedure on patient's chart. | _____ | 5 | |
| a. Initialed | _____ | 5 | |
| 21. Cleaned exam room; readied instruments for autoclave (regloved as necessary). | _____ | 5 | |

*EVALUATOR:* NOTE TIME COMPLETED _____

ADD POINTS OF STEPS CHECKED                                            _____ EARNED
TOTAL POINTS POSSIBLE                                                          185 POSSIBLE

Points assigned reflect importance of step to meeting objective:  Important  = (5)   Essential = (10)   Critical = (15)
Automatic failure results if any of the critical steps are omitted or performed incorrectly.

DETERMINE SCORE (divide points earned by total points possible, multiply results by 100)         _____ SCORE*

Evaluator's Name (print) _____ Signature _____

Comments _____

---

# DOCUMENTATION

Chart the procedure in the patient's medical record.

Date: _____

Charting: _____

_____

_____

_____

Student's Name: _____        Physician's Initials: __(____)__

Name _____

Date _____ Score* _____

## PROCEDURE 14-21   Administer Disposable Cleansing Enema

*PERFORMANCE OBJECTIVE*—Demonstrate each of the steps required in administering a cleansing enema.

| PROCEDURE STEPS | STEP PERFORMED | POINTS POSSIBLE | COMMENTS |
|---|---|---|---|
| *EVALUATOR:* Place check mark in space following each step performed satisfactorily | | | |
| NOTE TIME BEGAN _____ | | | |
| 1. Identified patient. | _____ | 5 | |
| a. Explained procedure to patient | _____ | 5 | |
| 2. Instructed patient to disrobe from waist down. | _____ | 5 | |
| a. Provided drape sheet | _____ | 5 | |
| b. Assisted patient onto exam table | _____ | 5 | |
| 3. Helped patient into Sims' position: | _____ | 10 | |
| a. Instructed patient to lie on left side | _____ | 10 | |
| b. Asked patient to bring right knee up to waist level | _____ | 15 | |
| c. Adjusted drape sheet over patient | _____ | 5 | |
| 4. Washed hands. | _____ | 5 | |
| a. Put on gloves | _____ | 5 | |
| 5. Removed protective covering from tip of enema container. | _____ | 10 | |
| a. Applied small amount of lubricant to the tip | _____ | 5 | |
| 6. Separated buttocks to expose anus. | _____ | 10 | |
| 7. Inserted tip of bottle into anus. | _____ | 10 | |
| a. Advised patient to breathe deeply and slowly through the mouth | _____ | 5 | |
| 8. Expressed entire contents into the anus. | _____ | 15 | |
| a. Advised patient to retain contents for as long as possible | _____ | 15 | |
| 9. Withdrew enema tip slowly. | _____ | 5 | |
| a. Provided tissues to patient | _____ | 5 | |
| b. Disposed of used tissues in biohazardous container | _____ | 5 | |
| 10. Directed patient to restroom. | _____ | 5 | |
| a. Asked patient to show results before flushing | _____ | 15 | |
| 11. Reported results to physician. | _____ | 10 | |

503

| PROCEDURE STEPS | STEP PERFORMED | POINTS POSSIBLE | COMMENTS |
|---|---|---|---|
| 12. Cleaned room | _____ | 5 | |
| a. Discarded disposables in appropriate waste containers | _____ | 5 | |
| 13. Removed gloves | _____ | 10 | |
| a. Washed hands | _____ | 10 | |
| 14. Initialed chart. | _____ | 5 | |

*EVALUATOR:* NOTE TIME COMPLETED _____

ADD POINTS OF STEPS CHECKED                                    _____ EARNED
TOTAL POINTS POSSIBLE                                          225 POSSIBLE

Points assigned reflect importance of step to meeting objective:  Important  = (5)   Essential = (10)   Critical = (15)
Automatic failure results if any of the critical steps are omitted or performed incorrectly.

DETERMINE SCORE (divide points earned by total points possible, multiply results by 100)        _____ SCORE*

Evaluator's Name (print) _____ Signature _____

Comments _____

---

# DOCUMENTATION

Chart the procedure in the patient's medical record.

Date: _____

Charting: _____

_____

_____

_____

Student's Name: _____          Physician's Initials: __( )__

Name _____

Date _____ Score* _____

## PROCEDURE 15-1   Use a Microscope

*PERFORMANCE OBJECTIVE*—Provided with all necessary equipment and supplies, demonstrate the use of the microscope following the steps in the procedure with the instructor observing each step.

| PROCEDURE STEPS | STEP PERFORMED | POINTS POSSIBLE | COMMENTS |
|---|---|---|---|
| *EVALUATOR:* Place check mark in space following each step performed satisfactorily | | | |
| NOTE TIME BEGAN _____ | | | |
| 1. Washed hands and put on gloves. | _____ | 5 | |
| 2. Assembled necessary equipment. | _____ | 5 | |
| 3. Labeled specimen on frosted end of slide with pencil. | _____ | 10 | |
| 4. Cleaned ocular lens with lens cleaning tissue. | _____ | 10 | |
| 5. Plugged light source into electrical outlet. | _____ | 15 | |
| 6. Turned light source on. | _____ | 10 | |
| 7. Placed specimen slide on stage with frosted side up between clips. | _____ | 10 | |
| 8. Secured slide over opening of stage. | _____ | 5 | |
| 9. Raised substage carefully. | _____ | 5 | |
| 10. Turned revolving nosepiece to 1pf (10X). | _____ | 5 | |
| 11. Began to focus until specimen was in view. | _____ | 10 | |
| 12. Turned fine adjustment until specimen was seen in detail. | _____ | 10 | |
| 13. Adjusted substage diaphragm lever for proper lighting. | _____ | 5 | |
| 14. Turned revolving nosepiece to intermediate (40X). | _____ | 5 | |
| 15. Adjusted fine focus for detail in viewing specimen. | _____ | 10 | |
| 16. Use hpf: | | | |
| a. Use cover slide | _____ | 10 | |
| b. Clean lens after use | _____ | 5 | |
| c. Adjust diaphragm lever | _____ | 5 | |
| 17. Identified specimen. | _____ | 5 | |
| 18. Turned light off. | _____ | 5 | |
| 19. Cleaned microscopic stage. | _____ | 5 | |
| 20. Disposed of clean slide(s). | _____ | 5 | |
| 21. Removed gloves and washed hands. | _____ | 5 | |

## PROCEDURE 15-1 Use a Microscope—continued

| PROCEDURE STEPS | STEP PERFORMED | POINTS POSSIBLE | COMMENTS |
|---|---|---|---|
| 22. Recorded findings of microscopic examination on chart | _____ | 15 | |
| a. Initialed | _____ | 5 | |
| *EVALUATOR:* NOTE TIME COMPLETED _____ | | | |

ADD POINTS OF STEPS CHECKED          _____ EARNED

TOTAL POINTS POSSIBLE          185 POSSIBLE

Points assigned reflect importance of step to meeting objective: Important = (5)   Essential = (10)   Critical = (15)
Automatic failure results if any of the critical steps are omitted or performed incorrectly.

DETERMINE SCORE (divide points earned by total points possible, multiply results by 100)          _____ SCORE*

Evaluator's Name (print) _____ Signature _____

Comments _____

Name _____

Date _____ Score* _____

## PROCEDURE 15-2   Puncture Skin with Sterile Lancet

*PERFORMANCE OBJECTIVE*—Demonstrate skin puncture procedure following all steps to obtain capillary blood for test(s) specified by physician/instructor.

| PROCEDURE STEPS | STEP PERFORMED | POINTS POSSIBLE | COMMENTS |
|---|---|---|---|
| *EVALUATOR:* Place check mark in space following each step performed satisfactorily | | | |
| NOTE TIME BEGAN _____ | | | |
| 1. Identified patient. | _____ | 5 | |
| 2. Explained procedure to patient. | _____ | 5 | |
| 3. Inspected patient's finger and selected puncture site. | _____ | 5 | |
| 4. Washed hands and put on gloves. | _____ | 5 | |
| 5. Assembled needed items next to patient. | _____ | 5 | |
| 6. Cleaned site with alcohol pad. | _____ | 5 | |
| 7. Allowed site to air dry. | _____ | 5 | |
| 8. Removed sterile lancet from package without contaminating it. | _____ | 10 | |
| 9. Secured puncture site between thumb and great finger. | _____ | 5 | |
| 10. Held lancet pointed downward between thumb and great finger of other hand. | _____ | 5 | |
| 11. Punctured site with a quick, firm, steady down-and-up motion. | _____ | 10 | |
| a. Approximately 2mm deep | _____ | 5 | |
| b. Control entry and exit of lancet to avoid ripping skin | _____ | 5 | |
| 12. Discarded first drop of blood by blotting with gauze square. | _____ | 10 | |
| 13. Applied gentle pressure on either side of puncture site to obtain desired amount of blood. | _____ | 15 | |
| 14. Wiped site with cotton ball/gauze square. | _____ | 10 | |
| 15. Asked patient to apply gentle pressure with gauze square over site to control bleeding. | _____ | 10 | |
| 16. Checked site and attended to patient. | _____ | 5 | |
| 17. Discarded disposables in proper receptacles. | _____ | 5 | |

| PROCEDURE STEPS | STEP PERFORMED | POINTS POSSIBLE | COMMENTS |
|---|---|---|---|
| 18. Removed gloves. | _____ | 5 | |
| 19. Washed hands. | _____ | 5 | |

*EVALUATOR:* NOTE TIME COMPLETED _____

ADD POINTS OF STEPS CHECKED                                          _____ EARNED
TOTAL POINTS POSSIBLE                                                      140 POSSIBLE

Points assigned reflect importance of step to meeting objective:  Important  = (5)   Essential = (10)   Critical = (15)
Automatic failure results if any of the critical steps are omitted or performed incorrectly.

DETERMINE SCORE (divide points earned by total points possible, multiply results by 100)        _____ SCORE*

Evaluator's Name (print) _____ Signature _____

Comments _____

---

## DOCUMENTATION

Chart the procedure in the patient's medical record.

Date: _____

Charting: _____

_____

_____

_____

Student's Name: _____          Physician's Initials:  _( )_

Name _____

Date _____ Score* _____

## PROCEDURE 15-3   Obtain Blood for PKU Test

*PERFORMANCE OBJECTIVE*—Demonstrate the steps of the procedure for obtaining a blood specimen for determination of phenylketonuria level in the blood.

| PROCEDURE STEPS | STEP PERFORMED | POINTS POSSIBLE | COMMENTS |
|---|---|---|---|
| *EVALUATOR:* Place check mark in space following each step performed satisfactorily | | | |
| NOTE TIME BEGAN _____ | | | |
| 1. Identified patient. | _____ | 5 | |
| 2. Explained procedure to patient. | _____ | 5 | |
| 3. Washed hands. | _____ | 5 | |
|   a. Put on gloves | _____ | 5 | |
| 4. Assembled all needed items. | _____ | 10 | |
| 5. Explained procedure to parent of patient. | _____ | 5 | |
| 6. Asked all necessary information. | _____ | 10 | |
| 7. Completed form. | _____ | 10 | |
| 8. Asked assistance of parent. | _____ | 5 | |
| 9. Performed skin puncture adequately. | _____ | 10 | |
| 10. Wiped first drop of blood from site. | _____ | 5 | |
| 11. Secured site between great finger and thumb. | _____ | 5 | |
| 12. Applied gentle pressure to produce large drop of blood. | _____ | 10 | |
| 13. Applied blood to the circles on the back of the form, saturating each circle completely. | _____ | 15 | |
| 14. Repeated steps 11 and 12 until all circles have been saturated. | _____ | 15 | |
| 15. Wiped puncture site with dry gauze square. | _____ | 5 | |
|   a. Asked patient to hold gently | _____ | 5 | |
|   b. Placed small round bandage over area | _____ | 5 | |
| 16. Placed completed PKU test form in protective paper envelope. | _____ | 10 | |
|   a. Then, into addressed envelope to health dept. | _____ | 10 | |
| 17. Discarded used items properly. | _____ | 5 | |
| 18. Removed gloves. | _____ | 5 | |
|   a. Washed hands | _____ | 5 | |

| PROCEDURE STEPS | STEP PERFORMED | POINTS POSSIBLE | COMMENTS |
|---|---|---|---|
| 19. Returned items to proper storage. | _____ | 5 | |
| 20. Recorded procedure on patient's chart. | _____ | 10 | |
|    a. Initialed | _____ | 5 | |
| *EVALUATOR:* NOTE TIME COMPLETED _____ | | | |

ADD POINTS OF STEPS CHECKED                                          _____ EARNED

TOTAL POINTS POSSIBLE                                                          190 POSSIBLE

Points assigned reflect importance of step to meeting objective:  Important  = (5)   Essential = (10)   Critical = (15)
Automatic failure results if any of the critical steps are omitted or performed incorrectly.

DETERMINE SCORE (divide points earned by total points possible, multiply results by 100)          _____ SCORE*

Evaluator's Name (print) _____ Signature _____

Comments _____

---

# DOCUMENTATION

Chart the procedure in the patient's medical record.

Date: _____

Charting: _____

_____

_____

_____

Student's Name: _____          Physician's Initials: __(     )__

Name _____

Date _____ Score* _____

## PROCEDURE 15-4   Determine Hematocrit (Hct) Using Microhematocrit Centrifuge

*PERFORMANCE OBJECTIVE*—Demonstrate the steps of the procedure for determining hematocrit (Hct) readings using the microhematocrit centrifuge.

| PROCEDURE STEPS | STEP PERFORMED | POINTS POSSIBLE | COMMENTS |
|---|---|---|---|
| *EVALUATOR:* Place check mark in space following each step performed satisfactorily | | | |
| NOTE TIME BEGAN _____ | | | |
| 1. Identified patient. | _____ | 5 | |
| 2. Explained procedure to patient. | _____ | 5 | |
| 3. Washed hands. | _____ | 5 | |
| a. Put on gloves | _____ | 5 | |
| 4. Assembled necessary items. | _____ | 5 | |
| 5. Followed desired skin puncture procedure. | _____ | 5 | |
| 6. Held microhematocrit tube horizontally. (There should be no bubbles in tube. Subtract points if bubbles are present.) | _____ | 10 | |
| 7. Filled tube(s) to line. | _____ | 15 | |
| 8. Wiped puncture site with cotton ball. | _____ | 5 | |
| 9. Wiped outside end of glass tube while holding horizontally. | _____ | 5 | |
| 10. Placed carefully into clay tray to seal end of tube. | _____ | 10 | |
| 11. Instructed patient to hold dry gauze over site gently. | _____ | 5 | |
| a. Make sure bleeding has stopped | _____ | 5 | |
| 12. Secured sealed end of tube against rubber padding of centrifuge. | _____ | 10 | |
| 13. Balanced centrifuge. | _____ | 10 | |
| 14. Noted number of placed tube in centrifuge. | _____ | 10 | |
| 15. Closed inside cover and locked by turning clockwise. | _____ | 10 | |
| 16. Closed and locked outside cover. | _____ | 10 | |
| 17. Listened for click to assure locking. | _____ | 5 | |
| 18. Turned timer switch past desired time and then to three minutes to set automatic timer. | _____ | 5 | |
| 19. Waited until completely stopped to unlock cover. | _____ | 15 | |
| 20. Placed bottom line of packed red cells up to buffy coat against calibrated chart (in centrifuge). | _____ | 15 | |
| 21. Used magnifying glass to read results. | _____ | 10 | |
| 22. Reclosed cover of centrifuge. | _____ | 5 | |

| PROCEDURE STEPS | STEP PERFORMED | POINTS POSSIBLE | COMMENTS |
|---|---|---|---|
| 23. Discarded used items in proper receptacle. | _____ | 5 | |
| 24. Removed gloves. | _____ | 5 | |
| a. Washed hands | _____ | 5 | |
| 25. Returned items to proper storage. | _____ | 5 | |
| 26. Recorded reading in patient's chart as percentage | _____ | 15 | |
| a. Initialed | _____ | 5 | |

*EVALUATOR:* NOTE TIME COMPLETED _____

ADD POINTS OF STEPS CHECKED                                                            _____ EARNED
TOTAL POINTS POSSIBLE                                                                        230 POSSIBLE

Points assigned reflect importance of step to meeting objective:  Important  = (5)   Essential = (10)   Critical = (15)
Automatic failure results if any of the critical steps are omitted or performed incorrectly.

DETERMINE SCORE (divide points earned by total points possible, multiply results by 100)         _____ SCORE*

Evaluator's Name (print) _____ Signature _____

Comments _____

---

## DOCUMENTATION

Chart the procedure in the patient's medical record.

Date: _____

Charting: _____

_____

_____

_____

Student's Name: _____          Physician's Initials: __(____)__

Name _____

Date _____ Score* _____

---

## PROCEDURE 15-5  Hemoglobin (Hb) Determination Using the Hemoglobinometer

*PERFORMANCE OBJECTIVE*—Demonstrate the steps of the procedure for determining hemoglobin (Hb) using the hemoglobinometer.

| PROCEDURE STEPS | STEP PERFORMED | POINTS POSSIBLE | COMMENTS |
|---|---|---|---|
| *EVALUATOR:* Place check mark in space following each step performed satisfactorily | | | |
| NOTE TIME BEGAN _____ | | | |
| 1. Identified patient. | _____ | 5 | |
| 2. Washed hands. | _____ | 5 | |
| a. Put on gloves | _____ | 5 | |
| 3. Assembled all necessary items. | _____ | 5 | |
| 4. Checked batteries and light bulb in hemoglobinometer. | _____ | 10 | |
| 5. Explained procedure to patient. | _____ | 5 | |
| 6. Followed desired skin puncture procedure. | _____ | 15 | |
| 7. Pulled glass chamber out of hemoglobinometer and fixed lower part of slide so that it was slightly offset. | _____ | 5 | |
| 8. Placed large drop of blood directly onto offset glass chamber. | _____ | 10 | |
| 9. Gave patient dry gauze to place over site gently. | _____ | 5 | |
| 10. Mixed blood on slide with hemolysis applicator. | _____ | 15 | |
| 11. Pushed chamber into clip and into slot on left side of hemoglobinometer. | _____ | 10 | |
| 12. Held hemoglobinometer in left hand at eye level. | _____ | 10 | |
| 13. Depressed light button on bottom of instrument. | _____ | 10 | |
| 14. Looked into hemoglobinometer to view green field. | _____ | 10 | |
| 15. Slid button on right of meter to match green field. | _____ | 15 | |
| 16. Left sliding scale lever where fields match. | _____ | 5 | |
| 17. Read hemoglobin level at top of calibrator scale. | _____ | 15 | |
| 18. Recorded reading on patient's chart. | _____ | 10 | |
| a. Initialed | _____ | 5 | |
| 19. Washed chambers, rinsed, dried and returned to hemoglobinometer | _____ | 5 | |

## PROCEDURE 15-5 Hemoglobin (Hb) Determination Using the Hemoglobinometer—continued

| PROCEDURE STEPS | STEP PERFORMED | POINTS POSSIBLE | COMMENTS |
|---|---|---|---|
| 20. Removed gloves. | _____ | 5 | |
|   a. Washed hands. | _____ | 5 | |
| 21. Discarded disposable items. | _____ | 5 | |
| 22. Returned items to proper storage. | _____ | 5 | |
| *EVALUATOR:* NOTE TIME COMPLETED _____ | | | |

ADD POINTS OF STEPS CHECKED          _____ EARNED

TOTAL POINTS POSSIBLE          200 POSSIBLE

Points assigned reflect importance of step to meeting objective: Important = (5) Essential = (10) Critical = (15)
Automatic failure results if any of the critical steps are omitted or performed incorrectly.

DETERMINE SCORE (divide points earned by total points possible, multiply results by 100)   _____ SCORE*

Evaluator's Name (print) _____ Signature _____

Comments _____

---

## DOCUMENTATION
Chart the procedure in the patient's medical record.

Date: _____

Charting: _____

_____

_____

_____

Student's Name: _____      Physician's Initials: __(_____)__

# PERFORMANCE EVALUATION CHECKLIST

Name _____

Date _____ Score* _____

## PROCEDURE 15-6   Screen Blood Sugar (Glucose) Level

*PERFORMANCE OBJECTIVE*—Demonstrate the steps required in the procedure for determining blood glucose level.

| PROCEDURE STEPS | STEP PERFORMED | POINTS POSSIBLE | COMMENTS |
|---|---|---|---|
| *EVALUATOR:* Place check mark in space following each step performed satisfactorily | | | |
| NOTE TIME BEGAN _____ | | | |
| 1. Identified patient. | _____ | 10 | |
| 2. Washed hands. | _____ | 5 | |
|    a. Put on gloves | _____ | 5 | |
| 3. Assembled all necessary items. | _____ | 5 | |
| 4. Calibrated instrument to be used (dextrometer). | _____ | 15 | |
| 5. Explained procedure to patient. | _____ | 5 | |
| 6. Followed desired skin puncture procedure. | _____ | 10 | |
| 7. Removed reagent strip from bottle without contaminating it. | _____ | 5 | |
| 8. Closed bottle. | _____ | 5 | |
| 9. Applied large drop of blood onto entire chemically treated surface of reagent strip. | _____ | 15 | |
| 10. Began timing immediately. | _____ | 15 | |
| 11. Wiped puncture site with cotton ball. | _____ | 5 | |
| 12. Gave patient dry gauze square to hold over site. | _____ | 5 | |
| 13. Blotted reagent strip after timing precisely. | _____ | 10 | |
| 14. Moved strip to clean area of tissue and blotted again. | _____ | 10 | |
| 15. Read strip by matching with color chart to determine glucose level of blood. | _____ | 15 | |
| 16. Recorded reading in patient's chart. | _____ | 15 | |
|    a. Initialed | _____ | 5 | |
| 17. Discarded used items. | _____ | 5 | |
| 18. Removed gloves. | _____ | 5 | |
|    a. Washed hands | _____ | 5 | |
| 19. Returned items to proper storage area. | _____ | 5 | |
| *EVALUATOR:* NOTE TIME COMPLETED _____ | | | |

ADD POINTS OF STEPS CHECKED         _____ EARNED

TOTAL POINTS POSSIBLE         180 POSSIBLE

Points assigned reflect importance of step to meeting objective: Important = (5)   Essential = (10)   Critical = (15)
Automatic failure results if any of the critical steps are omitted or performed incorrectly.

DETERMINE SCORE (divide points earned by total points possible, multiply results by 100)     _____ SCORE*

Evaluator's Name (print) _____ Signature _____

Comments _____

**DOCUMENTATION**

Chart the procedure in the patient's medical record.

Date: _____

Charting: _____

_____

_____

_____

Student's Name: _____     Physician's Initials: __(____)__

Name _____

Date _____ Score* _____

## PROCEDURE 15-7   Making a Blood Smear

*PERFORMANCE OBJECTIVE*—Demonstrate the steps required to make an adequate blood smear for a differential white blood cell count.

| PROCEDURE STEPS | STEP PERFORMED | POINTS POSSIBLE | COMMENTS |
|---|---|---|---|
| *EVALUATOR:* Place check mark in space following each step performed satisfactorily | | | |
| NOTE TIME BEGAN _____ | | | |
| 1. Identified patient. | _____ | 10 | |
| 2. Explained procedure to patient. | _____ | 5 | |
| 3. Completed lab request form. | _____ | 5 | |
| 4. Printed patient's name on frosted end of slide(s). | _____ | 10 | |
| 5. Assembled necessary items near patient. | _____ | 5 | |
| 6. Washed hands. | _____ | 5 | |
|   a. Put on gloves | _____ | 5 | |
| 7. Performed desired method of obtaining blood specimen. | _____ | 10 | |
| 8. Placed a small drop of blood on end of slide | _____ | 5 | |
|   a. ¼″ from frosted end | _____ | 10 | |
|   b. Approximately ⅛″ in diameter | _____ | 10 | |
| 9. Held corners of frosted end of glass slide down on flat surface. | _____ | 10 | |
|   a. Held second slide at 45° angle | _____ | 10 | |
| 10. Rested spreader slide against frosted slide. | _____ | 10 | |
|   a. Moved slide back carefully into the blood | _____ | 10 | |
|   b. Allowed blood to flow to edge of slide | _____ | 15 | |
|   c. Moved angled slide toward frosted end quickly and gently | _____ | 15 | |
|   d. Made feathered edge | _____ | 15 | |
| 11. Allowed smear to air dry/fan dry. | _____ | 5 | |
| 12. Placed blood smear in lab container. | _____ | 5 | |
|   a. Attached lab request form | _____ | 5 | |

| PROCEDURE STEPS | STEP PERFORMED | POINTS POSSIBLE | COMMENTS |
|---|---|---|---|
| 13. Removed gloves. | _____ | 5 | |
|    a. Washed hands | _____ | 5 | |
| 14. Discarded waste in appropriate containers. | _____ | 5 | |
| 15. Initialed procedure in patient's chart. | _____ | 5 | |
| *EVALUATOR:* NOTE TIME COMPLETED _____ | | | |

ADD POINTS OF STEPS CHECKED                  _____ EARNED
TOTAL POINTS POSSIBLE                             200 POSSIBLE

Points assigned reflect importance of step to meeting objective:  Important = (5)   Essential = (10)   Critical = (15)
Automatic failure results if any of the critical steps are omitted or performed incorrectly.

DETERMINE SCORE (divide points earned by total points possible, multiply results by 100)     _____ SCORE*

Evaluator's Name (print) _____ Signature _____

Comments _____

---

## DOCUMENTATION

Chart the procedure in the patient's medical record.

Date: _____

Charting: _____

_____

_____

_____

Student's Name: _____        Physician's Initials: __(____)__

Name _____

Date _____ Score* _____

## PROCEDURE 15-8  Obtain Venous Blood with Butterfly Needle Method

*PERFORMANCE OBJECTIVE*—Demonstrate the steps necessary for obtaining blood specimens using the butterfly needle method.

| PROCEDURE STEPS | STEP PERFORMED | POINTS POSSIBLE | COMMENTS |
|---|---|---|---|
| *EVALUATOR:* Place check mark in space following each step performed satisfactorily | | | |
| NOTE TIME BEGAN _____ | | | |
| 1. Identified patient. | _____ | 5 | |
| 2. Explained procedure to patient. | _____ | 5 | |
| 3. Completed lab request form. | _____ | 5 | |
| 4. Assembled necessary items near patient. | _____ | 5 | |
| 5. Attached butterfly needle to syringe. | _____ | 10 | |
| 6. Put on gloves. | _____ | 5 | |
| 7. Palpated vein. | _____ | 5 | |
|    a. Cleaned skin with alcohol | _____ | 5 | |
|    b. Dried excess alcohol with cottonball | _____ | 5 | |
| 8. Applied tourniquet properly. | _____ | 10 | |
| 9. Asked patient to make fist and hold. | _____ | 10 | |
| 10. Removed needle guard. | _____ | 5 | |
|    a. Pushed air out of syringe | _____ | 5 | |
|    b. Quickly inserted needle into vein | _____ | 5 | |
|    c. Pulled back on plunger slowly | _____ | 10 | |
|    d. Obtained sufficient amount of blood | _____ | 15 | |
|    e. Removed tourniquet | _____ | 5 | |
|    f. Withdrew needle quickly | _____ | 5 | |
| 11. Filled appropriate blood tubes. | _____ | 15 | |
|    a. Filled in correct order | _____ | 15 | |
| 12. Applied gentle pressure to site with cottonball. | _____ | 5 | |
|    a. Advised patient to hold arm slightly upward | _____ | 5 | |
| 13. Applied bandaid to puncture site. | _____ | 5 | |
|    a. Asked if patient is allergic to adhesive | _____ | 5 | |
| 14. Placed used needle in biohazard sharps container. | _____ | 5 | |
| 15. Placed used disposables in biohazard bag. | _____ | 5 | |
| 16. Removed gloves and placed in biohazard bag. | _____ | 5 | |
| 17. Washed hands. | _____ | 5 | |

| PROCEDURE STEPS | STEP PERFORMED | POINTS POSSIBLE | COMMENTS |
|---|---|---|---|
| 18. Recorded procedure in patient's chart. | _____ | 5 | |
|   a. Initialed | _____ | 5 | |
| *EVALUATOR:* NOTE TIME COMPLETED _____ | | | |

ADD POINTS OF STEPS CHECKED                                                    _____ EARNED
TOTAL POINTS POSSIBLE                                                         200 POSSIBLE

Points assigned reflect importance of step to meeting objective: Important = (5) Essential = (10) Critical = (15)
Automatic failure results if any of the critical steps are omitted or performed incorrectly.

DETERMINE SCORE (divide points earned by total points possible, multiply results by 100)        _____ SCORE*

Evaluator's Name (print) _____ Signature _____

Comments _____

---

## DOCUMENTATION

Chart the procedure in the patient's medical record.

Date: _____

Charting: _____

_____

_____

_____

Student's Name: _____           Physician's Initials: __(____)__

Name _____

Date _____ Score* _____

## PROCEDURE 15-9   Obtain Venous Blood with Sterile Needle and Syringe

*PERFORMANCE OBJECTIVE*—Demonstrate the steps necessary for obtaining venous blood using the sterile needle and syringe method.

| PROCEDURE STEPS | STEP PERFORMED | POINTS POSSIBLE | COMMENTS |
|---|---|---|---|
| *EVALUATOR:* Place check mark in space following each step performed satisfactorily | | | |
| NOTE TIME BEGAN _____ | | | |
| 1. Identified patient. | _____ | 10 | |
| 2. Washed hands. | _____ | 5 | |
|   a. Put on gloves | _____ | 5 | |
| 3. Assembled necessary items near patient. | _____ | 5 | |
| 4. Completed lab request form. | _____ | 5 | |
|   a. Labeled specimen tube(s) | _____ | 5 | |
| 5. Explained procedure to patient. | _____ | 5 | |
|   a. Asked patient for preferred venipuncture site | _____ | 5 | |
| 6. Positioned patient appropriately. | _____ | 5 | |
| 7. Secured needle into syringe. | _____ | 10 | |
|   a. Pushed in plunger to expel air from barrel | _____ | 10 | |
| 8. Applied tourniquet to patient's upper arm. | _____ | 5 | |
|   a. Placed 3″ above elbow | _____ | 10 | |
| 9. Cleansed site lightly with alcohol/cottonball. | _____ | 5 | |
|   a. Allowed alcohol to air dry/dried with cottonball | _____ | 5 | |
| 10. Asked patient to clench fist to make vein stand up. | _____ | 5 | |
| 11. Took needle guard off. | _____ | 5 | |
|   a. Pointed bevel of needle up | _____ | 10 | |
|   b. Inserted needle tip into vein with quick and steady motion | _____ | 10 | |
|   c. Inserted needle into vein at 15° angle | _____ | 10 | |
|   d. Held skin taut for easier insertion | _____ | 5 | |
|   e. Inserted needle between ¼″ and ½″ | _____ | 15 | |
| 12. Held barrel of syringe in one hand. | _____ | 5 | |
|   a. Pulled plunger back with other hand | _____ | 5 | |
|   b. Pulled plunger slowly/steadily | _____ | 5 | |
|   c. Allowed sufficient blood collection for specimen tube(s) | _____ | 15 | |
|   d. Asked patient to release clenched fist slowly | _____ | 5 | |
|   e. Released tourniquet within one minute | _____ | 10 | |
|   f. Pulled needle out in same path as inserted | _____ | 5 | |

| PROCEDURE STEPS | STEP PERFORMED | POINTS POSSIBLE | COMMENTS |
|---|---|---|---|
| g. Placed cottonball/gauze square over site | _____ | 5 | |
| 13. Instructed patient to apply gentle pressure to site and elevate arm slightly. | _____ | 5 | |
| 14. Filled specimen tube(s) quickly. | _____ | 10 | |
| a. Angled flow of blood to run down side of tube | _____ | 10 | |
| b. Filled tubes in correct order of draw | _____ | 15 | |
| c. Made blood smears as needed | _____ | 5 | |
| 15. Stood red-stoppered tubes vertically. | _____ | 5 | |
| a. Did not shake tubes/mixed additives carefully | _____ | 5 | |
| 16. Deposited needle/syringe in sharps container. | _____ | 5 | |
| 17. Assembled specimen tubes/lab form together in biobag. | _____ | 5 | |
| 18. Attended to patient's needs. | _____ | 5 | |
| a. Applied bandage | _____ | 5 | |
| 19. Discarded disposables in proper containers. | _____ | 5 | |
| 20. Removed gloves/placed in biobag. | _____ | 5 | |
| a. Washed hands | _____ | 5 | |
| 21. Returned items to proper storage. | _____ | 5 | |
| 22. Recorded procedure in patient's chart. | _____ | 10 | |
| a. Initialed | _____ | 5 | |

*EVALUATOR:* NOTE TIME COMPLETED _____

ADD POINTS OF STEPS CHECKED                                               _____ EARNED
TOTAL POINTS POSSIBLE                                                              320 POSSIBLE

Points assigned reflect importance of step to meeting objective:  Important  = (5)   Essential = (10)   Critical = (15)
Automatic failure results if any of the critical steps are omitted or performed incorrectly.

DETERMINE SCORE (divide points earned by total points possible, multiply results by 100)      _____ SCORE*

Evaluator's Name (print) _____ Signature _____

Comments _____

## DOCUMENTATION

Chart the procedure in the patient's medical record.

Date: _____

Charting: _____

_____

_____

_____

Student's Name: _____          Physician's Initials:  __( )__

Name _____

Date _____ Score* _____

## PROCEDURE 15-10   Obtain Venous Blood with Vacuum Tube

*PERFORMANCE OBJECTIVE*—Demonstrate the steps necessary for obtaining venous blood using the vacuum tube method.

| PROCEDURE STEPS | STEP PERFORMED | POINTS POSSIBLE | COMMENTS |
|---|---|---|---|
| *EVALUATOR:* Place check mark in space following each step performed satisfactorily | | | |
| NOTE TIME BEGAN _____ | | | |
| 1.  Identified patient. | _____ | 10 | |
| 2.  Washed hands. | _____ | 5 | |
| 3.  Assembled necessary items near patient. | _____ | 5 | |
| 4.  Completed lab request form. | _____ | 5 | |
| a.  Labeled specimen tube(s) | _____ | 5 | |
| 5.  Explained procedure to patient. | _____ | 5 | |
| a.  Asked patient for preferred venipuncture site | _____ | 5 | |
| 6.  Positioned patient appropriately. | _____ | 5 | |
| 7.  Put on gloves. | _____ | 5 | |
| 8.  Secured needle into adapter. | _____ | 10 | |
| 9.  Applied tourniquet to patient's upper arm. | _____ | 5 | |
| a.  Placed 3″ above elbow | _____ | 10 | |
| 10.  Cleansed site lightly with alcohol/cottonball. | _____ | 5 | |
| a.  Allowed alcohol to air dry/dried with cottonball | _____ | 5 | |
| 11.  Asked patient to clench fist to make vein stand up. | _____ | 5 | |
| 12.  Took needle guard off. | _____ | 5 | |
| a.  Pointed bevel of needle up | _____ | 10 | |
| b.  Inserted needle tip into vein with quick and steady motion | _____ | 10 | |
| c.  Inserted needle into vein at 15° angle | _____ | 10 | |
| d.  Held skin taut for easier insertion | _____ | 5 | |
| e.  Inserted needle between ¼″ and ½″ | _____ | 15 | |
| 13.  Held adapter with one hand. | _____ | 5 | |
| a.  Placed index and great fingers of other hand on either side of protruding edges of adapter | | 5 | |
| b.  Pushed vacuum tube completely into adapter with thumb | _____ | 10 | |
| c.  Allowed needle to puncture rubber stopper | _____ | 15 | |
| d.  Asked patient to release clenched fist slowly | _____ | 5 | |
| e.  Released tourniquet within one minute | _____ | 10 | |
| f.  Pulled filled tube out by holding it between | | | |

## PROCEDURE 15-10   Obtain Venous Blood with Vacuum Tube—continued

| PROCEDURE STEPS | STEP PERFORMED | POINTS POSSIBLE | COMMENTS |
|---|---|---|---|
| thumb and great finger and pushed against adapter with index finger | _____ | 5 | |
| g. Filled required number of tubes in correct order | _____ | 10 | |
| h. Pulled needle out in same path as inserted | _____ | 5 | |
| i. Placed cottonball/gauze square over site | _____ | 5 | |
| 14. Instructed patient to apply gentle pressure to site and elevate arm slightly. | _____ | 5 | |
| 15. Stood red-stoppered tubes vertically. | _____ | 5 | |
| a. Did not shake tubes/mixed additives carefully | _____ | 5 | |
| b. Made blood smear if ordered | _____ | 5 | |
| 16. Deposited needle/syringe in sharps container. | _____ | 5 | |
| 17. Assembled specimen tubes/lab form together in biobag. | _____ | 5 | |
| 18. Attended to patient's needs. | _____ | 5 | |
| a. Applied bandage | _____ | 5 | |
| 19. Discarded disposables in proper containers. | _____ | 5 | |
| 20. Removed gloves/placed in biobag. | _____ | 5 | |
| a. Washed hands | _____ | 5 | |
| 21. Returned items to proper storage. | _____ | 5 | |
| 22. Recorded procedure in patient's chart. | _____ | 5 | |
| a. Initialed | _____ | 5 | |
| | | | |
| *EVALUATOR:* NOTE TIME COMPLETED _____ | | | |

ADD POINTS OF STEPS CHECKED                                                      _____ EARNED
TOTAL POINTS POSSIBLE                                                                      290 POSSIBLE

Points assigned reflect importance of step to meeting objective:  Important  = (5)   Essential = (10)   Critical = (15)
Automatic failure results if any of the critical steps are omitted or performed incorrectly.

DETERMINE SCORE (divide points earned by total points possible, multiply results by 100)          _____ SCORE*

Evaluator's Name (print) _____ Signature _____

Comments _____

---

### DOCUMENTATION

Chart the procedure in the patient's medical record.

Date: _____

Charting: _____

_____

_____

_____

Student's Name: _____          Physician's Initials: __(____)__

Name _____

Date _____ Score* _____

## PROCEDURE 15-11   Catheterize Urinary Bladder

*PERFORMANCE OBJECTIVE*—Demonstrate all required steps to perform a urinary bladder catheterization.

| PROCEDURE STEPS | STEP PERFORMED | POINTS POSSIBLE | COMMENTS |
|---|---|---|---|
| *EVALUATOR:* Place check mark in space following each step performed satisfactorily | | | |
| NOTE TIME BEGAN _____ | | | |
| 1. Identify patient. | _____ | 5 | |
| 2. Placed catheter kit on Mayo table next to patient. | _____ | 5 | |
| 3. Explained procedure to patient. | _____ | 5 | |
| 4. a. Adjusted lamp | _____ | 5 | |
|    b. Turned lamp on | _____ | 5 | |
| 5. Asked patient to lie back on table. | _____ | 5 | |
|    a. Assisted patient into dorsal recumbent position | _____ | 10 | |
|    b. Assisted patient in positioning her feet in stirrups | _____ | 10 | |
| 6. Draped patient with sheet. | _____ | 5 | |
|    a. Exposed only external genitalia | _____ | 5 | |
| 7. Pulled out foot rest. | _____ | 5 | |
| 8. Opened outer wrapping of sterile kit. | _____ | 5 | |
| 9. Placed sterile towel between patient's knees. | _____ | 5 | |
| 10. Placed sterile plastic sheet under patient's buttocks. | _____ | 5 | |
| 11. Placed catheter kit on foot rest. | _____ | 5 | |
| 12. Asked patient to keep knees apart. | _____ | 5 | |
| 13. Washed and dried hands. | _____ | 5 | |
| 14. Put on sterile latex gloves. | _____ | 5 | |
| 15. Poured antiseptic solution over cotton balls in medicine cups. | _____ | 10 | |
| 16. Opened urine specimen container. | _____ | 5 | |
| 17. Applied sterile lubricant to one of the gauze squares. | _____ | 5 | |
| 18. Spread labia and wiped genitalia with each of the three antiseptic soaked cotton balls. | _____ | 10 | |
|    a. Used front to back motion | _____ | 10 | |
|    b. Discarded onto Mayo table | _____ | 5 | |
| 19. Placed tip of catheter in lubricant and other end of catheter into basin. | _____ | 5 | |
| 20. Held catheter about four inches from lubricated end. | _____ | 5 | |
| 21. Inserted lubricated tip of catheter into urinary meatus gently. | _____ | 15 | |
| 22. Instructed patient to breathe slowly and deeply. | _____ | 5 | |
| 23. Stopped urine flow by closing metal clamps attached to tubing. | _____ | 10 | |
| 24. Positioned end of tube into urine specimen container. | _____ | 10 | |

| PROCEDURE STEPS | STEP PERFORMED | POINTS POSSIBLE | COMMENTS |
|---|---|---|---|
| 25. Released clamp to collect specimen. | _____ | 10 | |
| 26. Allowed remainder of urine flow to collect in basin. | _____ | 5 | |
|    a. Measured amount of urine—both specimen and basin | _____ | 15 | |
| 27. Withdrew catheter tube gently. | _____ | 5 | |
| 28. Dried area with sterile gauze squares or cotton balls. | _____ | 5 | |
| 29. Secured lid onto urine specimen container. | _____ | 5 | |
| 30. Placed reusable items in cold water to soak. | _____ | 5 | |
| 31. Removed items from foot rest. | _____ | 5 | |
| 32. Cleaned exam table. | _____ | 5 | |
| 33. Discarded gloves and other disposables. | _____ | 5 | |
| 34. Washed hands. | _____ | 5 | |
| 35. Turned lamp off and returned to usual position. | _____ | 5 | |
| 36. Assisted patient in sitting up or relaxing in a horizontal recumbent position. | _____ | 5 | |
| 37. Labeled specimen (completed request form and attached). | _____ | 5 | |
| 38. Assisted patient from exam table. | _____ | 5 | |
| 39. Recorded procedure and measured amount of urine. | _____ | 5 | |
|    a. Observations and comments | _____ | 5 | |
|    b. Initialed | _____ | 5 | |

*EVALUATOR:* NOTE TIME COMPLETED _____

ADD POINTS OF STEPS CHECKED                  _____ EARNED

TOTAL POINTS POSSIBLE                           300 POSSIBLE

Points assigned reflect importance of step to meeting objective:  Important  = (5)    Essential = (10)    Critical = (15)
Automatic failure results if any of the critical steps are omitted or performed incorrectly.

DETERMINE SCORE (divide points earned by total points possible, multiply results by 100)     _____ SCORE*

Evaluator's Name (print) _____ Signature _____

Comments _____

---

## DOCUMENTATION

Chart the procedure in the patient's medical record.

Date: _____

Charting: _____

_____

_____

_____

Student's Name: _____       Physician's Initials: __(     )__

# PERFORMANCE EVALUATION CHECKLIST

Name _____

Date _____ Score* _____

---

## PROCEDURE 15-12   Test Urine with Multistix® 10   SG

*PERFORMANCE OBJECTIVE*—Demonstrate the steps required to perform the procedure for using Multistix® 10 SG.

| PROCEDURE STEPS | STEP PERFORMED | POINTS POSSIBLE | COMMENTS |
|---|---|---|---|
| *EVALUATOR:* Place check mark in space following each step performed satisfactorily | | | |
| NOTE TIME BEGAN _____ | | | |
| 1. Washed hands. | _____ | 5 | |
|   a. Put on gloves | _____ | 5 | |
| 2. Assembled all needed items. | _____ | 5 | |
| 3. Stirred urine with tongue depressor. | _____ | 10 | |
| 4. Removed cap from bottle. | _____ | 5 | |
| 5. Took reagent strip out without touching test paper end. | _____ | 5 | |
| 6. Placed cap back on bottle securely. | _____ | 5 | |
| 7. Reviewed times given for reading each test on bottle. | _____ | 5 | |
| 8. Dipped test paper end of reagent strip into urine specimen. | _____ | 5 | |
| 9. Removed strip by touching its edge against inside of container to remove excess urine. | _____ | 5 | |
| 10. Began timing test immediately. | _____ | 15 | |
| 11. Placed reagent strip next to color chart. | _____ | 10 | |
| 12. Read each test section at proper time. | _____ | 15 | |
| 13. Discarded disposables in proper receptacle. | _____ | 5 | |
| 14. Returned items to proper storage. | _____ | 5 | |
| 15. Removed gloves. | _____ | 5 | |
|   a. Washed hands | _____ | 5 | |
| 16. Recorded results of each test section on patient's chart. | _____ | 15 | |
| *EVALUATOR:* NOTE TIME COMPLETED _____ | | | |

ADD POINTS OF STEPS CHECKED             _____ EARNED

TOTAL POINTS POSSIBLE            130 POSSIBLE

Points assigned reflect importance of step to meeting objective: Important = (5)   Essential = (10)   Critical = (15)
Automatic failure results if any of the critical steps are omitted or performed incorrectly.

DETERMINE SCORE (divide points earned by total points possible, multiply results by 100)    _____ SCORE*

Evaluator's Name (print) _____ Signature _____

Comments _____

## DOCUMENTATION

Chart the procedure in the patient's medical record.

Date: _____

Charting: _____

_____

_____

_____

Student's Name: _____          Physician's Initials: __(___)__

## PROCEDURE 15-13    Determine Glucose Content of Urine with Clinitest Tablet

*PERFORMANCE OBJECTIVE*—Demonstrate the steps in the procedure for using Clinitest tablets to determine the glucose content of urine.

| PROCEDURE STEPS | STEP PERFORMED | POINTS POSSIBLE | COMMENTS |
|---|---|---|---|
| *EVALUATOR:* Place check mark in space following each step performed satisfactorily | | | |
| NOTE TIME BEGAN _____ | | | |
| 1. Washed hands. | _____ | 5 | |
|    a. Put on gloves | _____ | 5 | |
| 2. Assembled needed items. | _____ | 5 | |
| 3. Stirred urine with tongue depressor. | _____ | 5 | |
| 4. Filled dropper halfway with urine. | _____ | 5 | |
| 5. Held test tube near top between thumb and index finger. | _____ | 5 | |
| 6. Released five drops of urine into test tube. | _____ | 10 | |
| 7. Rinsed dropper. | _____ | 5 | |
| 8. Half filled dropper with water. | _____ | 10 | |
| 9. Released ten drops water into test tube. | _____ | 10 | |
| 10. Mixed gently. | _____ | 5 | |
| 11. Set test tube in rack. | _____ | 5 | |
| 12. Opened bottle. | _____ | 5 | |
| 13. Shook out one Clinitest tablet into bottle cap. | _____ | 10 | |
| 14. Dropped one tablet into test tube from cap. | _____ | 10 | |
| 15. Recapped bottle. | _____ | 5 | |
| 16. Watched reaction of tablet and urine-water mixture. | _____ | 15 | |
| 17. Began 15 second timing immediately when boiling stopped. | _____ | 15 | |
| 18. Held test tube at top. | _____ | 10 | |
| 19. Tilted test tube back and forth to mix contents. | _____ | 10 | |
| 20. Compared color of contents to color chart to read results. | _____ | 15 | |
| 21. Recorded results as % of milligrams/deciliter on patient's chart. | _____ | 15 | |
|    a. Initialed | _____ | 5 | |
| 22. Rinsed test tube with cold water. | _____ | 5 | |
| 23. Washed and dried test tube and dropper. | _____ | 5 | |

| PROCEDURE STEPS | STEP PERFORMED | POINTS POSSIBLE | COMMENTS |
|---|---|---|---|
| 24.  Discarded disposables in proper receptacle. | _____ | 5 | |
| 25.  Removed gloves. | _____ | 5 | |
|    a.  Washed hands | _____ | 5 | |
| 26.  Returned items to proper storage. | _____ | 5 | |
| *EVALUATOR:* NOTE TIME COMPLETED _____ | | | |

ADD POINTS OF STEPS CHECKED             _____ EARNED

TOTAL POINTS POSSIBLE             220 POSSIBLE

Points assigned reflect importance of step to meeting objective:  Important  = (5)   Essential = (10)   Critical = (15)
Automatic failure results if any of the critical steps are omitted or performed incorrectly.

DETERMINE SCORE (divide points earned by total points possible, multiply results by 100)    _____ SCORE*

Evaluator's Name (print) _____ Signature _____

Comments _____

---

## DOCUMENTATION

Chart the procedure in the patient's medical record.

Date: _____

Charting: _____

_____

_____

_____

Student's Name: _____        Physician's Initials:  _(     )_

Name _____

Date _____ Score* _____

## PROCEDURE 15-14   Obtain Urine Sediment for Microscopic Examination

*PERFORMANCE OBJECTIVE*—Demonstrate all steps required in the procedure for obtaining urine sediment for microscopic examination.

| PROCEDURE STEPS | STEP PERFORMED | POINTS POSSIBLE | COMMENTS |
|---|---|---|---|
| *EVALUATOR:* Place check mark in space following each step performed satisfactorily | | | |
| NOTE TIME BEGAN _____ | | | |
| 1. Washed hands. | _____ | 5 | |
| a. Put on gloves | _____ | 5 | |
| 2. Assembled all needed items near patient. | _____ | 5 | |
| a. Explained procedure | _____ | 5 | |
| 3. Identified patient. | _____ | 5 | |
| 4. Performed skin puncture. | _____ | 5 | |
| 5. Filled RBC unopette pipette and reservoir: | _____ | 10 | |
| a. Punctured diaphragm of reservoir | _____ | 10 | |
| b. Removed shield from pipette assembly with a twist | _____ | 5 | |
| c. Held pipette almost horizontally to touch tip of pipette to sample | _____ | 5 | |
| d. Wiped excess sample from pipette | _____ | 5 | |
| e. Squeezed reservoir slightly | _____ | 5 | |
| f. Covered opening of overflow chamber with index finger and seated pipette securely in reservoir neck | _____ | 5 | |
| g. Released pressure on reservoir | _____ | 5 | |
| h. Squeezed reservoir gently 2 to 3 times to rinse capillary bore | _____ | 5 | |
| i. Placed index finger over upper opening and gently inverted several times to mix well | _____ | 5 | |
| 6. Converted to dropper assembly: | | | |
| a. Withdrew pipette from reservoir and reseated securely in reverse position | _____ | 5 | |
| b. Inverted reservoir and gently squeezed sides to discard first 3 to 4 drops | _____ | 5 | |
| 7. Positioned cover glass onto hemocytometer. | _____ | 5 | |
| 8. Placed tip of pipette almost touching the "V" on the slide's chamber. | _____ | 10 | |
| 9. Released moderate drop of solution onto both sides of chamber. | _____ | 10 | |
| 10. Waited 2 to 3 minutes for cells to settle. | _____ | 5 | |
| 11. Placed slide on microscope stage. | _____ | 5 | |
| a. Turned light on | _____ | 5 | |

| PROCEDURE STEPS | STEP PERFORMED | POINTS POSSIBLE | COMMENTS |
|---|---|---|---|
| 22.  Removed gloves. | _____ | 5 | |
| a.  Washed hands | _____ | 5 | |
| 23.  Returned items to proper storage. | _____ | 5 | |

*EVALUATOR:* NOTE TIME COMPLETED _____

ADD POINTS OF STEPS CHECKED                                                    _____ EARNED
TOTAL POINTS POSSIBLE                                                              195 POSSIBLE

Points assigned reflect importance of step to meeting objective:  Important  = (5)   Essential = (10)   Critical = (15)
Automatic failure results if any of the critical steps are omitted or performed incorrectly.

DETERMINE SCORE (divide points earned by total points possible, multiply results by 100)          _____ SCORE*

Evaluator's Name (print) _____ Signature _____

Comments _____

---

## DOCUMENTATION

Chart the procedure in the patient's medical record.

Date: _____

Charting: _____

_____

_____

_____

Student's Name: _____        Physician's Initials: _(____)_

Name _____

Date _____ Score* _____

## PROCEDURE 15-15   Instruct Patient to Collect Sputum Specimen

*PERFORMANCE OBJECTIVE*—Demonstrate all steps required in the procedure for instructing a patient in the collection of a sputum specimen for analysis.

| PROCEDURE STEPS | STEP PERFORMED | POINTS POSSIBLE | COMMENTS |
|---|---|---|---|
| *EVALUATOR:* Place check mark in space following each step performed satisfactorily | | | |
| NOTE TIME BEGAN _____ | | | |
| 1. Assembled items next to patient. | _____ | 10 | |
| 2. Wrote patient's name on specimen cup label. | _____ | 10 | |
| 3. Completed lab request form. | _____ | 5 | |
| 4. Explained physician's orders to patient. | _____ | 10 | |
|    a. Wrote instructions out/gave printed instructions to patient | _____ | 15 | |
| 5. Instructed patient to: | | | |
|    a. Expel only those secretions of first AM coughing episode into center of cup | _____ | 15 | |
|    b. Fill cup one-half full | _____ | 10 | |
|    c. Seal with cover | _____ | 5 | |
|    d. Write time and date on label and request form | _____ | 10 | |
|    e. Take to lab/medical office as soon as possible | _____ | 10 | |
|    f. Secure lab request form to specimen container with tape or rubber band | _____ | 5 | |
|    g. Refrigerate if she/he cannot take within two hours | _____ | 10 | |
| 6. Record what instructions were given to patient. | _____ | 5 | |
|    a. Initialed | _____ | 5 | |
| *EVALUATOR:* NOTE TIME COMPLETED _____ | | | |

ADD POINTS OF STEPS CHECKED                  _____ EARNED
TOTAL POINTS POSSIBLE                                    125 POSSIBLE

Points assigned reflect importance of step to meeting objective: Important = (5)   Essential = (10)   Critical = (15)
Automatic failure results if any of the critical steps are omitted or performed incorrectly.

DETERMINE SCORE (divide points earned by total points possible, multiply results by 100)       _____ SCORE*

Evaluator's Name (print) _____ Signature _____

Comments _____

# DOCUMENTATION

Chart the procedure in the patient's medical record.

Date: _____

Charting: _____

_____

_____

_____

Student's Name: _____     Physician's Initials: __(_____)__

Name _____

Date _____ Score* _____

## PROCEDURE 15-16   Instruct Patient to Collect a Stool Specimen

*PERFORMANCE OBJECTIVE*—Demonstrate the steps required in the procedure for instructing a patient in the collection of an adequate stool specimen for laboratory analysis.

| PROCEDURE STEPS | STEP PERFORMED | POINTS POSSIBLE | COMMENTS |
|---|---|---|---|
| *EVALUATOR:* Place check mark in space following each step performed satisfactorily | | | |
| NOTE TIME BEGAN _____ | | | |
| 1. Assembled items next to patient. | _____ | 10 | |
| 2. Identified patient. | _____ | 10 | |
| 3. Explained physician's orders. | _____ | 10 | |
| 4. Gave printed instructions or wrote out. | _____ | 10 | |
| 5. Wrote information on label of specimen cups and lab request form. | _____ | 5 | |
| 6. Instructed patient to: | | | |
|   a. Obtain small amount of stool from next bowel movement with tongue depressor | _____ | 15 | |
|   b. Place specimen in container | _____ | 10 | |
|   c. Secure cup with cover | _____ | 5 | |
|   d. Write date and time of specimen on label | _____ | 5 | |
|   e. Write time and date on request form and attach request form to specimen container | _____ | 5 | |
|   f. Take to lab/medical office as soon as possible | _____ | 10 | |
|   g. Refrigerate specimen if she/he cannot take within two hours | _____ | 10 | |
| 7. Explained when report would be available. | _____ | 5 | |
| 8. Recorded that instructions were given on patient's chart. | _____ | 15 | |
|   a. Initialed | _____ | 5 | |

*EVALUATOR:* NOTE TIME COMPLETED _____

ADD POINTS OF STEPS CHECKED                                              _____ EARNED
TOTAL POINTS POSSIBLE                                                       130 POSSIBLE

Points assigned reflect importance of step to meeting objective: Important = (5)   Essential = (10)   Critical = (15)
Automatic failure results if any of the critical steps are omitted or performed incorrectly.

DETERMINE SCORE (divide points earned by total points possible, multiply results by 100)          _____ SCORE*

Evaluator's Name (print) _____ Signature _____

Comments _____

# DOCUMENTATION

Chart the procedure in the patient's medical record.

Date: _____

Charting: _____

_____

_____

_____

Student's Name: _____          Physician's Initials: __(_____)__

Name _____

Date _____ Score* _____

## PROCEDURE 15-17    Perform a Hemoccult® Sensa® Test

*PERFORMANCE OBJECTIVE*—Demonstrate each step required in the Hemoccult® Sensa® testing procedure.

| PROCEDURE STEPS | STEP PERFORMED | POINTS POSSIBLE | COMMENTS |
|---|---|---|---|
| *EVALUATOR:* Place check mark in space following each step performed satisfactorily | | | |
| NOTE TIME BEGAN _____ | | | |
| 1. Washed hands. | _____ | 5 | |
| 2. Put on gloves. | _____ | 5 | |
| 3. Assembled items needed for testing on counter. | _____ | 10 | |
| 4. Opened test slide of Hemoccult paper slide. | _____ | 10 | |
| 5. Removed cap from bottle of developer. | _____ | 5 | |
| 6. Placed 2 drops of developer on each of three sections: | | | |
| a. A | _____ | 15 | |
| b. B | _____ | 15 | |
| c. Control | _____ | 15 | |
| 7. Began timing immediately for 60 seconds. | _____ | 15 | |
| 8. Watched closely for any change of color at 30 seconds. | _____ | 5 | |
| 9. Compared test with control and read results after 60-second time period. | _____ | 15 | |
| 10. Recorded results on patient's chart. | _____ | 15 | |
| a. Initialed | _____ | 5 | |
| 11. Discarded disposables. | _____ | 5 | |
| 12. Returned items to proper storage. | _____ | 5 | |
| 13. Removed gloves. | _____ | 5 | |
| a. Washed hands | _____ | 5 | |
| *EVALUATOR:* NOTE TIME COMPLETED _____ | | | |

ADD POINTS OF STEPS CHECKED                                        _____ EARNED

TOTAL POINTS POSSIBLE                                                        155 POSSIBLE

Points assigned reflect importance of step to meeting objective: Important = (5)   Essential = (10)   Critical = (15)
Automatic failure results if any of the critical steps are omitted or performed incorrectly.

DETERMINE SCORE (divide points earned by total points possible, multiply results by 100)        _____ SCORE*

Evaluator's Name (print) _____ Signature _____

Comments _____

# DOCUMENTATION

Chart the procedure in the patient's medical record.

Date: _____

Charting: _____

_____

_____

_____

Student's Name: _____          Physician's Initials: __(____)__

Name _____

Date _____ Score* _____

## PROCEDURE 15-18   Prepare Bacteriological Smear

*PERFORMANCE OBJECTIVE*—Demonstrate the steps of the procedure for preparing a bacteriological smear for microscopic analysis.

| PROCEDURE STEPS | STEP PERFORMED | POINTS POSSIBLE | COMMENTS |
|---|---|---|---|
| *EVALUATOR:* Place check mark in space following each step performed satisfactorily | | | |
| NOTE TIME BEGAN _____ | | | |
| 1. Assembled all needed items. | _____ | 10 | |
| 2. Penciled patient's name on frosted end of glass slide. | _____ | 10 | |
| 3. Completed lab request form. | _____ | 5 | |
| 4. Washed hands. | _____ | 5 | |
| a. Put on gloves | _____ | 5 | |
| 5. Prepared smear(s): | _____ | 5 | |
| a. Held slide with thumb and great finger | _____ | 5 | |
| b. Rolled swab containing specimen evenly over two-thirds of slide | _____ | 15 | |
| 6. Lit bunsen burner. | _____ | 5 | |
| a. Adjusted flame | _____ | 5 | |
| 7. Held frosted part of slide with forceps or thumb and index finger. | _____ | 5 | |
| 8. Passed smear (side up) of slide through blue flame two or three times. | _____ | 15 | |
| 9. Turned burner off. | _____ | 5 | |
| 10. Placed heat-fixed smear on staining rack or Placed on stage of microscope for observation. | _____ | 10 | |
| 11. Discarded used disposables in proper receptacle. | _____ | 5 | |
| 12. Returned items to proper storage. | _____ | 5 | |
| 13. Removed gloves. | _____ | 5 | |
| a. Washed hands | _____ | 5 | |
| 14. Recorded procedure on patient's chart | _____ | 5 | |
| a. Initialed | _____ | 5 | |
| *EVALUATOR:* NOTE TIME COMPLETED _____ | | | |

ADD POINTS OF STEPS CHECKED                                   _____ EARNED

TOTAL POINTS POSSIBLE                                                135 POSSIBLE

Points assigned reflect importance of step to meeting objective: Important = (5)   Essential = (10)   Critical = (15)
Automatic failure results if any of the critical steps are omitted or performed incorrectly.

DETERMINE SCORE (divide points earned by total points possible, multiply results by 100)          _____ SCORE*

Evaluator's Name (print) _____ Signature _____

Comments _____

# DOCUMENTATION

Chart the procedure in the patient's medical record.

Date: _____

Charting: _____

_____

_____

_____

Student's Name: _____          Physician's Initials: __(____)__

Name _____

Date _____ Score* _____

## PROCEDURE 15-19   Obtain a Throat Culture

*PERFORMANCE OBJECTIVE*—Demonstrate the steps required to perform the procedure for obtaining a throat culture.

| PROCEDURE STEPS | STEP PERFORMED | POINTS POSSIBLE | COMMENTS |
|---|---|---|---|
| *EVALUATOR:* Place check mark in space following each step performed satisfactorily | | | |
| NOTE TIME BEGAN _____ | | | |
| 1. Identified patient. | _____ | 5 | |
| 2. Washed hands. | _____ | 10 | |
| a. Put on gloves | _____ | 5 | |
| b. Assembled needed items near patient | _____ | 5 | |
| 3. Labeled culture plate. | _____ | 5 | |
| a. Completed lab request form if required | _____ | 10 | |
| 4. Explained procedure to patient. | _____ | 5 | |
| 5. Assisted patient into comfortable position. | _____ | 5 | |
| a. Asked for assistance if child. | _____ | 5 | |
| 6. Opened sterile swab. | _____ | 5 | |
| 7. Asked patient to open mouth wide. | _____ | 5 | |
| 8. Examined patient's throat visually with light. | _____ | 10 | |
| 9. Depressed tongue with sterile tongue depressor. | _____ | 15 | |
| 10. Asked patient to say "ahh." | _____ | 15 | |
| 11. Inserted sterile swab to back of throat. | _____ | 5 | |
| 12. Rolled swab over area to obtain specimen. | _____ | 15 | |
| 13. Removed swab and depressor from patient's mouth. | _____ | 10 | |
| 14. Attended to patient; offered tissue. | _____ | 10 | |
| 15. Applied specimen to agar of petri dish in pattern. | _____ | 15 | |
| 16. Placed lid on dish. | _____ | 5 | |
| a. Secured with tape | _____ | 5 | |
| 17. Discarded disposables in proper receptacle. | _____ | 5 | |
| 18. Placed culture dish in incubator bottom up<br>or<br>Attached request form and sent to lab. | _____ | 5 | |
| 19. Removed gloves. | _____ | 5 | |
| a. Washed hands | _____ | 5 | |

| PROCEDURE STEPS | STEP PERFORMED | POINTS POSSIBLE | COMMENTS |
|---|---|---|---|
| 20. Recorded procedure in patient's chart. | _____ | 5 | |
|    a. Initialed | _____ | 5 | |

*EVALUATOR:* NOTE TIME COMPLETED _____

ADD POINTS OF STEPS CHECKED                                     _____ EARNED

TOTAL POINTS POSSIBLE                                             200 POSSIBLE

Points assigned reflect importance of step to meeting objective:  Important = (5)   Essential = (10)   Critical = (15)
Automatic failure results if any of the critical steps are omitted or performed incorrectly.

DETERMINE SCORE (divide points earned by total points possible, multiply results by 100)      _____ SCORE*

Evaluator's Name (print) _____ Signature _____

Comments _____

---

## DOCUMENTATION

Chart the procedure in the patient's medical record.

Date: _____

Charting: _____

_____

_____

_____

Student's Name: _____        Physician's Initials: __(_____)__

Name _____

Date _____ Score* _____

## PROCEDURE 15-20   Prepare Gram Stain

*PERFORMANCE OBJECTIVE*—Demonstrate the steps of the procedure for preparing a Gram stain.

| PROCEDURE STEPS | STEP PERFORMED | POINTS POSSIBLE | COMMENTS |
|---|---|---|---|
| *EVALUATOR:* Place check mark in space following each step performed satisfactorily | | | |
| NOTE TIME BEGAN _____ | | | |
| 1. Assembled all needed items on counter. | _____ | 10 | |
| 2. Washed hands. | _____ | 5 | |
|    a. Put apron/gloves on | _____ | 5 | |
| 3. Placed heat-fixed slide on staining rack. | _____ | 5 | |
| 4. Opened crystal violet dye. | _____ | 5 | |
| 5. Filled dropper. | _____ | 5 | |
| 6. Applied over entire specimen area of slide. | _____ | 10 | |
| 7. Timed for sixty seconds. | _____ | 10 | |
| 8. Held frosted end with forceps. | _____ | 5 | |
| 9. Tipped slide to allow stain to run off into tray. | _____ | 5 | |
| 10. Washed slide with water from top to bottom. | _____ | 10 | |
| 11. Placed slide flat on rack. | _____ | 5 | |
| 12. Filled dropper with Gram's iodine. | _____ | 10 | |
| 13. Applied over entire specimen area. | _____ | 10 | |
| 14. Tipped slide to allow stain to run off. | _____ | 5 | |
| 15. Refilled dropper with Gram's iodine. | _____ | 10 | |
| 16. Applied to entire specimen area. | _____ | 10 | |
|    a. Timed for sixty seconds | _____ | 5 | |
| 17. Tipped slide to allow stain to run off. | _____ | 5 | |
| 18. Washed slide with water. | _____ | 10 | |
| 19. Applied alcohol/acetone with dropper until purple color in excess runoff was gone. | _____ | 15 | |
| 20. Washed with water immediately. | _____ | 10 | |
| 21. Applied Safranin solution with dropper. | _____ | 10 | |
| 22. Immediately washed with water. | _____ | 10 | |
| 23. Held slide by frosted end. | _____ | 5 | |
| 24. Wiped excess solution from underneath. | _____ | 5 | |

| PROCEDURE STEPS | STEP PERFORMED | POINTS POSSIBLE | COMMENTS |
|---|---|---|---|
| 25. Held slide on its side and tapped onto paper towel to remove excess. | _____ | 5 | |
| 26. Allowed slide to air dry<br>or<br>Blotted slide carefully between two paper towels. | _____ | 5 | |
| 27. Applied small drop of immersion oil to specimen. | _____ | 5 | |
|    a. Placed cover glass on slide | _____ | 5 | |
| 28. Placed slide on stage of microscope to view. | _____ | 5 | |
|    a. Turned light source on to view | _____ | 5 | |
| 29. Discarded disposables in proper receptacle. | _____ | 5 | |
| 30. Washed used items. | _____ | 5 | |
| 31. Returned items to proper storage. | _____ | 5 | |
|    a. Replaced caps on bottles immediately after use | _____ | 5 | |
| 32. Removed gloves. | _____ | 5 | |
|    a. Washed hands | _____ | 5 | |
| 33. Recorded procedure and results on patient's chart. | _____ | 5 | |
|    a. Initialed | _____ | 15 | |

*EVALUATOR:* NOTE TIME COMPLETED _____

ADD POINTS OF STEPS CHECKED                             _____ EARNED

TOTAL POINTS POSSIBLE                                       280 POSSIBLE

Points assigned reflect importance of step to meeting objective: Important = (5)  Essential = (10)  Critical = (15)

Automatic failure results if any of the critical steps are omitted or performed incorrectly.

DETERMINE SCORE (divide points earned by total points possible, multiply results by 100)     _____ SCORE*

Evaluator's Name (print) _____ Signature _____

Comments _____

---

## DOCUMENTATION

Chart the procedure in the patient's medical record.

Date: _____

Charting: _____

_____

_____

_____

Student's Name: _____        Physician's Initials: __(_____)__

Name _____

Date _____ Score* _____

## PROCEDURE 16-1   Perform a Scratch Test

*PERFORMANCE OBJECTIVE*—Demonstrate each of the steps required in the scratch test procedure.

| PROCEDURE STEPS | STEP PERFORMED | POINTS POSSIBLE | COMMENTS |
|---|---|---|---|
| *EVALUATOR:* Place check mark in space following each step performed satisfactorily | | | |
| NOTE TIME BEGAN _____ | | | |
| 1. Identified patient. | _____ | 10 | |
| 2. Assembled all needed items next to patient. | _____ | 10 | |
| 3. Washed hands. | _____ | 5 | |
| 4. Put on gloves. | _____ | 5 | |
| 5. Explained procedure to patient. | _____ | 5 | |
| 6. Assisted patient into comfortable position. | _____ | 5 | |
| 7. Prepared test site with alcohol pad. | _____ | 5 | |
|    a. Allowed to air dry | _____ | 5 | |
| 8. Marked site(s) with initials or number of extract in pen. | _____ | 10 | |
|    a. Spaced adequately (about 1½″ to 2″ between each) | _____ | 10 | |
| 9. Applied small drop of extract onto site. | _____ | 10 | |
|    a. Repeated for each extract ordered | _____ | 10 | |
| 10. Removed sterile needle or lancet without contaminating it. | _____ | 15 | |
|    a. Made one-eighth inch scratch in surface of skin at site. | _____ | 15 | |
| 11. Began timing for 20 minutes. | _____ | 15 | |
| 12. Checked each site as soon as 20-minute period was up. | _____ | 15 | |
|    a. Cleaned each site with alcohol pad | _____ | 10 | |
|    b. Did not wash off extract identification | _____ | 15 | |
| 13. Washed hands. | _____ | 5 | |
| 14. Compared reaction sites with package insert drawing or measured reaction sites in centimeters. | _____ | 15 | |
| 15. Recorded test results on patient's chart. | _____ | 15 | |
|    a. Initialed | _____ | 5 | |
|    b. Attended to patient | _____ | 5 | |
| 16. Discarded disposables in proper receptacle. | _____ | 5 | |

| PROCEDURE STEPS | STEP PERFORMED | POINTS POSSIBLE | COMMENTS |
|---|---|---|---|
| 17. Returned items to proper storage area. | _____ | 5 | |
| 18. Removed gloves. | _____ | 5 | |
|   a. Washed hands | _____ | 5 | |

*EVALUATOR:* NOTE TIME COMPLETED _____

ADD POINTS OF STEPS CHECKED _____ EARNED

TOTAL POINTS POSSIBLE 240 POSSIBLE

Points assigned reflect importance of step to meeting objective: Important = (5)  Essential = (10)  Critical = (15)
Automatic failure results if any of the critical steps are omitted or performed incorrectly.

DETERMINE SCORE (divide points earned by total points possible, multiply results by 100) _____ SCORE*

Evaluator's Name (print) _____ Signature _____

Comments _____

---

## DOCUMENTATION

Chart the procedure in the patient's medical record.

Date: _____

Charting: _____

_____

_____

_____

Student's Name: _____  Physician's Initials: __(____)__

Name _____

Date _____ Score* _____

## PROCEDURE 16-2   Apply a Patch Test

*PERFORMANCE OBJECTIVE*—Demonstrate each of the steps required in carrying out the skin patch test, including the 48 hour recheck.

| PROCEDURE STEPS | STEP PERFORMED | POINTS POSSIBLE | COMMENTS |
|---|---|---|---|
| *EVALUATOR:* Place check mark in space following each step performed satisfactorily | | | |
| NOTE TIME BEGAN _____ | | | |
| 1. Identified patient. | _____ | 10 | |
| 2. Assembled items next to patient. | _____ | 10 | |
| 3. Washed hands. | _____ | 5 | |
| 4. Put on gloves. | _____ | 5 | |
| 5. Explained procedure to patient. | _____ | 5 | |
| 6. Assisted patient into comfortable sitting position. | _____ | 5 | |
| 7. Cleaned test site with alcohol pad. | _____ | 5 | |
|   a. Allowed to air dry | _____ | 5 | |
| 8. Applied substance to test site. | _____ | 10 | |
| 9. Secured substance to test site with non-allergic tape. | _____ | 15 | |
| 10. Recorded date, time, substance, and area tested on patient's chart. | _____ | 15 | |
|   a. Initialed | _____ | 5 | |
| 11. Scheduled patient to return in 48 hours for check. | _____ | 5 | |
| 12. Instructed patient to keep test area clean and dry. | _____ | 10 | |
| 13. Removed gloves. | _____ | 5 | |
|   a. Washed hands | _____ | 5 | |
| **When patient returned after 48 hours:** | | | |
| 14. Washed hands. | _____ | 5 | |
|   a. Put on gloves | _____ | 5 | |
| 15. Removed patch. | _____ | 5 | |
| 16. Read results of test. | _____ | 15 | |
| 17. Removed gloves. | _____ | 5 | |
|   a. Washed hands | _____ | 5 | |

| PROCEDURE STEPS | STEP PERFORMED | POINTS POSSIBLE | COMMENTS |
|---|---|---|---|
| Recorded results on patient's chart. | _____ | 5 | |
| a. Initialed | _____ | 5 | |
| *EVALUATOR:* NOTE TIME COMPLETED _____ | | | |

ADD POINTS OF STEPS CHECKED                                     _____ EARNED
TOTAL POINTS POSSIBLE                                                    170 POSSIBLE

Points assigned reflect importance of step to meeting objective: Important = (5)   Essential = (10)   Critical = (15)
Automatic failure results if any of the critical steps are omitted or performed incorrectly.

DETERMINE SCORE (divide points earned by total points possible, multiply results by 100)     _____ SCORE*

Evaluator's Name (print) _____ Signature _____

Comments _____

---

## DOCUMENTATION

Chart the procedure in the patient's medical record.

Date: _____

Charting: _____

_____

_____

_____

Student's Name: _____          Physician's Initials: __(____)__

Name _____

Date _____ Score* _____

## PROCEDURE 16-3   Obtain a Standard 12-Lead Electrocardiogram

*PERFORMANCE OBJECTIVE*—Demonstrate each of the steps required in obtaining a standard 12-lead ECG reading.

| PROCEDURE STEPS | STEP PERFORMED | POINTS POSSIBLE | COMMENTS |
|---|---|---|---|
| *EVALUATOR:* Place check mark in space following each step performed satisfactorily | | | |
| NOTE TIME BEGAN _____ | | | |
| 1.  Identified patient. | _____ | 5 | |
| 2.  Plugged in ECG machine to electrical outlet, away from known electrical interference. | _____ | 5 | |
| 3.  Assembled electrodes. | _____ | 5 | |
|     a.  Attached to straps | _____ | 5 | |
|     b.  Applied electrolyte pads | _____ | 5 | |
| 4.  Turned machine on. | _____ | 5 | |
| 5.  Washed hands. | _____ | 5 | |
| 6.  Asked patient to disrobe from waist up and remove clothing from lower legs. | _____ | 5 | |
| 7.  Explained procedure to patient. | _____ | 5 | |
| 8.  Assisted patient to table. | _____ | 5 | |
|     a.  Asked patient to lie down. | _____ | 5 | |
|     b.  Covered patient with drape sheet. | _____ | 5 | |
|     c.  Pulled out foot rest. | _____ | 5 | |
|     d.  Adjusted pillow under patient's head. | _____ | 5 | |
| Note: For computerized electrocardiographs: | | | |
|     a.  Applied limb and chest lead wires by clipping to disposable electrodes. | _____ | 15 | |
|     b.  Pressed "auto" to run complete 12-lead recording. | _____ | 10 | |
|     c.  Removed patient cable and proceeded with step 28. | _____ | 5 | |
| 9.  Placed chest strap with hard plastic end under left side of patient's back. | _____ | 5 | |
|     a.  Weighed end at patient's right side. | _____ | 5 | |
| 10.  Placed upper limb electrodes on outer fleshy area of upper arms. | _____ | 10 | |
|     a.  Pointed connectors of electrodes toward shoulders. | _____ | 5 | |
|     b.  Moved straps one space tighter than relaxed. | _____ | 5 | |
| 11.  Placed lower limb electrodes on inner fleshy area of lower legs. | _____ | 5 | |
|     a.  Pointed connectors toward upper part of body | _____ | 5 | |

| PROCEDURE STEPS | STEP PERFORMED | POINTS POSSIBLE | COMMENTS |
|---|---|---|---|
| 12. Connected lead wire tips to electrodes, all pointing downward. | _____ | 5 | |
| 13. Placed power cord directed away from patient. | _____ | 5 | |
| 14. Placed chest electrode under chest strap. | _____ | 5 | |
|    a. Placed electrolyte side up | _____ | 5 | |
| 15. Turned lead selector switch to STD. | _____ | 5 | |
|    a. Adjusted stylus to center of graph paper. | _____ | 5 | |
| 16. Moved record switch to 25 mm/second position. | _____ | 10 | |
|    a. Ran for a few seconds to adjust centering | _____ | 5 | |
|    b. Made standardization mark correctly | _____ | 5 | |
|    c. Turned off | _____ | 5 | |
| 17. Turned lead selector switch to Lead I. | _____ | 15 | |
|    a. Ran 8″–12″ of tracing. | _____ | 15 | |
|    b. Proceeded to run 8″–12″ of Leads II and III. | _____ | 15 | |
| 18. Ran 4″–6″ of leads aVR, aVL and aVF. | _____ | 15 | |
| 19. Paused between leads to allow machine to adjust automatically. | _____ | 5 | |
| 20. Made standardization mark at the beginning of each lead. | _____ | 5 | |
| 21. Marked each lead appropriately with correct code marking. | _____ | 15 | |
| 22. Placed chest electrode in proper positions, V1–V6. | _____ | 15 | |
|    a. Standardized each lead | _____ | 5 | |
|    b. Ran 4″–6″ of each | _____ | 5 | |
|    c. Marked each lead correctly | _____ | 15 | |
|    d. Turned switch to AMP off when changing electrode position | _____ | 5 | |
|    e. Paused a few seconds between leads to allow stylus to adjust | _____ | 5 | |
| 23. Turned lead selector switch back to STD slowly. | _____ | 5 | |
|    a. Ran tracing out until only baseline appears | _____ | 5 | |
| 24. Turned machine off. | _____ | 5 | |
| 25. Tore tracing from machine. | _____ | 5 | |
|    a. Marked immediately with patient's name, age, date | _____ | 10 | |
|    b. Initialed | _____ | 5 | |
| 26. Rolled or loosely overlapped tracing and secured with paper clip. | _____ | 5 | |
| 27. Removed tips of lead wires from limb electrodes. | _____ | 5 | |
|    a. Removed chest electrode and strap | _____ | 5 | |
|    b. Removed limb straps from patient | _____ | 5 | |

| PROCEDURE STEPS | STEP PERFORMED | POINTS POSSIBLE | COMMENTS |
|---|---|---|---|
| c. Instructed patient to wash areas well | _____ | 5 | |
| 28. Removed electrolyte from areas with warmed towel; dried area. | _____ | 5 | |
| a. Discarded in proper receptacle | _____ | 5 | |
| 29. Assisted patient to sitting position. | _____ | 5 | |
| a. Assisted patient down from table | _____ | 5 | |
| b. Assisted to dress PRN | _____ | 5 | |
| 30. Changed table paper and pillow cover. | _____ | 5 | |
| a. Discarded disposables | _____ | 5 | |
| 31. Washed hands. | _____ | 5 | |
| 32. Placed tracing in patient's chart. | _____ | 5 | |
| a. Initialed ECG order in chart | _____ | 5 | |
| b. Placed tracing in appropriate area for physician to read<br>or<br>Mounted tracing/placed in patient's chart for physician to read. | _____ | 5 | |
| 33. Recorded any unusual findings or observations on patient's chart. | _____ | 10 | |

*EVALUATOR:* NOTE TIME COMPLETED _____

ADD POINTS OF STEPS CHECKED                                     _____ EARNED
TOTAL POINTS POSSIBLE                                           455  POSSIBLE Steps 1–33
                                                               140  *Steps 1–8; 28–33

Points assigned reflect importance of step to meeting objective:  Important = (5)   Essential = (10)   Critical = (15)
Automatic failure results if any of the critical steps are omitted or performed incorrectly.

DETERMINE SCORE (divide points earned by total points possible, multiply results by 100)        _____ SCORE*

Evaluator's Name (print) _____ Signature _____

Comments _____

---

**DOCUMENTATION**

Chart the procedure in the patient's medical record.

Date: _____

Charting: _____

_____

_____

_____

Student's Name: _____          Physician's Initials: __(    )__

Name _____

Date _____ Score* _____

# PROCEDURE 16-4   Holter Monitoring

*PERFORMANCE OBJECTIVE*—Demonstrate the steps of the procedure for hooking up a patient for the Holter monitor.

| PROCEDURE STEPS | STEP PERFORMED | POINTS POSSIBLE | COMMENTS |
|---|---|---|---|
| *EVALUATOR:* Place check mark in space following each step performed satisfactorily | | | |
| NOTE TIME BEGAN _____ | | | |
| 1. Identified patient. | _____ | 5 | |
| 2. Explained procedure to patient. | _____ | 5 | |
| 3. Asked patient to remove clothing from the waist up. | _____ | 5 | |
| 4. Provided drape sheet. | _____ | 5 | |
| 5. Assisted patient to end of exam table. | _____ | 5 | |
| 6. Washed hands. | _____ | 5 | |
| 7. Assembled equipment and supplies near patient. | _____ | 5 | |
| 8. Tested Holter monitor for proper function. | _____ | 15 | |
| 9. Used shaving cream and razor to remove excess hair from patient's chest. | _____ | 10 | |
| 10. Rinsed, dried, and used alcohol on electrode sites. | _____ | 5 | |
| 11. Rubbed each site vigorously with gauze squares. | _____ | 10 | |
| 12. Applied electrodes/lead wires. | _____ | 15 | |
|    a. Made good contact | _____ | 15 | |
|    b. Secured electrodes with tape | _____ | 10 | |
| 13. Placed belt with recorder around patient's waist. | _____ | 10 | |
|    a. Advised patient in care of recorder | _____ | 10 | |
| 14. Assisted patient in dressing. | _____ | 5 | |
| 15. Instructed patient to perform routine activities. | _____ | 5 | |
|    a. Advised not to bathe in tub or shower | _____ | 10 | |
| 16. Recorded date and time monitor began on patient's chart. | _____ | 15 | |
|    a. Recorded in patient's diary | _____ | 10 | |
| 17. Instructed patient to record symptoms in diary. | _____ | 10 | |
| 18. Gave patient return appointment time in 24 hours. | _____ | 10 | |
| 19. When patient returned: | | | |
|    a. Assisted patient in disrobing | _____ | 5 | |
|    b. Removed electrodes and wires | _____ | 5 | |

| PROCEDURE STEPS | STEP PERFORMED | POINTS POSSIBLE | COMMENTS |
|---|---|---|---|
| c. Placed cassette in computerized ECG for printout of tracing | _____ | 15 | |
| d. Placed diary and recording of ECG in patient's chart | _____ | 10 | |
| e. Initialed | _____ | 5 | |
| *EVALUATOR:* NOTE TIME COMPLETED _____ | | | |

ADD POINTS OF STEPS CHECKED      _____ EARNED

TOTAL POINTS POSSIBLE      240 POSSIBLE

Points assigned reflect importance of step to meeting objective: Important = (5) Essential = (10) Critical = (15)
Automatic failure results if any of the critical steps are omitted or performed incorrectly.

DETERMINE SCORE (divide points earned by total points possible, multiply results by 100)      _____ SCORE*

Evaluator's Name (print) _____ Signature _____

Comments _____

---

## DOCUMENTATION

Chart the procedure in the patient's medical record.

Date: _____

Charting: _____

_____

_____

_____

Student's Name: _____      Physician's Initials: _(    )_

# PERFORMANCE EVALUATION CHECKLIST

Name _____

Date _____ Score* _____

---

## PROCEDURE 17-1   Prepare Skin for Minor Surgery

*PERFORMANCE OBJECTIVE*—Demonstrate each of the steps required in the skin prep procedure for minor surgery.

| PROCEDURE STEPS | STEP PERFORMED | POINTS POSSIBLE | COMMENTS |
|---|---|---|---|
| *EVALUATOR:* Place check mark in space following each step performed satisfactorily | | | |
| NOTE TIME BEGAN _____ | | | |
| 1. Washed hands. | _____ | 5 | |
| 2. Assembled all necessary items. | _____ | 10 | |
| 3. Identified patient. | _____ | 5 | |
|    a. Explained procedure to patient | _____ | 5 | |
| 4. Asked patient to remove necessary clothing. | _____ | 5 | |
|    a. Instructed patient where to put clothing | _____ | 5 | |
|    b. Assisted patient as necessary | _____ | 5 | |
| 5. Positioned patient appropriately. | _____ | 5 | |
|    a. Draped patient appropriately | _____ | 5 | |
| 6. Positioned Mayo table over patient near surgical site. | _____ | 5 | |
| 7. Positioned gooseneck lamp over site. | _____ | 5 | |
| 8. Placed gauze squares in soapy solution. | _____ | 10 | |
|    a. Used one at a time to soap area to be shaved. | _____ | 10 | |
|    b. Discarded each in basin after use | _____ | 10 | |
| 9. Used scissors to clip hair as necessary. | _____ | 10 | |
| 10. Shaved hair placing razor at 30° angle. | _____ | 10 | |
|    a. Held skin taut while shaving | _____ | 10 | |
|    b. Shaved in direction hair grows | _____ | 15 | |
|    c. Wiped hair and soap from razor with tissues | _____ | 10 | |
|    d. Swished razor through soapy water | _____ | 5 | |
|    e. Shook excess water from razor | _____ | 5 | |
|    f. Repeated steps 10 a through e as necessary | _____ | 15 | |
| 11. Removed all soap and hair from site with sterile gauze and water. | _____ | 10 | |
|    a. Dried area with sterile gauze squares | _____ | 5 | |
| 12. Applied antiseptic solution to site with sterile gauze. | _____ | 15 | |
|    a. Applied in a circular motion from center outward | _____ | 10 | |

| PROCEDURE STEPS | STEP PERFORMED | POINTS POSSIBLE | COMMENTS |
|---|---|---|---|
| 13. Covered skin prep area with sterile drape sheet. | _____ | 10 | |
| a. Instructed patient not to touch site/tray | _____ | 5 | |
| 14. Discarded disposable items in proper container. | _____ | 5 | |
| 15. Returned reusable items to proper storage. | _____ | 5 | |
| 16. Removed gloves and discarded properly. | _____ | 5 | |
| 17. Washed hands. | _____ | 5 | |
| 18. Initialed procedure completed. | _____ | 5 | |
| 19. Attended to patient comfort. | _____ | 5 | |

*EVALUATOR:* NOTE TIME COMPLETED _____

ADD POINTS OF STEPS CHECKED ........................................................................................ _____ EARNED

TOTAL POINTS POSSIBLE .................................................................................................... 255 POSSIBLE

Points assigned reflect importance of step to meeting objective:  Important  = (5)   Essential = (10)   Critical = (15)
Automatic failure results if any of the critical steps are omitted or performed incorrectly.

DETERMINE SCORE (divide points earned by total points possible, multiply results by 100) _____ SCORE*

Evaluator's Name (print) _____ Signature _____

Comments _____

---

## DOCUMENTATION

Chart the procedure in the patient's medical record.

Date: _____

Charting: _____

_____

_____

_____

Student's Name: _____        Physician's Initials: __(      )__

Name _____

Date _____ Score* _____

## PROCEDURE 17-2   Put on Sterile Gloves

*PERFORMANCE OBJECTIVE*—Demonstrate the correct method of putting on sterile gloves.

| PROCEDURE STEPS | STEP PERFORMED | POINTS POSSIBLE | COMMENTS |
|---|---|---|---|
| *EVALUATOR:* Place check mark in space following each step performed satisfactorily | | | |
| NOTE TIME BEGAN _____ | | | |
| 1. Selected appropriate size gloves. | _____ | 10 | |
| 2. Removed jewelry. | _____ | 5 | |
| 3. Performed surgical scrub. | _____ | 10 | |
| a. Used nail brush | _____ | 5 | |
| b. Thoroughly dried hands | _____ | 5 | |
| 4. Opened sterile gloves without contaminating them. | _____ | 15 | |
| a. Placed package on counter with cuffs of gloves toward body | _____ | 10 | |
| 5. Grasped cuff with finger and thumb of non-dominant hand. | _____ | 10 | |
| a. Inserted dominant hand in glove | _____ | 10 | |
| b. Pulled glove onto dominant hand by pulling cuff with non-dominant hand | _____ | 10 | |
| 6. Placed gloved fingers under cuff of other glove. | _____ | 15 | |
| a. Inserted hand into glove | _____ | 10 | |
| b. Pushed up on folded cuff | _____ | 10 | |
| 7. Placed gloved fingers under each cuff to smooth gloves over wrists | _____ | 15 | |
| a. Checked gloves for tears and holes. | _____ | 10 | |
| 8. Kept hands above waist level. | _____ | 10 | |
| a. Did not touch anything other than sterile items. | _____ | 10 | |
| 9. Removed gloves by pulling outside cuff with thumb and fingers. | _____ | 10 | |
| a. Pulled gloves off inside out | _____ | 5 | |
| b. Did not touch contaminated side | _____ | 5 | |

# PROCEDURE 17-2  Put on Sterile Gloves—continued

| PROCEDURE STEPS | STEP PERFORMED | POINTS POSSIBLE | COMMENTS |
|---|---|---|---|
| 10.  Placed gloves in biohazard bag. | _____ | 5 | |
| *EVALUATOR:* NOTE TIME COMPLETED _____ | | | |

ADD POINTS OF STEPS CHECKED                                             _____ EARNED

TOTAL POINTS POSSIBLE                                                          195 POSSIBLE

Points assigned reflect importance of step to meeting objective:  Important  = (5)   Essential = (10)   Critical = (15)
Automatic failure results if any of the critical steps are omitted or performed incorrectly.

DETERMINE SCORE (divide points earned by total points possible, multiply results by 100)        _____ SCORE*

Evaluator's Name (print) _____ Signature _____

Comments _____

Name _____

Date _____ Score* _____

## PROCEDURE 17-3   Assist with Minor Surgery

*PERFORMANCE OBJECTIVE*—Demonstrate each of the steps required in assisting with minor surgery.

| PROCEDURE STEPS | STEP PERFORMED | POINTS POSSIBLE | COMMENTS |
|---|---|---|---|
| *EVALUATOR:* Place check mark in space following each step performed satisfactorily | | | |
| NOTE TIME BEGAN _____ | | | |
| 1. Identified patient. | _____ | 10 | |
| 2. Washed hands. | _____ | 5 | |
| 3. Assembled appropriate items on Mayo tray (sterile packs). | _____ | 15 | |
| a. Positioned next to treatment table | _____ | 10 | |
| b. Checked expiration dates of items | _____ | 10 | |
| 4. Explained procedure to patient. | _____ | 5 | |
| a. Obtained signature on consent form | _____ | 5 | |
| b. Advised patient to empty bladder | _____ | 5 | |
| c. Took vital signs and recorded | _____ | 5 | |
| d. Instructed patient to disrobe as indicated for procedure | _____ | 10 | |
| e. Advised where to put belongings | _____ | 5 | |
| 5. Assisted patient to treatment table. | _____ | 5 | |
| a. Positioned patient | _____ | 10 | |
| 6. Performed skin prep procedure. | _____ | 10 | |
| 7. Draped patient appropriately. | _____ | 5 | |
| 8. Placed sterile towel on Mayo tray. | _____ | 5 | |
| a. Put sterile gloves on | _____ | 10 | |
| b. Opened sterile items at tabs | _____ | 10 | |
| c. Placed items in order of use | _____ | 10 | |
| d. Covered with sterile towel | _____ | 10 | |
| e. Removed gloves | _____ | 5 | |
| f. Washed hands | _____ | 5 | |
| 9. When physician was ready to begin: | | | |
| a. Removed cover | _____ | 5 | |
| b. Handed physician sterile gloves | _____ | 5 | |
| c. Wiped top of vial with alcohol | _____ | 5 | |
| d. Held anesthetic vial for doctor | _____ | 5 | |
| 10. Washed hands and regloved to assist. | _____ | 10 | |
| a. Mopped with sterile gauze | _____ | 15 | |
| b. Handed sterile items to physician PRN | _____ | 15 | |

| PROCEDURE STEPS | STEP PERFORMED | POINTS POSSIBLE | COMMENTS |
|---|---|---|---|
| c. Opened specimen container for biopsy | _____ | 15 | |
| d. Clipped suture PRN | _____ | 10 | |
| 11. Cleaned and bandaged surgery site. | _____ | 5 | |
| a. Asked patient if allergic to adhesive | _____ | 5 | |
| 12. Removed gloves. | _____ | 5 | |
| a. Washed hands | _____ | 5 | |
| 13. Assisted patient to sitting position. | _____ | 5 | |
| a. And then from table | _____ | 5 | |
| 14. Provided patient education. | _____ | 5 | |
| a. Care of site | _____ | 5 | |
| b. Return visit appointment given | _____ | 5 | |
| 15. Regloved to clean up room. | _____ | 5 | |
| a. Discarded disposables in biohazardous waste container | _____ | 5 | |
| b. Rinsed instruments in cool water and placed in detergent solution to soak | _____ | 5 | |
| 16. Removed gloves. | _____ | 5 | |
| a. Washed hands | _____ | 5 | |
| 17. Restocked room | _____ | 5 | |

*EVALUATOR:* NOTE TIME COMPLETED _____

ADD POINTS OF STEPS CHECKED _____ EARNED

TOTAL POINTS POSSIBLE                                    330  POSSIBLE

Points assigned reflect importance of step to meeting objective:  Important = (5)    Essential = (10)    Critical = (15)
Automatic failure results if any of the critical steps are omitted or performed incorrectly.

DETERMINE SCORE (divide points earned by total points possible, multiply results by 100) _____ SCORE*

Evaluator's Name (print) _____ Signature _____

Comments _____

## DOCUMENTATION

Chart the procedure in the patient's medical record.

Date: _____

Charting: _____

_____

_____

_____

Student's Name: _____        Physician's Initials: __(____)__

Name _____

Date _____ Score* _____

## PROCEDURE 17-4   Assisting with Suturing a Laceration

*PERFORMANCE OBJECTIVE*—Demonstrate each of the steps required in the procedure to assist with suturing a laceration.

| PROCEDURE STEPS | STEP PERFORMED | POINTS POSSIBLE | COMMENTS |
|---|---|---|---|
| *EVALUATOR:* Place check mark in space following each step performed satisfactorily | | | |
| NOTE TIME BEGAN _____ | | | |
| 1. Washed hands. | _____ | 5 | |
| 2. Assembled all necessary items. | _____ | 10 | |
| 3. Identified patient. | _____ | 5 | |
| a. Explained procedure to patient | _____ | 5 | |
| b. Advised patient to empty bladder | _____ | 5 | |
| 4. Took and recorded patient's vital signs. | _____ | 5 | |
| 5. Asked/assisted patient in removing clothing. | _____ | 5 | |
| a. Explained where to store clothing | _____ | 5 | |
| 6. Positioned patient appropriately. | _____ | 10 | |
| 7. Performed skin prep of site. | _____ | 15 | |
| 8. Draped patient appropriately. | _____ | 10 | |
| 9. Assembled unsterile items on Mayo tray. | _____ | 10 | |
| 10. Answered patient's questions. | _____ | 5 | |
| 11. Opened sterile pack on Mayo tray. | _____ | 5 | |
| a. Handled sterile towel from underneath | _____ | 10 | |
| b. Dropped sterile items on sterile field as appropriate | _____ | 15 | |
| 12. Put PPE and sterile gloves on. | _____ | 15 | |
| 13. Arranged sterile items in order of use. | _____ | 15 | |
| a. Covered sterile field with sterile towel | _____ | 5 | |
| 14. Removed gloves. | _____ | 5 | |
| a. Washed hands | _____ | 5 | |
| Assisting physician with actual procedure: | | | |
| 15. Removed cover from set-up. | _____ | 5 | |
| 16. Handed sterile gloves to physician. | _____ | 10 | |
| 17. Held vial of anesthetic for physician. | _____ | 5 | |
| a. Wiped top of vial with alcohol pad | _____ | 5 | |
| 18. Washed hands. | _____ | 5 | |
| a. Put on sterile gloves | _____ | 15 | |
| 19. Handed sterile items to physician as needed. | _____ | 15 | |
| 20. Mopped excess blood from site/sterile gauze. | _____ | 15 | |
| 21. Clipped sutures as directed by physician. | _____ | 15 | |

| PROCEDURE STEPS | STEP PERFORMED | POINTS POSSIBLE | COMMENTS |
|---|---|---|---|
| 22. Assisted with cleaning site. | _____ | 15 | |
| a. Bandaged site appropriately | _____ | 10 | |
| b. Asked if patient has adhesive allergy | _____ | 10 | |
| c. Regloved as necessary | _____ | 5 | |
| d. Disposed of soiled items in biohazardous bag | _____ | 5 | |
| e. Washed hands | _____ | 5 | |
| 23. Administered tetanus toxoid as directed by physician. | _____ | 5 | |
| 24. Assisted patient in sitting. | _____ | 5 | |
| a. Assisted patient in dressing | _____ | 5 | |
| b. Assisted patient from exam table | _____ | 5 | |
| 25. Instructed patient in caring for suture site. | _____ | 5 | |
| 26. Provided return appointment. | _____ | 10 | |
| 27. Put on gloves to clean up room. | _____ | 5 | |
| a. Placed disposables in biobag/sharps | _____ | 10 | |
| b. Rinsed instruments in cool water | _____ | 5 | |
| c. Placed instruments in detergent solution | _____ | 5 | |
| 28. Removed gloves/PPE. | _____ | 5 | |
| a. Placed soiled disposables in biobag | _____ | 5 | |
| b. Washed hands | _____ | 5 | |
| 29. Restocked treatment room. | _____ | 5 | |
| 30. Recorded procedure in patient's chart. | _____ | 5 | |
| a. Initialed | _____ | 5 | |

*EVALUATOR:* NOTE TIME COMPLETED _____

ADD POINTS OF STEPS CHECKED                                                          _____ EARNED
TOTAL POINTS POSSIBLE                                                                          400 POSSIBLE

Points assigned reflect importance of step to meeting objective:  Important = (5)   Essential = (10)   Critical = (15)
Automatic failure results if any of the critical steps are omitted or performed incorrectly.

DETERMINE SCORE (divide points earned by total points possible, multiply results by 100)      _____ SCORE*

Evaluator's Name (print) _____ Signature _____

Comments _____

**DOCUMENTATION**

Chart the procedure in the patient's medical record.

Date: _____

Charting: _____

_____

_____

_____

Student's Name: _____          Physician's Initials: __(____)__

Name _____

Date _____ Score* _____

## PROCEDURE 17-5   Remove Sutures

*PERFORMANCE OBJECTIVE*—Demonstrate the steps required in removing sutures.

| PROCEDURE STEPS | STEP PERFORMED | POINTS POSSIBLE | COMMENTS |
|---|---|---|---|
| *EVALUATOR:* Place check mark in space following each step performed satisfactorily | | | |
| NOTE TIME BEGAN _____ | | | |
| 1. Identified patient. | _____ | 5 | |
| 2. Washed hands. | _____ | 5 | |
| 3. Placed Mayo tray next to treatment table. | _____ | 5 | |
|   a. Assembled items on tray | _____ | 5 | |
| 4. Asked about condition of suture site. | _____ | 5 | |
|   a. If laceration/ask about booster | _____ | 5 | |
|   b. Took vital signs and recorded | _____ | 5 | |
|   c. Recorded other information | _____ | 5 | |
| 5. Asked patient to remove appropriate clothing if necessary. | _____ | 10 | |
| 6. Assisted patient to treatment table. | _____ | 5 | |
|   a. Into position and draped as necessary | _____ | 10 | |
|   b. Explained procedure | _____ | 5 | |
| 7. Washed hands. | _____ | 5 | |
|   a. Put gloves on | _____ | 5 | |
| 8. Removed bandage/inspected site. | _____ | 10 | |
| 9. Soaked to remove bandage if stuck. | _____ | 10 | |
| 10. Advised physician to check the site. | _____ | 10 | |
| 11. Followed doctor's orders to remove sutures. | _____ | 15 | |
|   a. Opened sterile pack of instruments | _____ | 15 | |
|   b. Used thumb forceps to grasp knot of suture and pull up | _____ | 15 | |
|   c. Placed tip of suture removal scissors next to skin to clip suture | _____ | 15 | |
|   d. Pulled suture toward the incision | _____ | 15 | |
|   e. Continued until all sutures were removed. | _____ | 15 | |
| 12. Applied antiseptic solution to site. | _____ | 10 | |
|   a. Allowed to air dry | _____ | 5 | |
|   b. Applied steri-strips or butterfly closures PRN. | _____ | 15 | |

| PROCEDURE STEPS | STEP PERFORMED | POINTS POSSIBLE | COMMENTS |
|---|---|---|---|
| c. Bandaged as necessary. | _____ | 10 | |
| d. Asked patient if allergic to adhesive | _____ | 10 | |
| 13. Removed gloves. | _____ | 5 | |
| a. Washed hands | _____ | 5 | |
| 14. Provided patient education. | _____ | 5 | |
| 15. Cleaned room. | _____ | 5 | |
| a. Cared for instruments  (gloves PRN) | _____ | 5 | |
| 16. Recorded information on patient's chart. | _____ | 5 | |
| a. Initialed | _____ | 5 | |

*EVALUATOR:* NOTE TIME COMPLETED _____

ADD POINTS OF STEPS CHECKED                                                                     _____ EARNED

TOTAL POINTS POSSIBLE                                                                                     285 POSSIBLE

Points assigned reflect importance of step to meeting objective:  Important  = (5)   Essential = (10)   Critical = (15)
Automatic failure results if any of the critical steps are omitted or performed incorrectly.

DETERMINE SCORE (divide points earned by total points possible, multiply results by 100)           _____ SCORE*

Evaluator's Name (print) _____ Signature _____

Comments _____

---

## DOCUMENTATION

Chart the procedure in the patient's medical record.

Date: _____

Charting: _____

_____

_____

_____

Student's Name: _____          Physician's Initials:  _(_____)_

Name _____

Date _____ Score* _____

## PROCEDURE 18-1   Obtain and Administer Oral Medication

*PERFORMANCE OBJECTIVE*—Demonstrate the steps required to obtain the ordered oral medication and administer it to the patient.

| PROCEDURE STEPS | STEP PERFORMED | POINTS POSSIBLE | COMMENTS |
|---|---|---|---|
| *EVALUATOR:* Place check mark in space following each step performed satisfactorily | | | |
| NOTE TIME BEGAN _____ | | | |
| 1. Read order of medication and compared it with medication in storage area. | _____ | 10 | |
| a. Obtained ordered medication | _____ | 15 | |
| 2. Calculated dosage if necessary. | _____ | 15 | |
| 3. Washed hands. | _____ | 5 | |
| 4. Removed bottle cap. | _____ | 5 | |
| a. Placed cap inside-up on counter | _____ | 5 | |
| b. Poured desired amount into cap and then into medicine cup | _____ | 15 | |
| or | | | |
| If liquid; poured desired amount directly into medicine cup at eye level. | _____ | 15 | |
| 5. Placed medicine on tray. | _____ | 5 | |
| a. Placed cup of water on tray (if medicine is in pill or capsule form) | _____ | 5 | |
| 6. Read label of medicine container again. | _____ | 10 | |
| a. Took medicine to patient | _____ | 10 | |
| 7. Identified patient. | _____ | 5 | |
| 8. Explained procedure to patient. | _____ | 15 | |
| 9. Observed patient taking medication. | _____ | 15 | |
| a. Reported any reaction or problem to the physician | _____ | 10 | |
| 10. Read label of medication container again. | _____ | 10 | |
| 11. Discarded disposables. | _____ | 5 | |
| 12. Returned items to proper storage. | _____ | 5 | |
| 13. Recorded medication information on patient's chart. | _____ | 15 | |
| a. Initialed | _____ | 5 | |
| *EVALUATOR:* NOTE TIME COMPLETED _____ | | | |

ADD POINTS OF STEPS CHECKED                                    _____ EARNED

TOTAL POINTS POSSIBLE                                              185 POSSIBLE

Points assigned reflect importance of step to meeting objective:  Important = (5)   Essential = (10)   Critical = (15)
Automatic failure results if any of the critical steps are omitted or performed incorrectly.

DETERMINE SCORE (divide points earned by total points possible, multiply results by 100)        _____ SCORE*

Evaluator's Name (print) _____   Signature _____

Comments _____

## DOCUMENTATION

Chart the procedure in the patient's medical record.

Date: _____

Charting: _____

_____

_____

_____

Student's Name: _____          Physician's Initials: __(_____)__

Name _____

Date _____ Score* _____

## PROCEDURE 18-2   Withdraw Medication from Ampule

*PERFORMANCE OBJECTIVE*—Demonstrate each of the steps required to withdraw medication from an ampule.

| PROCEDURE STEPS | STEP PERFORMED | POINTS POSSIBLE | COMMENTS |
|---|---|---|---|
| *EVALUATOR:* Place check mark in space following each step performed satisfactorily | | | |
| NOTE TIME BEGAN _____ | | | |
| 1. Washed hands. | _____ | 5 | |
| 2. Placed sterile gauze square over middle of ampule. | _____ | 5 | |
| 3. Held ampule between thumb and index finger of one hand. | _____ | 10 | |
| 4. Flicked pointed end of ampule with index finger to release medicine into bottom of ampule. | _____ | 15 | |
| 5. Grasped tip of ampule and snapped off. | _____ | 15 | |
| a. Discarded tip of ampule | _____ | 10 | |
| 6. Secured needle and syringe by turning barrel to right while holding guard. | _____ | 10 | |
| 7. Expelled air from syringe. | _____ | 10 | |
| 8. Inserted tip of needle below line of liquid in ampule without touching sides. | _____ | 15 | |
| 9. Drew ordered amount of medicine into barrel of syringe. | _____ | 15 | |
| a. Avoided air from entering by keeping tip of needle below line of liquid | _____ | 15 | |
| 10. Removed needle without touching sides of ampule. | _____ | 15 | |
| 11. Replaced needle guard without contaminating needle (scoop method). | _____ | 5 | |
| 12. Placed filled syringe on medicine tray. | _____ | 5 | |
| 13. Discarded disposables in proper receptacle. | _____ | 5 | |

*EVALUATOR:* NOTE TIME COMPLETED _____

ADD POINTS OF STEPS CHECKED                                         _____ EARNED
TOTAL POINTS POSSIBLE                                                      155 POSSIBLE

Points assigned reflect importance of step to meeting objective:  Important = (5)   Essential = (10)   Critical = (15)
Automatic failure results if any of the critical steps are omitted or performed incorrectly.

DETERMINE SCORE (divide points earned by total points possible, multiply results by 100)        _____ SCORE*

Evaluator's Name (print) _____  Signature _____

Comments _____

## PROCEDURE 18-3  Withdraw Medication from Vial

*PERFORMANCE OBJECTIVE*—Demonstrate each of the steps required to withdraw medication from a vial.

| PROCEDURE STEPS | STEP PERFORMED | POINTS POSSIBLE | COMMENTS |
|---|---|---|---|
| *EVALUATOR:* Place check mark in space following each step performed satisfactorily | | | |
| NOTE TIME BEGAN _____ | | | |
| 1. Washed hands. | _____ | 5 | |
| 2. Calculated dosage. | _____ | 15 | |
| 3. Cleaned rubber-topped vial with alcohol pad. | _____ | 10 | |
| 4. Secured needle onto syringe by holding needle guard and turning barrel of syringe to the right. | _____ | 10 | |
| 5. Removed needle guard without contaminating the needle. | _____ | 10 | |
| 6. Pulled back on plunger to fill syringe with same amount of air as medication ordered. | _____ | 10 | |
| 7. Held syringe at barrel. | _____ | 10 | |
| 8. Held vial upside down. | _____ | 10 | |
| 9. Inserted needle into rubber top and pushed plunger in, expelling air into vial. | _____ | 15 | |
| 10. Pulled back plunger to allow desired amount of medication to enter syringe. | _____ | 15 | |
| a. Kept needle below level of medication in vial to avoid air bubbles | _____ | 15 | |
| b. Flicked barrel of syringe to release air bubbles into hub of syringe and pushed plunger to release | _____ | 15 | |
| 11. Pulled needle out of vial without contaminating it. | _____ | 10 | |
| 12. Replaced needle guard. | _____ | 5 | |
| 13. Placed filled syringe on medicine tray. | _____ | 5 | |
| a. Placed alcohol on tray | _____ | 5 | |
| *EVALUATOR:* NOTE TIME COMPLETED _____ | | | |

ADD POINTS OF STEPS CHECKED                                                           _____ EARNED
TOTAL POINTS POSSIBLE                                                                   165 POSSIBLE

Points assigned reflect importance of step to meeting objective:  Important = (5)   Essential = (10)   Critical = (15)
Automatic failure results if any of the critical steps are omitted or performed incorrectly.

DETERMINE SCORE (divide points earned by total points possible, multiply results by 100)      _____ SCORE*

Evaluator's Name (print) _____ Signature _____

Comments _____

Name _____

Date _____ Score* _____

## PROCEDURE 18-4    Administer Intradermal Injection

*PERFORMANCE OBJECTIVE*—Demonstrate each of the steps required in administering an intradermal injection.

| PROCEDURE STEPS | STEP PERFORMED | POINTS POSSIBLE | COMMENTS |
|---|---|---|---|
| *EVALUATOR:* Place check mark in space following each step performed satisfactorily | | | |
| NOTE TIME BEGAN _____ | | | |
| 1. Washed hands. | _____ | 5 | |
| 2. Read order. | _____ | 5 | |
| 3. Prepared syringe with ordered amount of medicine. | _____ | 15 | |
| 4. Replaced needle guard. | _____ | 10 | |
| 5. Placed medicine on tray. | _____ | 5 | |
| 6. Compared medicine order with patient's chart. | _____ | 15 | |
| 7. Identified patient. | _____ | 5 | |
| 8. Explained procedure to patient. | _____ | 5 | |
| 9. Placed medicine tray near patient. | _____ | 5 | |
| 10. Used alcohol pad to clean injection site. | _____ | 10 | |
|    a. Allowed alcohol to air dry | _____ | 5 | |
| 11. Removed needle guard without contaminating it. | _____ | 15 | |
| 12. Held patient's skin taut between thumb and index finger to steady area to be injected. | _____ | 5 | |
| 13. Inserted needle at 10°–15° angle. | _____ | 10 | |
|    a. Held bevel of needle up | _____ | 15 | |
| 14. Expelled medicine from syringe. | _____ | 15 | |
|    a. Caused wheal to develop | _____ | 15 | |
| 15. Removed needle quickly. | _____ | 10 | |
|    a. At same angle as insertion | _____ | 10 | |
|    b. Wiped site with gauze pad | _____ | 5 | |
|    c. Did not massage site | _____ | 10 | |
| 16. Observed patient. | _____ | 10 | |
|    a. Timed reaction | _____ | 15 | |
| 17. Gave patient instructions/answered questions. | _____ | 5 | |
| 18. Applied bandage. | _____ | 5 | |
| 19. Discarded disposables in sharps container including intact syringe and needle. | _____ | 5 | |

| PROCEDURE STEPS | STEP PERFORMED | POINTS POSSIBLE | COMMENTS |
|---|---|---|---|
| 20. Returned items to proper storage. | _____ | 5 | |
| 21. Recorded information on patient's chart. | _____ | 15 | |
| a. Initialed | _____ | 5 | |
| *EVALUATOR:* NOTE TIME COMPLETED _____ | | | |

ADD POINTS OF STEPS CHECKED                                                          _____ EARNED
TOTAL POINTS POSSIBLE                                                                      260 POSSIBLE

Points assigned reflect importance of step to meeting objective:  Important = (5)   Essential = (10)   Critical = (15)
Automatic failure results if any of the critical steps are omitted or performed incorrectly.

DETERMINE SCORE (divide points earned by total points possible, multiply results by 100)        _____ SCORE*

Evaluator's Name (print) _____ Signature _____

Comments _____

---

# DOCUMENTATION

Chart the procedure in the patient's medical record.

Date: _____

Charting: _____

_____

_____

_____

Student's Name: _____          Physician's Initials: __( __ )__

Name _____

Date _____ Score* _____

## PROCEDURE 18-5   Administer Subcutaneous Injection

*PERFORMANCE OBJECTIVE*—Demonstrate each of the steps required in administering a subcutaneous injection.

| PROCEDURE STEPS | STEP PERFORMED | POINTS POSSIBLE | COMMENTS |
|---|---|---|---|
| *EVALUATOR:* Place check mark in space following each step performed satisfactorily | | | |
| NOTE TIME BEGAN _____ | | | |
| 1. Compared orders with medication. | _____ | 10 | |
| 2. Washed hands. | _____ | 5 | |
| 3. Prepared syringe. | _____ | 10 | |
|    a. Replaced needle guard | _____ | 5 | |
| 4. Placed filled syringe on medicine tray. | _____ | 10 | |
| 5. Compared medication order with patient's chart. | _____ | 15 | |
| 6. Identified patient. | _____ | 5 | |
| 7. Explained procedure to patient. | _____ | 5 | |
| 8. Asked patient to remove necessary clothing. | _____ | 10 | |
| 9. Used alcohol pad to clean injection site. | _____ | 10 | |
| 10. Removed needle guard without contaminating it. | _____ | 15 | |
| 11. Held skin at injection site taut. | _____ | 5 | |
| 12. Held syringe securely with bevel of needle down. | _____ | 10 | |
| 13. Inserted needle at 45° angle. | _____ | 15 | |
| 14. Held barrel of syringe with one hand. | _____ | 10 | |
|    a. Aspirated with other hand | _____ | 15 | |
|    b. Determined if in a blood vessel | _____ | 15 | |
| 15. Pushed plunger of syringe to release medication. | _____ | 15 | |
| 16. Pulled needle out at same angle as insertion. | _____ | 10 | |
| 17. Wiped site with alcohol pad. | _____ | 5 | |
| 18. Placed dry cotton ball on site. | _____ | 5 | |
|    a. Massaged area gently | _____ | 5 | |
| 19. Observed patient for possible reaction. | _____ | 5 | |
| 20. Reported any reaction to physician. | _____ | 10 | |
| 21. Advised patient to remain for 20 minutes. | _____ | 10 | |
| 22. Answered questions from patient. | _____ | 5 | |
| 23. Applied bandage. | _____ | 5 | |
| 24. Discarded disposables including intact syringe and needle in sharps container. | _____ | 5 | |

| PROCEDURE STEPS | STEP PERFORMED | POINTS POSSIBLE | COMMENTS |
|---|---|---|---|
| 25. Returned items to proper storage. | _____ | 5 | |
| 26. Recorded information on patient's chart. | _____ | 5 | |
|    a. Initialed | _____ | 5 | |

*EVALUATOR:* NOTE TIME COMPLETED _____

ADD POINTS OF STEPS CHECKED                                                   _____ EARNED
TOTAL POINTS POSSIBLE                                                              265 POSSIBLE

Points assigned reflect importance of step to meeting objective:  Important = (5)   Essential = (10)   Critical = (15)
Automatic failure results if any of the critical steps are omitted or performed incorrectly.

DETERMINE SCORE (divide points earned by total points possible, multiply results by 100)          _____ SCORE*

Evaluator's Name (print) _____ Signature _____
Comments _____

---

## DOCUMENTATION

Chart the procedure in the patient's medical record.

Date: _____

Charting: _____
_____
_____
_____

Student's Name: _____          Physician's Initials: __(        )__

Name _____

Date _____ Score* _____

## PROCEDURE 18-6   Administer Intramuscular Injection

*PERFORMANCE OBJECTIVE*—Demonstrate each of the steps required in administering an intramuscular injection.

| PROCEDURE STEPS | STEP PERFORMED | POINTS POSSIBLE | COMMENTS |
|---|---|---|---|
| *EVALUATOR:* Place check mark in space following each step performed satisfactorily | | | |
| NOTE TIME BEGAN _____ | | | |
| 1.  Washed hands. | _____ | 5 | |
| 2.  Read label of medication. | _____ | 5 | |
| 3.  Compared with order. | _____ | 10 | |
| 4.  Prepared syringe with ordered amount of medication. | _____ | 15 | |
| 5.  Replaced needle guard. | _____ | 5 | |
| 6.  Placed filled syringe on medicine tray. | _____ | 10 | |
| 7.  Compared medication order with patient's chart. | _____ | 15 | |
| 8.  Identified patient. | _____ | 5 | |
| 9.  Explained procedure to patient. | _____ | 5 | |
| 10.  Asked patient to remove necessary clothing. | _____ | 5 | |
| 11.  Cleaned injection site with alcohol pad. | _____ | 10 | |
| a.  Allowed to air dry | _____ | 5 | |
| 12.  Removed needle guard. | _____ | 10 | |
| 13.  Secured injection site between thumb and index finger. | _____ | 10 | |
| 14.  Grasped syringe as a dart. | _____ | 10 | |
| 15.  Inserted needle at 90° angle. | _____ | 15 | |
| 16.  Aspirated syringe. | _____ | 15 | |
| a.  Determined if in a blood vessel | _____ | 15 | |
| 17.  Pushed plunger of syringe to release medication. | _____ | 15 | |
| 18.  Pulled needle out at angle of insertion. | _____ | 10 | |
| 19.  Wiped injection site with alcohol pads. | _____ | 5 | |
| 20.  Gently massaged area with dry cotton ball. | _____ | 5 | |
| 21.  Observed patient for reaction. | _____ | 10 | |
| 22.  Reported any reaction to physician. | _____ | 10 | |
| 23.  Applied bandage. | _____ | 5 | |
| 24.  Discarded disposables including intact syringe and needle in sharps container. | _____ | 5 | |

## PROCEDURE 18-6 Administer Intramuscular Injection—continued

| PROCEDURE STEPS | STEP PERFORMED | POINTS POSSIBLE | COMMENTS |
|---|---|---|---|
| 25. Washed and sterilized reusable items. | _____ | 5 | |
| 26. Returned items to proper storage. | _____ | 5 | |
| 27. Recorded information on patient's chart. | _____ | 5 | |
|    a. Initialed | _____ | 5 | |
| *EVALUATOR:* NOTE TIME COMPLETED _____ | | | |

ADD POINTS OF STEPS CHECKED                                                 _____ EARNED
TOTAL POINTS POSSIBLE                                                 255 POSSIBLE

Points assigned reflect importance of step to meeting objective: Important = (5) Essential = (10) Critical = (15)
Automatic failure results if any of the critical steps are omitted or performed incorrectly.

DETERMINE SCORE (divide points earned by total points possible, multiply results by 100)     _____ SCORE*

Evaluator's Name (print) _____ Signature _____

Comments _____

---

## DOCUMENTATION

Chart the procedure in the patient's medical record.

Date: _____

Charting: _____

_____

_____

_____

Student's Name: _____       Physician's Initials: __(_____)__

## PROCEDURE 18-7   Administer Intramuscular Injection by Z-Tract Method

*PERFORMANCE OBJECTIVE*—Demonstrate each of the steps required in administering an intramuscular injection by Z-tract method.

| PROCEDURE STEPS | STEP PERFORMED | POINTS POSSIBLE | COMMENTS |
|---|---|---|---|
| *EVALUATOR:* Place check mark in space following each step performed satisfactorily | | | |
| NOTE TIME BEGAN _____ | | | |
| 1. Washed hands. | _____ | 5 | |
| 2. Read label of medication. | _____ | 10 | |
| 3. Compared with order. | _____ | 15 | |
| 4. Prepared syringe with ordered amount of medication. | _____ | 15 | |
| 5. Replaced needle guard. | _____ | 5 | |
| 6. Placed filled syringe on medicine tray. | _____ | 5 | |
| 7. Compared medication order with patient's chart. | _____ | 15 | |
| 8. Identified patient. | _____ | 5 | |
| 9. Explained procedure to patient. | _____ | 5 | |
| 10. Asked patient to remove necessary clothing. | _____ | 10 | |
| 11. Cleaned injection site with alcohol pad. | _____ | 10 | |
|    a. Allowed to air dry | _____ | 5 | |
| 12. Removed needle guard. | _____ | 5 | |
| 13. Read package insert instructions of medication. | _____ | 10 | |
| 14. Used sterile gauze square to displace skin/tissues throughout injection. | _____ | 10 | |
| 15. Inserted needle at 90° angle. | _____ | 15 | |
| 16. Used fingers to pull back on plunger to aspirate while holding barrel of syringe with thumb and ring finger. | _____ | 15 | |
| 17. Pushed plunger of syringe to slowly expel medication. | _____ | 15 | |
| 18. Waited a few seconds before withdrawing needle. | _____ | 15 | |
| 19. Removed needle quickly in same path as entered. | _____ | 10 | |
| 20. Let go of displaced skin/tissue immediately after needle is withdrawn to cover needle path. | _____ | 15 | |
| 21. Covered injection site with alcohol pad. | _____ | 5 | |
|    a. Held in place a few seconds | _____ | 5 | |
|    b. Did not massage injection site | _____ | 10 | |
| 22. Observed patient for reaction. | _____ | 10 | |

| PROCEDURE STEPS | STEP PERFORMED | POINTS POSSIBLE | COMMENTS |
|---|---|---|---|
| 23. Reported any reaction to physician. | _____ | 5 | |
| 24. Applied bandage. | _____ | 5 | |
| 25. Discarded disposables including intact syringe and needle in sharps container. | _____ | 5 | |
| 26. Washed and sterilized reusable items. | _____ | 5 | |
| 27. Returned items to proper storage. | _____ | 5 | |
| 28. Recorded information on patient's chart. | _____ | 5 | |
|    a. Initialed | _____ | 5 | |

*EVALUATOR:* NOTE TIME COMPLETED _____

ADD POINTS OF STEPS CHECKED                                     _____ EARNED
TOTAL POINTS POSSIBLE                                              280 POSSIBLE

Points assigned reflect importance of step to meeting objective:  Important = (5)   Essential = (10)   Critical = (15)
Automatic failure results if any of the critical steps are omitted or performed incorrectly.

DETERMINE SCORE (divide points earned by total points possible, multiply results by 100)     _____ SCORE*

Evaluator's Name (print) _____ Signature _____

Comments _____

**DOCUMENTATION**

Chart the procedure in the patient's medical record.

Date: _____

Charting: _____

_____

_____

_____

Student's Name: _____        Physician's Initials: __(_____)__

Name _____

Date _____ Score* _____

## PROCEDURE 19-1   Give Mouth-to-Mouth Resuscitation

*PERFORMANCE OBJECTIVE*—In a course taught by a certified instructor, using a training mannequin, demonstrate mouth-to-mouth resuscitation. Perform the steps as instructed following recommended standard precautions.

| PROCEDURE STEPS | STEP PERFORMED | POINTS POSSIBLE | COMMENTS |
|---|---|---|---|
| *EVALUATOR:* Place check mark in space following each step performed satisfactorily | | | |
| NOTE TIME BEGAN _____ | | | |
| 1. Determined whether unresponsive victim is breathing. | _____ | 15 | |
| 2. Positioned victim on back on firm surface. | _____ | 5 | |
| 3. Rescuer was positioned at victim's side near head and shoulders. | _____ | 5 | |
| 4. Opened airway. If not effective, continued with procedure. | _____ | 15 | |
| 5. Checked for mouth obstruction. | _____ | 10 | |
| 6. Demonstrated procedure to remove obstruction. | _____ | 15 | |
| 7. Used head tilt-chin lift maneuver, thereby moving tongue from back of throat. If not effective, continued with procedure. | _____ | 15 | |
| 8. Pinched victim's nostrils together with fingers of one hand while placing heel of hand on forehead to keep the head tilted. | _____ | 10 | |
| 9. Took a deep breath and then sealed mouth over victim's. Breathed two slow breaths into the victim's mouth. Took a breath after each ventilation. | _____ | 15 | |
| 10. Turned head to one side, felt and listened for return of air. Watched chest for movement. If not effective, lifted chin, tilted head, tried again. | _____ | 15 | |
| 11. If inflation had not occurred, gave cycles of 12 breaths per minute. Watched for return of breathing. | _____ | 15 | |
| 12. Continued cycles until breathing restored, assistance arrived, or resuscitation was no longer possible. | _____ | 10 | |
| 13. Recorded and signed procedure on patient's chart. | _____ | | |
| *EVALUATOR:* NOTE TIME COMPLETED _____ | | | |

ADD POINTS OF STEPS CHECKED                                           _____ EARNED
TOTAL POINTS POSSIBLE                                                          155 POSSIBLE

Points assigned reflect importance of step to meeting objective: Important = (5)   Essential = (10)   Critical = (15)
Automatic failure results if any of the critical steps are omitted or performed incorrectly.

DETERMINE SCORE (divide points earned by total points possible, multiply results by 100)            _____ SCORE*

Evaluator's Name (print) _____   Signature _____

Comments _____

## DOCUMENTATION

Chart the procedure in the patient's medical record.

Date: _____

Charting: _____

_____

_____

_____

Student's Name: _____     Physician's Initials: _( ___ )_

Name _____

Date _____ Score* _____

## PROCEDURE 19-2   Give Cardiopulmonary Resuscitation (CPR) to Adults

*PERFORMANCE OBJECTIVE*—In a course taught by a certified instructor, and using a training mannequin, demonstrate the procedure performing each step, following recommended precautions.

| PROCEDURE STEPS | STEP PERFORMED | POINTS POSSIBLE | COMMENTS |
|---|---|---|---|
| *EVALUATOR:* Place check mark in space following each step performed satisfactorily | | | |
| NOTE TIME BEGAN _____ | | | |
| 1. Gently shook victim and asked "Are you OK?" | _____ | 10 | |
| 2. If no response, called or sent someone for help. | _____ | 15 | |
| 3. Positioned mannequin on floor. | _____ | 5 | |
| 4. Rescuer was positioned at victim's side near head. | _____ | 5 | |
| 5. Opened airway. If not effective, continued with procedure. | _____ | 15 | |
| 6. Checked for mouth obstruction. | _____ | 5 | |
| 7. Positioned victim to open airway; pinched nostrils together with fingers while placing heel of hand on forehead to maintain head tilt. | _____ | 10 | |
| 8. Took a deep breath, sealed mouth over victim's, and breathed two slow breaths into victim's mouth. Took a breath after each ventilation. | _____ | 15 | |
| 9. Turned head to one side, listened, and felt for return of air. Watched chest for movement. | _____ | 5 | |
| 10. Checked for carotid pulse; allowed up to 10 seconds. | _____ | 15 | |
| 11. If victim had a pulse, continued mouth-to-mouth respiration at rate of one breath every five seconds, if no pulse, began chest compressions. | _____ | — | |
| 12. Identified location for chest compressions and positioned hands. | | | |
| a. Located lower rib cage | _____ | 5 | |
| b. Followed up to sternum | _____ | 5 | |
| c. Placed two index fingers at lower end of sternum | _____ | 5 | |
| d. Placed heel of hand nearest head next to fingers | _____ | 5 | |
| e. Positioned other hand over hand on sternum, locked fingers | _____ | 10 | |
| f. Held fingers away from body | _____ | 10 | |
| 13. Rose on knees, shoulder width apart. | _____ | 5 | |
| a. Directly over sternum | _____ | 5 | |
| b. Locked elbows | _____ | 5 | |

| PROCEDURE STEPS | STEP PERFORMED | POINTS POSSIBLE | COMMENTS |
|---|---|---|---|
| 14. Used a smooth, even motion to push straight down on chest and compressed about 1½″ to 2″ for a count of fifteen compressions. | _____ | 15 | |
| 15. Gave two ventilations. | _____ | 15 | |
| 16. Repeated four cycles: Pause, checked for signs of circulation. | _____ | 15 | |
| 17. If no pulse, resumed compressions and ventilations. | _____ | — | |
| 18. Paused every few minutes to check for pulse and respirations. | _____ | — | |
| 19. Continued CPR until victim recovered, help arrived, victim was pronounced dead, or after 15 minutes, no signs of life have occurred. | _____ | — | |
| 20. Cleaned mannequin as instructed. | _____ | 10 | |
| 21. Recorded and signed procedure on patient's chart. | _____ | 10 | |

*EVALUATOR:* NOTE TIME COMPLETED _____

ADD POINTS OF STEPS CHECKED                                                           _____ EARNED
TOTAL POINTS POSSIBLE                                                                      220 POSSIBLE

Points assigned reflect importance of step to meeting objective: Important = (5)   Essential = (10)   Critical = (15)
Automatic failure results if any of the critical steps are omitted or performed incorrectly.

DETERMINE SCORE (divide points earned by total points possible, multiply results by 100)     _____ SCORE*

Evaluator's Name (print) _____ Signature _____

Comments _____

---

## DOCUMENTATION

Chart the procedure in the patient's medical record.

Date: _____

Charting: _____

_____

_____

_____

Student's Name: _____          Physician's Initials: _(_____)_

Name _____

Date _____ Score* _____

## PROCEDURE 19-3   Give Cardiopulmonary Resuscitation (CPR) to Infants and Children

*PERFORMANCE OBJECTIVE*—In a course taught by a certified instructor, using a training mannequin, demonstrate the procedure as instructed, performing each step, and following standard precautions.

| PROCEDURE STEPS | STEP PERFORMED | POINTS POSSIBLE | COMMENTS |
|---|---|---|---|
| *EVALUATOR:* Place check mark in space following each step performed satisfactorily | | | |
| NOTE TIME BEGAN _____ | | | |
| 1. Gently shook and called to a child or flicked bottom of foot of an infant to check for consciousness. | _____ | 5 | |
| 2. Called to another person to phone 911 or local emergency service and began resuscitation. | _____ | 15 | |
| 3. Placed infant or child on back on firm surface. | _____ | 5 | |
| 4. Tipped victim's head back and lifted chin to open airway. | _____ | 15 | |
| 5. Listened and watched and felt for breathing. | _____ | 10 | |
| 6. If no breathing was observed, gave two slow breaths, one to two seconds each. | _____ | 15 | |
| 7. Checked carotid pulse and signs of circulation for up to 10 seconds. | _____ | 15 | |
|   a. Child at carotid location | _____ | 10 | |
|   b. Infants at mid upper arm over brachial | _____ | 10 | |
| 8. If pulse, continue one ventilation. | _____ | 10 | |
|   a. Every 3 seconds for infant | | | |
|   b. Every 4 seconds for child | | | |
| 9. If no pulse was present, started cardiac compression. | | | |
|   a. Infant—Two fingers, mid sternum, depress ½"–1"; not less than 100 times per minute. | _____ | 15 | |
|   b. Child—Adult position, one hand, depressed 1 inch to 1½ inches, 100 times per minute. | _____ | 15 | |
| 10. Did ten cycles of compressions and breaths. | _____ | 15 | |
| 11. Checked for pulse and signs of circulation for up to 5 seconds. | _____ | 5 | |
| 12. If alone, summoned help. | _____ | 15 | |

## PROCEDURE 19-3   Give Cardiopulmonary Resuscitation (CPR) to Infants and Children—continued

| PROCEDURE STEPS | STEP PERFORMED | POINTS POSSIBLE | COMMENTS |
|---|---|---|---|
| 13. If there was no pulse, gave one breath and continued cycle until help arrived. | _____ | 10 | |
| 14. Sanitized the mannequin. | _____ | 5 | |
| 15. Recorded and signed procedure on patient's chart. | _____ | 10 | |

*EVALUATOR:* NOTE TIME COMPLETED _____

ADD POINTS OF STEPS CHECKED                                                              _____ EARNED
TOTAL POINTS POSSIBLE                                                                             200 POSSIBLE

Points assigned reflect importance of step to meeting objective:  Important = (5)   Essential = (10)   Critical = (15)
Automatic failure results if any of the critical steps are omitted or performed incorrectly.

DETERMINE SCORE (divide points earned by total points possible, multiply results by 100)          _____ SCORE*

Evaluator's Name (print) _____ Signature _____

Comments _____

---

## DOCUMENTATION

Chart the procedure in the patient's medical record.

Date: _____

Charting: _____

_____

_____

_____

Student's Name: _____          Physician's Initials: __(____)__

Name _____

Date _____ Score* _____

## PROCEDURE 19-4    Clean Wound Areas

*PERFORMANCE OBJECTIVE*—Provided with all necessary equipment and supplies, demonstrate cleaning wounds, following procedure steps and standard precautions.

| PROCEDURE STEPS | STEP PERFORMED | POINTS POSSIBLE | COMMENTS |
|---|---|---|---|
| *EVALUATOR:* Place check mark in space following each step performed satisfactorily | | | |
| NOTE TIME BEGAN _____ | | | |
| 1. Assembled equipment and materials. | _____ | 5 | |
| 2. Washed hands and put on gloves. | _____ | 10 | |
| 3. Grasped gauze sponges with sponge forceps. | _____ | 5 | |
| 4. Dipped into warm detergent water. | _____ | 5 | |
| 5. Washed wound and wound area to remove microorganisms and any foreign matter. | | | |
| a. Avoided further injury from instrument | _____ | 10 | |
| b. Worked from inner to outer area, 2" to 3" beyond wound | _____ | 15 | |
| 6. Discarded sponges in biohazardous waste container. | _____ | 10 | |
| 7. Irrigated wound thoroughly with sterile water. | _____ | 15 | |
| 8. Blotted wound dry with sterile gauze and discarded gauze in biohazardous waste container. | _____ | 10 | |
| 9. Covered with dry sterile dressing and bandaged in place. | _____ | 15 | |
| 10. Instructed patient to call physician immediately if evidence of infection developed. | _____ | 15 | |
| 11. Cleaned up work area. Placed all used materials and gloves in the biohazardous waste bag and into proper receptacle for safe disposal. | _____ | 5 | |
| 12. Washed hands. | _____ | 5 | |
| 13. Recorded and signed procedure on patient's chart. | _____ | 10 | |
| *EVALUATOR:* NOTE TIME COMPLETED _____ | | | |

ADD POINTS OF STEPS CHECKED                                                          _____ EARNED
TOTAL POINTS POSSIBLE                                                                      135 POSSIBLE

Points assigned reflect importance of step to meeting objective: Important = (5)   Essential = (10)   Critical = (15)
Automatic failure results if any of the critical steps are omitted or performed incorrectly.

DETERMINE SCORE (divide points earned by total points possible, multiply results by 100)    _____ SCORE*

Evaluator's Name (print) _____ Signature _____

Comments _____

## DOCUMENTATION

Chart the procedure in the patient's medical record.

Date: _____

Charting: _____

_____

_____

_____

Student's Name: _____          Physician's Initials: __(_____)__

Name _____

Date _____ Score* _____

## PROCEDURE 19-5   Apply Bandage in Recurrent Turn to Finger

*PERFORMANCE OBJECTIVE*—Provided with all necessary equipment and supplies, apply recurrent turn bandage following procedure steps and standard precautions.

| PROCEDURE STEPS | STEP PERFORMED | POINTS POSSIBLE | COMMENTS |
|---|---|---|---|
| *EVALUATOR:* Place check mark in space following each step performed satisfactorily | | | |
| NOTE TIME BEGAN _____ | | | |
| 1. Washed hands. Put on gloves if appropriate. | _____ | 5 | |
| 2. Assembled supplies. | _____ | 5 | |
| 3. Covered injury with dressing. | _____ | 10 | |
| 4. Secured dressing with bandage of gauze. | | | |
|    a. Start at proximal end, palm side | _____ | 5 | |
|    b. Go to proximal end, back of hand | _____ | 5 | |
|    c. Repeat desired times | _____ | 5 | |
| 5. Held recurrent turns in place with spiral turns. | _____ | 10 | |
| 6. Secured by tying off gauze at proximal end of finger. | _____ | 10 | |
| 7. Discarded contaminated materials and gloves, if used, in biohazardous waste bag. | _____ | 15 | |
| 8. Washed hands. | _____ | 5 | |
| 9. Recorded and signed procedure in patient's chart. | _____ | 10 | |
| *EVALUATOR:* NOTE TIME COMPLETED _____ | | | |

ADD POINTS OF STEPS CHECKED                                                                 _____ EARNED

TOTAL POINTS POSSIBLE                                                                               85 POSSIBLE

Points assigned reflect importance of step to meeting objective: Important = (5)   Essential = (10)   Critical = (15)
Automatic failure results if any of the critical steps are omitted or performed incorrectly.

DETERMINE SCORE (divide points earned by total points possible, multiply results by 100)        _____ SCORE*

Evaluator's Name (print) _____ Signature _____

Comments _____

## DOCUMENTATION

Chart the procedure in the patient's medical record.

Date: _____

Charting: _____

_____

_____

_____

Student's Name: _____          Physician's Initials: __(_____)__

Name _____

Date _____ Score* _____

## PROCEDURE 19-6   Apply Bandage in Open or Closed Spiral

*PERFORMANCE OBJECTIVE*—Provided with all necessary equipment and supplies, apply open and closed spiral bandage so dressing is secure, following procedure steps and standard precautions.

| PROCEDURE STEPS | STEP PERFORMED | POINTS POSSIBLE | COMMENTS |
|---|---|---|---|
| *EVALUATOR:* Place check mark in space following each step performed satisfactorily | | | |
| NOTE TIME BEGAN _____ | | | |
| 1. Washed hands. Put on gloves if appropriate. | _____ | 5 | |
| 2. Assembled needed supplies. | _____ | 5 | |
| 3. Carefully opened dressing, without contaminating, and placed over wound area. | _____ | 10 | |
| 4. Anchored bandage by placing end of bandage on bias at starting point. | _____ | 5 | |
| 5. Encircled part, allowing corner of bandage end to protrude. | _____ | 5 | |
| 6. Turned down protruding tip of bandage. | _____ | 5 | |
| 7. Encircled part again. | _____ | 5 | |
| 8. Continued to encircle area to be covered with spiral turns spaced so that they do not overlap. *OR* Formed closed spiral by continuing to encircle with overlapping spiral turns until all open spaces were covered. | _____ | 5 | |
|    a. Subtract 10 pts. if wrapped straight around. | _____ | | |
| 9. Completed bandage by tying off or taping in place. | _____ | 5 | |
|    a. Tape if used, must be in opposite direction to body movement. Subtract 10 pts. if applied incorrectly | _____ | | |
| 10. Discarded contaminated materials and gloves, if used, in biohazardous waste bag. | _____ | 15 | |
| 11. Washed hands. | _____ | 5 | |
| 12. Recorded and signed procedure on patient's chart. | _____ | 10 | |
| *EVALUATOR:* NOTE TIME COMPLETED _____ | | | |

ADD POINTS OF STEPS CHECKED                                                     _____ EARNED
TOTAL POINTS POSSIBLE                                                                   80 POSSIBLE

Points assigned reflect importance of step to meeting objective: Important = (5)   Essential = (10)   Critical = (15)
Automatic failure results if any of the critical steps are omitted or performed incorrectly.

DETERMINE SCORE (divide points earned by total points possible, multiply results by 100)         _____ SCORE*

Evaluator's Name (print) _____ Signature _____

Comments _____

## DOCUMENTATION

Chart the procedure in the patient's medical record.

Date: _____

Charting: _____

_____

_____

_____

Student's Name: _____          Physician's Initials: __(_____)__

Name _____

Date _____ Score* _____

## PROCEDURE 19-7  Apply Figure-Eight Bandage to Hand and Wrist

*PERFORMANCE OBJECTIVE*—Provided with all necessary equipment and materials, apply a figure-eight bandage to the hand and
wrist neatly to secure dressing following procedure steps and standard precautions.

| PROCEDURE STEPS | STEP PERFORMED | POINTS POSSIBLE | COMMENTS |
|---|---|---|---|
| *EVALUATOR:* Place check mark in space following each step performed satisfactorily | | | |
| NOTE TIME BEGAN _____ | | | |
| 1. Washed hands. Put on gloves if appropriate. | _____ | 5 | |
| 2. Assembled needed supplies. | _____ | 5 | |
| 3. Applied dressing. Did not contaminate any part that would touch wound area. | _____ | 10 | |
| 4. Anchored bandage with one or two turns around palm of hand. | _____ | 5 | |
| 5. Rolled gauze diagonally across front of wrist and in figure-eight pattern around the hand. | _____ | 10 | |
| 6. Tied off at the wrist. Avoided constricting circulation. | _____ | 15 | |
| 7. Discarded contaminated materials and gloves, if used, in biohazardous waste bag. | _____ | 15 | |
| 8. Washed hands. | _____ | 5 | |
| 9. Recorded and signed procedure on patient's chart. | _____ | 10 | |
| *EVALUATOR:* NOTE TIME COMPLETED _____ | | | |

ADD POINTS OF STEPS CHECKED                                            _____ EARNED
TOTAL POINTS POSSIBLE                                                           80 POSSIBLE

Points assigned reflect importance of step to meeting objective:  Important = (5)   Essential = (10)   Critical = (15)
Automatic failure results if any of the critical steps are omitted or performed incorrectly.

DETERMINE SCORE (divide points earned by total points possible, multiply results by 100)          _____ SCORE*

Evaluator's Name (print) _____ Signature _____

Comments _____

# DOCUMENTATION

Chart the procedure in the patient's medical record.

Date: _____

Charting: _____

_____

_____

_____

Student's Name: _____          Physician's Initials: __( ___ )__

## PROCEDURE 19-8   Apply Cravat Bandage to Forehead, Ear, or Eyes

*PERFORMANCE OBJECTIVE*—Provided with all necessary equipment and supplies, apply a cravat bandage to the head following procedure steps and standard precautions.

| PROCEDURE STEPS | STEP PERFORMED | POINTS POSSIBLE | COMMENTS |
|---|---|---|---|
| *EVALUATOR:* Place check mark in space following each step performed satisfactorily | | | |
| NOTE TIME BEGAN _____ | | | |
| 1. Washed hands. Put on gloves if appropriate. | _____ | 5 | |
| 2. Assembled needed supplies. | _____ | 5 | |
| 3. Carefully placed dressing over wound, taking care not to contaminate area over wound. | _____ | 15 | |
| 4. Placed center of cravat over dressing. | _____ | 5 | |
| 5. Took ends around to opposite side of head and crossed them. Did not tie. | _____ | 5 | |
| 6. Brought ends back to starting point and tied. | _____ | 10 | |
| 7. Discarded contaminated materials and gloves, if used, in biohazardous waste bag. | _____ | 15 | |
| 8. Washed hands. | _____ | 5 | |
| 9. Recorded and signed procedure on patient's chart. | _____ | 10 | |

*EVALUATOR:* NOTE TIME COMPLETED _____

ADD POINTS OF STEPS CHECKED                                           _____ EARNED
TOTAL POINTS POSSIBLE                                                        75 POSSIBLE

Points assigned reflect importance of step to meeting objective:  Important = (5)   Essential = (10)   Critical = (15)
Automatic failure results if any of the critical steps are omitted or performed incorrectly.

DETERMINE SCORE (divide points earned by total points possible, multiply results by 100)          _____ SCORE*

Evaluator's Name (print) _____ Signature _____

Comments _____

## DOCUMENTATION

Chart the procedure in the patient's medical record.

Date: _____

Charting: _____

_____

_____

_____

Student's Name: _____          Physician's Initials: __(____)__

Name _____

Date _____ Score* _____

## PROCEDURE 19-9   Apply Triangular Bandage to Head

*PERFORMANCE OBJECTIVE*—Provided with all necessary equipment and supplies, apply a triangular bandage to the head following procedure steps and standard precautions so the dressing is neat and secure.

| PROCEDURE STEPS | STEP PERFORMED | POINTS POSSIBLE | COMMENTS |
|---|---|---|---|
| *EVALUATOR:* Place check mark in space following each step performed satisfactorily | | | |
| NOTE TIME BEGAN _____ | | | |
| 1. Washed hands. Put on gloves if appropriate. | _____ | 5 | |
| 2. Assembled needed supplies. | _____ | 5 | |
| 3. Carefully placed dressing over wound area without contaminating. | _____ | 15 | |
| 4. Folded a hem about two inches wide along base of bandage. | _____ | 10 | |
| 5. With hem on outside, placed bandage on head so that middle of base was on forehead close to eyebrows and point hangs down back. | _____ | 10 | |
| 6. Brought two ends around head above ears and crossed them just below occipital prominence at back of head. | _____ | 10 | |
| 7. Drew ends snugly around head and tied them in center of forehead. | _____ | 5 | |
| 8. Steadied head with one hand and with other hand drew point down firmly behind to hold dressing securely against head. | _____ | 10 | |
| 9. Grasped point and tucked it into area where bandage ends crossed. | _____ | 5 | |
| 10. Discarded contaminated materials and gloves, if used, in biohazardous waste bag. | _____ | 15 | |
| 11. Washed hands. | _____ | 5 | |
| 12. Recorded and signed procedure on patient's chart. | _____ | 10 | |

*EVALUATOR:* NOTE TIME COMPLETED _____

ADD POINTS OF STEPS CHECKED                        _____ EARNED
TOTAL POINTS POSSIBLE                                   105 POSSIBLE

Points assigned reflect importance of step to meeting objective: Important = (5)   Essential = (10)   Critical = (15)
Automatic failure results if any of the critical steps are omitted or performed incorrectly.

DETERMINE SCORE (divide points earned by total points possible, multiply results by 100)          _____ SCORE*

Evaluator's Name (print) _____  Signature _____

Comments _____

## DOCUMENTATION

Chart the procedure in the patient's medical record.

Date: _____

Charting: _____

_____

_____

_____

Student's Name: _____     Physician's Initials: __(____)__

Name _____

Date _____ Score* _____

# PROCEDURE 19-10   Apply Arm Sling

*PERFORMANCE OBJECTIVE*—Provided with the necessary equipment, demonstrate the steps in the procedure for applying an arm sling so that the arm is supported properly and the sling is correctly tied.

| PROCEDURE STEPS | STEP PERFORMED | POINTS POSSIBLE | COMMENTS |
|---|---|---|---|
| *EVALUATOR:* Place check mark in space following each step performed satisfactorily | | | |
| NOTE TIME BEGAN _____ | | | |
| 1. Washed hands. | _____ | 5 | |
| 2. Placed one end of triangle bandage over shoulder on uninjured side and let other end hang down over chest. | _____ | 15 | |
| 3. Pulled point behind elbow of injured arm. | _____ | 5 | |
| 4. Pulled end of bandage which was hanging down up around injured arm and over shoulder. | _____ | 5 | |
| 5. Raised end until hand rested 4″ to 5″ above elbow. | _____ | 15 | |
| 6. Tied ends at side of neck; checked hand. | _____ | 15 | |
| 7. Closed point end at elbow. | _____ | 15 | |
|   a. Folded neatly and pinned or | | | |
|   b. Tied knot in cloth to make sling snug at elbow | | | |
| 8. Extended fingers slightly beyond edge of sling. | _____ | 15 | |
| 9. Recorded and signed procedure on patient's chart. | _____ | 10 | |
| *EVALUATOR:* NOTE TIME COMPLETED _____ | | | |

ADD POINTS OF STEPS CHECKED                                  _____ EARNED
TOTAL POINTS POSSIBLE                                       100 POSSIBLE

Points assigned reflect importance of step to meeting objective: Important = (5)   Essential = (10)   Critical = (15)
Automatic failure results if any of the critical steps are omitted or performed incorrectly.

DETERMINE SCORE (divide points earned by total points possible, multiply results by 100)      _____ SCORE*

Evaluator's Name (print) _____   Signature _____

Comments _____

## DOCUMENTATION

Chart the procedure in the patient's medical record.

Date: _____

Charting: _____

_____

_____

_____

Student's Name: _____     Physician's Initials: __(_____)__

# PERFORMANCE EVALUATION CHECKLIST

Name _____

Date _____ Score* _____

## PROCEDURE 19-11    Use a Cane

*PERFORMANCE OBJECTIVE*—Provided with a cane, demonstrate adjusting the length of a cane and provide patient with instruction to properly and safely use a cane. The cane will be the appropriate length and the patient will demonstrate correct usage.

| PROCEDURE STEPS | STEP PERFORMED | POINTS POSSIBLE | COMMENTS |
|---|---|---|---|
| *EVALUATOR:* Place check mark in space following each step performed satisfactorily | | | |
| NOTE TIME BEGAN _____ | | | |
| 1. Identified patient and confirmed physician's orders. | _____ | 5 | |
| 2. Assembled equipment. Checked cane for intact rubber tip. | _____ | 10 | |
| 3. Adjusted height of cane. | | | |
|   a. Elbow flexed at 25° to 30° angle | _____ | 15 | |
|   b. Handle just below hip on strong side | _____ | 15 | |
| 4. Demonstrated use of cane—moving cane forward with injured extremity. | _____ | 15 | |
| 5. Allowed patient to practice the procedure. | _____ | 5 | |
| 6. Demonstrated going up stairs and had patient practice (Uninjured extremity up first). | _____ | 15 | |
| 7. Demonstrate going down stairs and had patient practice (Uninjured extremity down first). | _____ | 15 | |
| 8. Rechecked cane height. | _____ | 5 | |
| 9. Ensured correct usage. | _____ | 15 | |
| 10. Recorded and signed procedure on patient's chart. | _____ | 10 | |
| *EVALUATOR:* NOTE TIME COMPLETED _____ | | | |

ADD POINTS OF STEPS CHECKED

TOTAL POINTS POSSIBLE

_____ EARNED

125 POSSIBLE

Points assigned reflect importance of step to meeting objective:  Important = (5)   Essential = (10)   Critical = (15)

Automatic failure results if any of the critical steps are omitted or performed incorrectly.

DETERMINE SCORE (divide points earned by total points possible, multiply results by 100)     _____ SCORE*

Evaluator's Name (print) _____    Signature _____

Comments _____

# DOCUMENTATION

Chart the procedure in the patient's medical record.

Date: _____

Charting: _____

_____

_____

_____

Student's Name: _____          Physician's Initials: _( _____ )_

Name _____

Date _____ Score* _____

# PROCEDURE 19-12   Use Crutches

*PERFORMANCE OBJECTIVE*—Provided with all necessary equipment and supplies, adjust the length of the crutches and demonstrate the steps of this procedure to instruct a patient in the correct use of crutches. The crutches will be the correct length and the patient will be able to demonstrate the proper and safe use of crutches.

| PROCEDURE STEPS | STEP PERFORMED | POINTS POSSIBLE | COMMENTS |
|---|---|---|---|
| *EVALUATOR:* Place check mark in space following each step performed satisfactorily | | | |
| NOTE TIME BEGAN _____ | | | |
| 1. Identified patient and confirmed physician's orders. | _____ | 5 | |
| 2. Assembled equipment. Made sure crutches were intact (hand pads and rubber tips) and stable. | _____ | 5 | |
| 3. Stabilized patient upright near wall or chair for support. | _____ | 10 | |
| 4. Adjusted length of crutches. | | | |
| a. Elbows with 30° bend | _____ | 15 | |
| b. Pads 2″ below axilla | _____ | 15 | |
| 5. Explained proper usage to patient. | | | |
| a. Supported weight on hands | _____ | 15 | |
| b. Took small steps | _____ | 10 | |
| c. Stood on uninjured extremity, swung injured extremity with crutches | _____ | 15 | |
| 6. Demonstrated proper use of crutches for gait ordered. | _____ | 15 | |
| 7. Allowed patient to practice the procedure to ensure correct use. | _____ | 10 | |
| 8. Recorded and signed procedure on patient's chart. | _____ | 10 | |

*EVALUATOR:* NOTE TIME COMPLETED _____

ADD POINTS OF STEPS CHECKED                      _____ EARNED
TOTAL POINTS POSSIBLE                              125 POSSIBLE

Points assigned reflect importance of step to meeting objective: Important = (5)   Essential = (10)   Critical = (15)
Automatic failure results if any of the critical steps are omitted or performed incorrectly.

DETERMINE SCORE (divide points earned by total points possible, multiply results by 100)      _____ SCORE*

Evaluator's Name (print) _____ Signature _____

Comments _____

## DOCUMENTATION

Chart the procedure in the patient's medical record.

Date: _____

Charting: _____

_____

_____

_____

Student's Name: _____     Physician's Initials: __( )__

Name _____

Date _____ Score* _____

# PROCEDURE 19-13   Use a Walker

*PERFORMANCE OBJECTIVE*—Provided with a walker, adjust it to the appropriate height and demonstrate the steps in the procedure to instruct a patient in the proper use of a walker. The patient will be able to demonstrate the safe and correct use of a walker.

| PROCEDURE STEPS | STEP PERFORMED | POINTS POSSIBLE | COMMENTS |
|---|---|---|---|
| *EVALUATOR:* Place check mark in space following each step performed satisfactorily | | | |
| NOTE TIME BEGAN _____ | | | |
| 1. Identified patient and confirmed physician's orders. | _____ | 5 | |
| 2. Assembled equipment. Checked walker for rubber tips, pads at handles, and stability. | _____ | 10 | |
| 3. Stabilized patient upright near wall or chair for support. | _____ | 10 | |
| 4. Adjusted walker to fit patient. | | | |
| a. Handles at hip level | _____ | 15 | |
| b. Elbows bent 25° to 30° | _____ | 15 | |
| 5. Positioned the walker around the patient. | _____ | 5 | |
| 6. Instructed patient to pick up the walker and move it slightly forward and walk into it. | _____ | 10 | |
| 7. Demonstrated the correct use of a walker. | _____ | 15 | |
| 8. Had patient practice the procedure. | _____ | 5 | |
| 9. Observed patient and was ready to assist in case of possible fall until able to use safely and correctly. | _____ | 10 | |
| 10. Recorded and signed procedure on patient's chart. | _____ | 10 | |
| *EVALUATOR:* NOTE TIME COMPLETED _____ | | | |

ADD POINTS OF STEPS CHECKED _____ EARNED

TOTAL POINTS POSSIBLE 110 POSSIBLE

Points assigned reflect importance of step to meeting objective: Important = (5)   Essential = (10)   Critical = (15)
Automatic failure results if any of the critical steps are omitted or performed incorrectly.

DETERMINE SCORE (divide points earned by total points possible, multiply results by 100) _____ SCORE*

Evaluator's Name (print) _____ Signature _____

Comments _____

**DOCUMENTATION**

Chart the procedure in the patient's medical record.

Date: _____

Charting: _____

_____

_____

_____

Student's Name: _____          **Physician's Initials:** __(____)__

## PROCEDURE 19-14  Assist Patient from Wheelchair to Examination Table

*PERFORMANCE OBJECTIVE*—Provided with necessary equipment, demonstrate the steps in the procedure for assisting a patient from wheelchair to examination table in a safe manner.

| PROCEDURE STEPS | STEP PERFORMED | POINTS POSSIBLE | COMMENTS |
|---|---|---|---|
| *EVALUATOR:* Place check mark in space following each step performed satisfactorily | | | |
| NOTE TIME BEGAN _____ | | | |
| 1. Unlocked wheels of chair and wheeled patient to examination room. | _____ | 5 | |
| 2. Positioned chair as near as possible to place where patient should sit on table. | _____ | 5 | |
| 3. Lowered table to chair level or provided stool. | _____ | 5 | |
| 4. Locked wheels on chair. | _____ | 15 | |
| 5. Folded footrests back. | _____ | 10 | |
| 6. Assumed stable position in front of patient. | _____ | 10 | |
| 7. Assisted patient to stand; side step or pivot to front of table. | _____ | 15 | |
| 8. Assisted patient to sitting position on table. | _____ | 10 | |
| 9. Helped adjust position and recline for examination. | _____ | 5 | |
| 10. Placed pillow under head. | _____ | 5 | |
| 11. Draped as appropriate. | _____ | 5 | |
| 12. Unlocked chair wheels and moved chair out of way. | _____ | 5 | |

*EVALUATOR:* NOTE TIME COMPLETED _____

ADD POINTS OF STEPS CHECKED                    _____ EARNED
TOTAL POINTS POSSIBLE                                    95 POSSIBLE

Points assigned reflect importance of step to meeting objective: Important = (5)  Essential = (10)  Critical = (15)
Automatic failure results if any of the critical steps are omitted or performed incorrectly.

DETERMINE SCORE (divide points earned by total points possible, multiply results by 100)     _____ SCORE*

Evaluator's Name (print) _____ Signature _____

Comments _____

## PROCEDURE 19-15   Assist Patient from Examination Table to Wheelchair

*PERFORMANCE OBJECTIVE*—Provided with a wheelchair and an examination table, demonstrate the steps in the procedure, in order, to assist the patient from examination table to wheelchair in a safe manner.

| PROCEDURE STEPS | STEP PERFORMED | POINTS POSSIBLE | COMMENTS |
|---|---|---|---|
| *EVALUATOR:* Place check mark in space following each step performed satisfactorily | | | |
| NOTE TIME BEGAN _____ | | | |
| 1. Repositioned chair and locked wheels. | _____ | 15 | |
| 2. Assisted patient to sitting position on table. | _____ | 10 | |
| 3. Assisted to redress as needed. | _____ | 5 | |
| 4. Supported patient while assisting to step onto floor or stepstool (if stool—assisted to step onto floor). | _____ | 15 | |
| 5. Side-stepped or pivoted patient to position in front of chair. | _____ | 15 | |
| 6. Instructed patient to reach back to chair arms while helping lower patient into chair. | _____ | 15 | |
| 7. Adjusted footrests. | _____ | 10 | |
| 8. Unlocked wheels and returned patient to consultation or reception room. | _____ | 5 | |
| *EVALUATOR:* NOTE TIME COMPLETED _____ | | | |

ADD POINTS OF STEPS CHECKED                                        _____ EARNED

TOTAL POINTS POSSIBLE                                                      90 POSSIBLE

Points assigned reflect importance of step to meeting objective: Important = (5)   Essential = (10)   Critical = (15)
Automatic failure results if any of the critical steps are omitted or performed incorrectly.

DETERMINE SCORE (divide points earned by total points possible, multiply results by 100)        _____ SCORE*

Evaluator's Name (print) _____   Signature _____

Comments _____

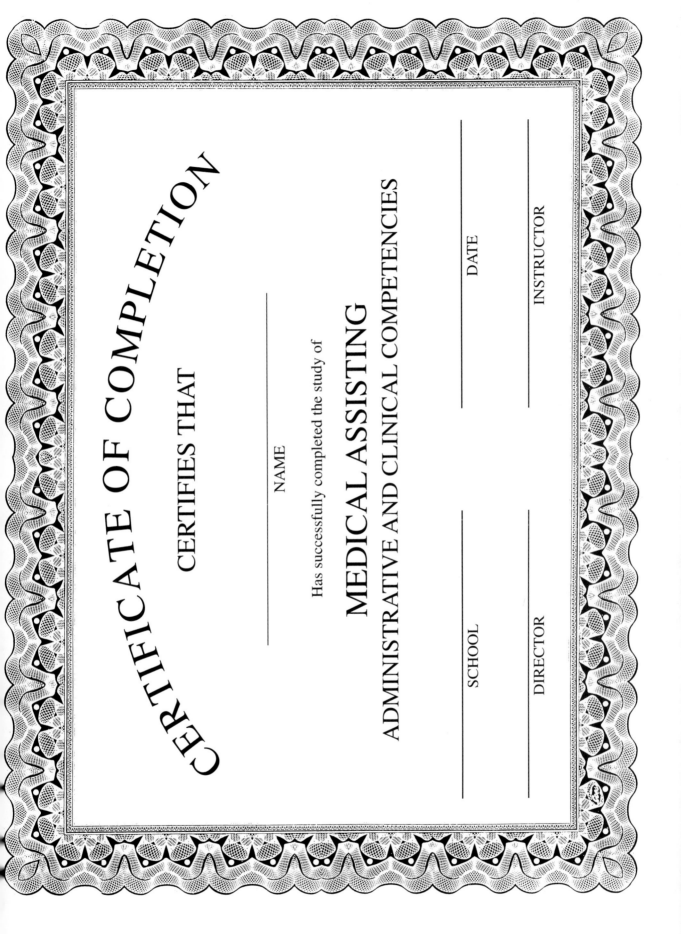

CERTIFICATE OF COMPLETION

CERTIFIES THAT

_____

NAME

Has successfully completed the study of

MEDICAL ASSISTING

ADMINISTRATIVE AND CLINICAL COMPETENCIES

_____          _____

SCHOOL                                                          DATE

_____          _____

DIRECTOR                                                     INSTRUCTOR